LAZY F*CKS
DON'T LIVE TO 100

LAZY F*CKS
DON'T LIVE TO 100

TOM BROADWELL

LAZY F*CKS DON'T LIVE TO 100
Copyright © Tom Broadwell, 2020

www.TomBroadwell.com
ISBN: 9798644027576

MEDICAL DISCLAIMER

This book is not intended as a substitute for the medical advice of physicians. The reader should regularly consult a physician in matters relating to his/her health and particularly with respect to any symptoms that may require diagnosis or medical attention.

This book details the author's personal experiences with and opinions about health and fitness. The author is not a healthcare provider. The author and publisher are providing this book and its contents on an "as is" basis and make no representations or warranties of any kind with respect to this book or its contents.

The author and publisher disclaim all such representations and warranties, including for example warranties of merchantability and healthcare for a particular purpose. In addition, the author and publisher do not represent or warrant that the information accessible via this book is accurate, complete or current.

The statements made about products and services have not been evaluated by the U.S. Food and Drug Administration. They are not intended to diagnose, treat, cure, or prevent any condition or disease. Please consult with your own physician or healthcare specialist regarding the suggestions and recommendations made in this book.

Except as specifically stated in this book, neither the author or publisher, nor any authors, contributors, or other representatives will be liable for damages arising out of or in connection with the use of this book. This is a comprehensive limitation of liability that applies to all damages of any kind, including (without limitation) compensatory; direct, indirect or consequential damages; loss of data, income or profit; loss of or damage to property and claims of third parties. You understand that this book is not intended as a substitute for consultation with a licensed healthcare practitioner, such as your physician. Before you begin any healthcare program, or change your lifestyle in any way, you will consult your physician or another licensed healthcare practitioner to ensure that you are in good health and that the examples contained in this book will not harm you.

This book provides content related to physical and/or mental health issues. As such, use of this book implies your acceptance of this disclaimer.

To Mum and Dad,

Even though I'm sure you think I'm a little bit crazy sometimes, thank you for standing by me in whatever I choose to do (and say!). For all the support you've given me throughout my rather eventful life, I dedicate this book to you. Thank you from the bottom of my heart.

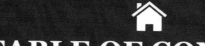

TABLE OF CONTENTS

Introduction

Firstly, sorry if I offended you in some way, shape or form with the title of this book. I had to grab your attention somehow. Secondly, we all have our lazy days, which can be very good for you. Thirdly, you can't really argue that it's not true! Being a lazy fuck is *not* going to get you to live a long life full of health, vitality with full mobility, is it? And it certainly won't help you look better naked! True, you can lose drastic amounts of weight sitting on your ass, eating nothing but lettuce and celery, but it won't build the lean, toned physique that I imagine most people want when they think of looking better naked.

Why does any of this matter? You might currently be reading this in a young, fit, and healthy body with no end in sight for when this might change. Or you may be on the opposite end of the scale, in such a broken-down body that you think you're either too old or too far gone to make the necessary changes. You might be somewhere in between, thinking I've heard and seen it all before, nothing works, it's all *bullshit*.

No matter where you stand on the *ever-changing*, sliding scale of your health, at the end of the day, you owe it to yourself to be as healthy as you possibly can. Why? Because health should always be your *number one* priority.

I know most people see sense in that, but day in, day out over the last 18 years of me being a professional in the Health & Fitness Industry I see people putting everything *but* their health first. Their careers, their children, their families, their homes, and even their freaking cars! People literally take more care of their house and their car than they do their own *body*.

But it's all okay. It's all good. That is until the day their health disappears...

"A healthy man has a thousand wishes, a sick man, only one." - Indian Proverb

Some people see it as selfish if they don't put their children or grandchildren first. Just take a moment to think about that, because if you don't have your health, then your children don't have *you* in the capacity that they do now. Pretty much every person in the world would much rather have a healthy parent or grandparent than one who gives them too much and doesn't take care of themselves and ends up sick, or worse, *dead*.

What I mean by all this is, rather than just focusing on cooking and feeding your children healthy meals, take the time to do it for *yourself* too. Rather than spending all your money on things for the grandchildren, invest in your health *first*.

When I say invest in your health first, I don't mean going out and buying the latest Ab Crunch Machine that promises Six Pack Abs in 30 days — or buying the newest Magic Pill that shows you the science behind how to burn fat without moving a muscle. Or signing up to the latest fad diet where you eat 500 calories a day of food that you hate, that is sent directly to your house and is as easy as throwing it in the microwave and nuking the fuck out of every nutrient that was in there in the first place...how *healthy*.

Let's clear this up once and for all. Health doesn't happen with quick fixes; we all know that. And neither does *permanent* weight loss. However, with health comes permanent weight loss.

So, let's all vouch right now, together, to ditch the diets, never to buy another magic pill, and to stop relying on expensive exercise equipment.

Maybe you did vouch. Perhaps you have your doubts. The choice, of course, is yours, but first, let me present all my *evidence* that the above is a good idea. Throughout this entire book, I will give you so much evidence that I'm sure I will leave you without an ounce of doubt in your mind.

As mentioned, some of you will still be thinking, BULLLLLLSHIIIIIT! I've tried it. *All* of it. Nothing works! It's my genetics; it's a medical predisposition; I was always meant to be fat! I was always meant to be sick. It runs in the family!

The thing is, *maybe*. But probably not. It's shown that 90-99% of disease comes down to lifestyle. But you see, if that *massive* amount comes down to lifestyle, that means only a fraction of what we are led to believe actually comes down to *genetics*. That means yes, you *can* be more predisposed to have a certain disease, but if 90-99% of all disease comes down to *lifestyle*, then you don't *have* to get that disease!

It means 90-99% of disease comes down to *choice*. I'm grouping being overweight and being obese under the disease umbrella. *Don't blame me!* The American Medical Association said so. Obesity is a now a disease. *Of course,* it is, because it means someone can profit from treating it with the latest pill or surgery. It's a disease just like a child acting like a child and losing concentration in a boring math class and daydreaming about running around outside in the sunshine is now a disease...but that's a story for another chapter! All I'm saying, and this should make you so excited to hear;

Being overweight and sick comes down to *choice*.

Why get so excited over this? Well, *whatever* your reason is for reading this book, whether you want to heal your body or lose weight, ask yourself; if a doctor turns round to you and says *it runs in the family*, what does that do to your power?

It *takes it away*. Exactly. You are now on a high blood pressure pill every day for the rest of your life, or you're overweight because it's all down to genetics, and there is *nothing* you can do about it. So, you give up. And carry on taking your pill. Or you book in for your expensive surgery. Both of these have severe side effects you're not really thinking about right now. You might do when your doctor recommends the seventh pill you have to take every day, and you can barely get out of a chair because of the joint pain brought about by your cholesterol medication...

I know this to be true. Not only because of the many medical research papers I've read, but mainly because of the people I meet almost every day. I once met an older lady who was one of six children; she was the oldest of them all, but the only one who takes care of herself eating a healthy balanced diet and exercising daily. It just turns out she's the only one who doesn't have diabetes. In fact, she has no health issues, whereas her five siblings all have diabetes, plus the usual high blood pressure and cholesterol problems shared out between them.

I've also met my own father (unbelievable I know), who has lived to an older age than both his father and grandfather who died from heart attacks, even though at one point over a decade ago a doctor put him on cholesterol medication stating; "It runs in the family." When it became so difficult for him to walk, he had to give up his much-beloved crown green bowling (barely a hardcore sport) because of the side effects, he changed his nutrition and did a proper detoxification program. Today he is on no prescription medication and gets around absolutely fine, finding the energy and mobility to play crown green bowling every single day!

Now I don't know your goal is as I write these words. But I can guarantee you one thing. I can help you. If you follow the Action Steps in this book, you can go a long way to achieving everything you are thinking and even more! In less than one week, you can be feeling better. In 21 days, you will have created some new life-changing habits and could have lost considerable amounts of fat. In just 66 days, you will have a brand new healthy *lifestyle*, significantly reducing your risk of *all* lifestyle diseases, and more importantly, you will look better naked. Joking about the more important thing...maybe...

Whether your goal is as simple as being able to tie your own shoelaces or walking up a flight of stairs without getting out of breath OR as big as losing 100lbs (+) or seeing your grandchildren grow up, it *all* comes down to *choice*. Do you *choose* to lead a life of better health? Or in true 'No Bullshit' fashion (I told you on the front cover!), do you *choose* to be fat and sick?

Talking of goals, do yourself a favour and *write* your goals down. It is proven that you are 42% more likely to achieve a goal if you write it down. Follow the Action Steps at the end of this introduction to get the best out of goal setting, and we will also go into much more detail on goal setting in a chapter later.

What I ask you to do within the pages of this book are not unachievable Action Steps of epic proportions. No, they are simple, small, easy to do lifestyle changes. I'm not going to be asking you to exercise like a fitness freak, running marathons and lifting obscene amounts of weight over your head. No, I'm looking at getting you to walk for twenty minutes per day and if, if you are ready, stepping up to simple, fun exercise routines you can do at home in less than twenty minutes, with little or no equipment, 3x per week.

I am looking at taking you on a journey, that will be both full of fun and profound success. This book is a step-by-step guide with small, easy to make changes that you can make every day or every week if you so wish. The journey might take you a week to complete, or a month or even a year. That bits up to you. Go at a pace that makes *you* happy but understand that by the end of it you will have a whole new lifestyle and a whole new body, with a completely new outlook on life.

It will be a journey *full* of positive change for both your body and your mind. What I urge you to consider right now is one thing;

Everything that you need is right here in your hands.

You do not *need* another book, or another course, or another seminar. I know that sounds egotistical of me to say, but I mean it. Stop trying to learn more. *Now is the time to do.*

I'm not saying I know everything, and I will never say that for that is the perfect way to stop growing. However, the information in these pages has taken almost two decades to compile. Having brought it all together into one easy to understand, simple complete step-by-step guide, I know right now in your life, you need nothing else. It is *all* here. I have read countless books and medical papers and spent *thousands* of dollars trying different products and services and having done all that I've put everything that worked into *one* place, which is this book. I've done the hard work, so *you* don't have to.

After going through this journey, you might want more. I could go into some of the subjects in this book in *far* more detail, and I probably will in further books, but right now, that is information overload. It's simply not needed as the information in this book is enough to get you to where you want to be. Now is the time for *action*.

This journey will not be an expensive one, nor one that takes too much time. There is now *no excuse* to get into the shape of your life. Just follow me, and I will show you the way.

By the way, who am I? I am Tom Broadwell. I have of this day worked in the Health & Fitness Industry for 18 years on three different continents, most of the years as a qualified Personal Trainer. I studied in England, hailing from Leeds in Yorkshire.

I have taught thousands of people around the world in Health Seminars how to get in shape and improve their health. And many more in one-on-one sessions. I built my Personal Training business from scratch in Sydney, Australia, to teaching around 100 PT and Nutrition sessions per week. Yes, you read that right, *per week*. I may have been the busiest PT in the world at the time; I sure hope so because that workweek was slowly killing me!

I have to tell you this; If I taught you what I got taught to teach people in terms of what to eat and how to exercise, you would all end up fatter, sicker and more bored of it than you are now.

My real learning started 12 years ago when I developed such bad eczema as an adult that I had to change my bedsheets daily because they were covered in blood and puss. I had to get out of bed at least one hour early every morning (try that as a Personal Trainer!), because I needed that long to mentally prepare myself to take a shower. As the water hit my skin it felt like I was on fire.

I remember literally begging my doctor to send me to see a specialist because I was in so much pain. He had offered me very little way in terms of advice, simply resorting to giving me a different steroid cream and tablet each time I went back. Which I used, saw an immediate difference, but just a few days later, I would be back to scratching at night, causing more wounds to open up and ending up back at square one. Frustrating, to say the least.

His response was this; "The specialist is only going to give you a stronger steroid, but you can go." Basically, telling me, I was wasting my time. I couldn't believe this, surely a specialist would advise me about what to eat, tell me what the root cause of all this was and what I could do to cure the eczema that riddled my face and my entire body.

Oh, how naive I was! I literally knew *nothing*. Nothing that I will teach you in this book anyway.

Then an older lady came into my life who was a member of the gym, from Spain, by the name of Aida. She asked me why I had not used Apple Cider Vinegar to treat my ailment. I said, "What is that!?" Again, I knew nothing. I started using it in the way she described, one tablespoon on a morning in a cup of warm water that I drank and then two cups in a warm bath to soak in on a night-time.

It was slowly working for me. Aida told me to cut out dairy and wheat, which worked wonders. I asked her how she knew all of this because I don't ever remember getting taught any of this in school. In fact, we used to drink a pint of milk every day in school while growing up. Knowing what I know now...Yuck!

She told me of a book to read, which lead me to devour every book on health, natural remedies, nutrition, and detoxification I could get my hand on. I didn't read all these books while doing nothing about it, no I *implemented* everything that made sense to me, and I urge you to do the same while going through this book. Take the Action Steps at the end of each chapter. It took a while, but after a journey of discovery, I now have little to no eczema, and I am in a far better place both physically and mentally. So, if you are ready to heal your body and to look better naked, follow me...

I have to say if at this point you are taken aback by how brash my language is, and how straight to the point I am, don't worry, I understand a lot of what I am saying will come across as the opinions of an overly confident asshole, and I admit, I can be that person sometimes. However, everything I say, I have backed up with scientific studies from all over the world. You will find all the references at the end of this book. Besides, that's all science is; the current opinions of (sometimes) overconfident assholes...but some people need to see that stuff, and I completely understand that, so it's all there for you to check out for yourself.

As you go through the book, I will be talking about different nations, cultures, and people from all over the world. And so, if I'm talking about facts and figures from the US, for example, this is not to bash Americans and it doesn't mean it doesn't apply to you. It's simply where my research took me at that time. Just so you know, if you are from the Western world (and sadly it's beginning to be the rest of the world too), the facts and figures I'm representing will more than likely also relate to your nation, if not now, then in the near future!

Before you get to the references, let's start at the beginning. The first step will be building the foundations of what I call our Health House. These are all the things you need to put into place first, in order for the other stuff to work. There's no point in building a house on weak foundations, because we all know at some point it's going to fall! Then we will go onto the walls of our health house because again there's no point having a roof without any walls in place. And so on from there, until your Health House has windows, doors and even a garden path to call your own.

Simply take the Action Steps described at the end of each chapter. This book, however, as you'll soon find out is not about being *perfect*. I'm not perfect and would never pretend to be. I follow a simple ratio of 80% being good, and the other 20% I'm living life to the max. Let's strive for *progress* and not perfection. Having said that, the sooner you take the Action Steps in each chapter, the more likely you are to succeed. Remember that just reading, or just knowing this information is *not* enough. The 80/20 rule does not mean you get to procrastinate, hoping and wishing things will get better. You HAVE to take ACTION. As I said, the Action Steps are easy to do. So, get them done. In order. Step by simple step. Brick by brick, until your Health House is complete.

To make life easier for you, I also include a Resources section at the end of each chapter too. This is a link to a complementary portion of my website that is up to date with the latest gadgets, products, apps, videos, recipes, workouts, etc. that I currently recommend as the best things to help you achieve your goals. I've done this for two reasons, firstly as much as I talk down magic bullets and instant gratification, I know that in today's day and age people need an instant solution to their problem. If I said okay, now go and find your car keys, after a struggle, get in your car, drive through the traffic across town to 2 or 3 stores in the hope they have the exact product I'm talking about...most of you wouldn't even bother!

As mentioned, I need you to take action *right now* in the moment, or it's highly unlikely to happen! So, a link to a page that has everything you need seems like a much easier way to go. Secondly, things might change in years to come and what I believe to be currently the best thing since sliced bread may not be so good in the future, as a better version of it might come along, or I might develop digestive issues and work out it was the sliced breads fault all along! And so now I recommend gluten free sprouted grain bread...Get my drift? Rather than updating my book and charging you for a copy every time I change my mind about something, I'll simply update the Resources page on my website and let you know about it via email.

At this point, I need to point out that this is why I love technology as it makes life far easier. I openly admit that advancements in science and technology have made life better in many ways. However, as you go through the book, you'll also realise that I think technology and science can be terrible for our health and wellbeing if it is used in the wrong way. So, this is me telling you I am not a hypocrite. I know that technology and science is an awesome thing. But we need to use it in the correct way, so it doesn't start to hurt us. I'd go as far as to say that I think the future is looking bleaker and bleaker for humanity and that science, technology, and modern medicine is largely to blame. All of these subjects will be discussed in-depth in this book.

For now, there is no need to buy another book on health or nutrition, until you've completed this one. I believe this to be the most complete but easy-to-follow book on health ever written. You tell me if that's the case or not. I wouldn't even buy another one upon completing this one. I'd urge you to go back and reread it. Until you are following all the Action Steps, and fully comprehend what you are doing. The more you understand why it is you are doing what you are doing, the more powerful the information will be, and the more likely you will continue to do this for the rest of your life.

Again, there are no magic pills within these pages and no quick fixes. These are changes you will make as part of a new *lifestyle*, and it is something you will (or should at least) keep up for the rest of your life.

First, take the following Action Steps, and then I'll see you in Chapter One...

Action Steps

- You have just 30 seconds. - Quickly write down your three most important goals regarding your health, fitness and body.

- Now we have what you truly want; let's go into more detail. - Write down exactly what you want; each goal must be clear, specific and measurable.

- Set deadlines for each goal.

- Make a list of everything you need to achieve your goal, including obstacles to overcome (including your own limiting beliefs), equipment, people, knowledge and skills. As new items come up (from gaining more insight) add them to your list.

- Put the list into a plan. Break your plan down into daily, weekly and monthly goals. At the beginning of each week and month plan it out, prioritising your list, getting the most important (not the easiest) thing done first. Plan each day the night before in the same way.

- The more careful and detailed your plan is the more time you will save in the long run. It is said that every minute spent planning saves ten minutes in execution. That's a 1000% return on investment!

Section One

The Foundations of Your Health House

*"The foundation of success in life is good health: that is the substratum fortune; it is also the basis of happiness. A person cannot accumulate a fortune very well when he is sick." – **P. T. Barnum***

Chapter One
Mindset Mastery Matters Most
"The mind is everything. What you think you become." – **Buddha**

Everyone could see the pain on her face.

Every time she breathed a breath, she almost panicked.

I asked her, "Are you okay?"

"Yeah, I'm fine." she quickly answered.

It was clear to see that she was not telling the truth.

Trying to hide the fact,

she was uncomfortable with every breath she took.

I didn't press the matter further as so not to embarrass her.

As we continued the conversation, I could see,

she was holding her breath as much as possible.

Limiting the amount of air she took in.

As the girl went to the toilet, her friend told us, "She doesn't like the air in here."

"But it's like the air in any cafe," I said.

"No, she says the air is much denser in here than the cafe she usually goes too."

As she returned from the bathroom, you could see the colour had drained from her face.

She'd been hyperventilating to remove the old air from her lungs,

possibly using a handheld pure oxygen tank that all the young women seemed to carry nowadays.

Now she was back to holding her breath.

Looking like she might pass out at any moment.

How did someone become so obsessed with the air that they were breathing?

Imagine a world where this is how we treated air! Now understand this is how a lot of people treat food. We need to come to terms with one underlying concept that can forever change your relationship with food for the better.

Food is simply fuel.

It's needed to keep us alive. Just like oxygen. When it comes to food and when it comes to losing weight, it comes down to one thing. Well, four actually...

Four Choices

I know, it's a *big* statement to start and no it's not whether you choose to eat less cake than the next person, or even choosing a salad over a burger. I mean it would be a lie to say this doesn't come into it, but no it's not the *biggest* factor. The biggest thing that no one in the mainstream is talking about is your mindset when you eat. It blows my mind when I see people who lead the health & fitness industry still talking about calories in versus calories out. Seriously, what the hell? Do they believe this, are they stupid, or are they pushing another agenda? Food for thought, literally...

Okay, I love breaking things down into simple logic, so what I am saying makes sense to anyone. Today there is so much differing information out there if you are not trained in the field of health and weight loss, then how do you know what to believe? You will see a lot of examples of it throughout this book of simple, somewhat undeniable logic, but let's start with something to dispel the popular myth of calories in versus calories out for being the reason people put weight on;

If the same person ate 2000 calories per day of only ice cream for one week and then they ate 2000 calories of only lean chicken breast per day the next week, is the same thing going to happen to their body when it comes down to gaining fat?

Your answer should be a resounding NO! But people who have millions of views on YouTube and millions of followers on Twitter pedal this shit. I'm happy for everyone to spread the good word of health but damn it keep up to date with your information! This school of thought was old in the 1990s!

Now for the interesting thing. Think about the following question long and hard because this could be the *one* key to you losing weight forever or extending your health span by decades. By the way, I don't think about lifespans, people might be living longer but would you really call it living? People pilled up to their eyeballs for the last 20 years of their lives unable to wipe their own arse? Wouldn't you prefer first to extend your health span where you live life to the max, full of vitality and in a constant state of optimal health for as long as possible?

So now for the question;

Imagine if the same person ate the exact same meal plan and had the exact same activity levels one week to the next. However, one week they were feeling emotions of content, they got a promotion at work, and they just met their dream partner, and everything seemed to be going right for them.

Then the next week their life went to shit, they lost their job, their dog got run over by their neighbour, and their dream partner pissed on the toilet seat. Would the exact same thing happen to their body? Not only in terms of weight gain (or loss) but also their health?

Hopefully, you are getting my point and realise the same thing would absolutely not happen. Mindset truly does matter most. Now, that will be a new concept to most people, which is shocking when you think about it because most people would agree that stress is a massive contributor if not the biggest killer in the world. I know they say its heart attacks, but you're not telling me stress doesn't contribute to them! So, if large amounts of stress can cause massive reactions in the human body such as hair loss, hair growth in unwanted areas, depression, premature ageing, stroke, neuromuscular diseases, eczema etc. Then why in our day to day lives might stress not be *the* leading factor as to why you can't lose weight?

I mean think about it, if over a period of time when it comes to you eating, you're stressed, not just about day to day life but by the food itself, then what's going to happen? What do I mean by that? 'The food itself'...What I mean is that when a lot of people eat chocolate cake, they are thinking; "Fuck I'm going to get fat, oh man I'm fat, holy shit I can already see it on my hips. Oh man, that tastes good, I'll have some more, but shit I'm fat. Everyone will think I'm fat if I have another little bit, but fuck it I want more, no I need more!"

Then that person reaches for some more chocolate cake stressed out of their minds. The stress hormone cortisol is flowing like a river, which prevents the body not only from burning fat but when you're stressed your body wants to protect you and so stores fat to do that, namely visceral fat in the abdominal area. Fat storage is both a survival and defence mechanism. Do you want a 'flatter stomach'? You *have* to stress less.

Studies prove this time and again, linking cortisol to the storage of fat in the abdominal area (which is visceral fat and the most dangerous area to store fat as it intertwines around your vital organs leading to all sorts of health problems). Cortisol also leads to further poor food choices and cravings. In 2013 researchers at the University of Athens, Greece did one such study. They had subjects split into two groups, with one intervention group taking part in an 8-week stress management program and the other group just receiving standard lifestyle instructions. They found the group on the stress management program lost significantly more weight, had lower stress levels and lower cortisol levels. They lost more weight in the abdominal region to the point that the researchers stated that links between cortisol and visceral fat are undeniable.

Another such study was performed in 2011 at the University of California. Researchers found that obese women on a mindfulness program showed significant reductions in the cortisol awakening response (CAR) and maintained their body weight over four months, while the control group showed no difference in CAR and gained weight. The study showed that improvements in mindfulness, CAR and chronic stress could reduce abdominal fat over time.

We will be looking at various relaxation techniques you can utilise to bring about a better mindset not only around food but life in general in the next chapter. However, for now, when it comes to eating chocolate cake, drinking a beer or consuming any other 'treat' that you like, you have **Four Choices**.

- **The *worst* choice** you can make is to eat the cake and stress about it. Think about this, somewhere between 30-60% of the time someone is given a placebo, it works. In a 2002 paper published in the Oxford University Press, clinical oncologist and professor of medicine Robert Buckman is quoted as saying that 'Placebos are extraordinary drugs. They seem to have some effect on almost every symptom known to mankind, and work in at least a third of patients and sometimes in up to 60 percent. They have no serious side-effects and cannot be given in overdose. In short, they hold the prize for the most adaptable, protean, effective, safe and cheap drugs in the world's pharmacopeia.' And so, if your mind is so strong it can cure cancer, thinking that you are fat or worrying about your High Blood Pressure is only going to make the situation worse, much worse. Whatever you focus on expands. Focusing on your waistline while consuming sugar will only make it grow!

- **The second worst choice** is surprising to most. It's *not* to eat the cake and then stress about it. Thinking; "Man I want some cake, but I can't because I'm fat and going to get fatter...plus my blood pressure is through the roof...damn, I'm fat..." This will only make you fatter and sicker. It's only cake for fuck's sake...Haha! Damn, that's good! I'm definitely making T-shirts with that on! Check your emails for your chance to win a free 'It's Only Cake for Fuck's Sake' T-shirt! Haha. Anyway sorry, back to the subject at hand, your body will eventually process the food, but the stress, however, will kill you far quicker than the cake.

- **The second best choice** is to eat some cake and be happy with your decision. Move on in life; it's only cake for fuck's sake. Haha, I love that. Sorry, blowing my own whistle here but that's epic. But seriously it is only cake. Go back to eating healthy a little later, and your body will love you more for not stressing than hate you for eating some cake.

- **The best choice**, of course, is not to eat the cake and be happy with your decision. But the moral of the story here is to be happy. Proof of this is in multiple interviews with centenarians (people who live to 100) from all over the world. When asked what their secret was for their longevity, only one thing is mentioned in almost every single interview. They all eat different diets, do various forms of exercise, lead different lifestyles, but the one thing they all agreed upon and that was to have a positive mindset. They mention to avoid too much stress and basically 'to care, but not too much.' Don't worry, be happy...A lot more on centenarians and Positive Mental Attitude in a later chapter too.

So, the start of our journey together is for you to change your mindset around food.

Food is *not* the enemy.

If people treated breathing as they do eating, they would also stress about oxygen. That's the truth of it. Food is fuel; it's nutrition for your body; it's also something to enjoy. Imagine being stressed out about every breath you take. That's crazy, but it is precisely how people treat food. Having said that there are some foods, I would never put in my body, and I will cover that in a later chapter. But even if I did eat some of these Frankenfoods, I wouldn't stress about it. I'd move on with life and quickly. Because stress is a killer and we will cover it in more detail now. In the next chapter, I'm going to show you not only how to limit the stress in your life but how to deal with the unavoidable stress that arrives in everyone's experience with some simple techniques that anybody can do. As I say, stress is a massive contributor to many people's health issues and weight gain. The information in the next few pages is something everybody needs to hear. For now, let's take the relevant Action Steps regarding what we have already learned in Chapter 1: Mindset Mastery Matters Most.

Action Steps

- Take five deep breaths before you eat or drink anything to calm the body, but especially before food that usually makes you feel bad. Instead, decide to enjoy the experience of eating such wonderful food or drink.

- Stop eating with people who put you down about the way you look or comment negatively on what you eat.

- Start making choices number 3 or 4 every time you eat or drink something.

Chapter Two
Stress Less
"The time to relax is when you don't have time for it."– **Sydney J. Harris**

I once knew of a super successful guy, fought for every penny he earned.

Started at the bottom of the corporate ladder and worked his way to the top.

Was always the first to arrive at work and the last to leave.

He put in the hard slog that was necessary for him to rise to the top, even in the beginning when his pay was peanuts.

He had only five years left before he could retire early and spend the time with his family that he had missed out on while putting everything into his career.

He had the large house, expensive cars, and a beautiful watch collection that so many people crave who are on the same path.

Soon it was his time to relax and watch his grandchildren grow up.

He was preparing to walk his daughter down the aisle later that year.

Then one day he had a massive heart attack and died.

The End.

We all know of someone like this because according to The Centers for Disease Control and Prevention (CDC) it happens every 40 seconds in the US alone. Someone has a heart attack.

The average age of males first heart attack, according to the American Heart Association is 65.6 years old.

Hence the tag on the cartoon corpses toe on the front cover. That means the average male gets to enjoy retirement for not even a single year before suffering either life-changing health problems or even worse, death. That's the average by the way, for some, it happens far sooner. And it's not too much better for females with the average first heart attack happening at 72.

Question is why didn't they do something about it earlier? The answer is because they didn't know. They didn't know the information you are learning in this book. They didn't know what was happening in their body that then leads to a heart attack. You, my friend, are now in a very, very powerful position. If you choose to read this entire book, you will have the information you need to never, ever suffer from a heart attack or in fact become a statistic of any of the lifestyle diseases that claim so many lives in the Western world. Or if you have already had that happen to you, or indeed any life-changing health issues, understand that it's okay, we can get your body back to as close to optimal health as humanly possible.

I have people's experiences in these very pages that point to the fact that most diseases can be nullified to the point that it may seem to some that they never really happened. My eczema story is one of them, but there are far more powerful stories than mine. Obviously, as already discussed, that information has to be put into action, but all you need to do is follow the simple, logical steps laid out on this book. So, what's my point?

My point is, what are you doing to limit the stress in your life? Consider these facts before you state you are too busy or don't have the time to do something to deal with your stress.

- Workplace stress alone contributes to over 120,000 deaths each year in the US, according to researchers at the Harvard Business School and Stanford's Graduate School of Business.

- 83% of US workers suffer from work-related stress according to a comprehensive survey done by Everest College in 2013

- Seven people die worldwide from stress every 2 seconds, according to the CDC.

- The World Health Organisation has called stress the "health epidemic of the 21st century."

It's called The Silent Killer for a reason. People don't realise that when they have depression, coronary heart disease, high blood pressure, fears, phobias, irritable bowel syndrome, fibromyalgia, ulcers, eczema and self-destructive habits like overeating, smoking, alcohol and other drug use, it is all brought on or made worse by stress.

An Average Day

Think now for a minute on the average person's day to day stress. We are only really designed for the fight or flight type of stress. That quick surge of adrenaline and cortisol can save your life, and so is a good thing. But the overproduction of adrenaline and cortisol without the physical offset of fight or flight leads them to build up in the blood causing major problems with both the body and mind.

Let's take a quick look at the average person's day;

The very first second of your day has you waking up to an alarm that scares the crap out of you.

There's the usual race against time due to hitting the snooze button 3 or 4 times. You not only have to get yourself ready for work, but the children prepared for school. This race against time means you miss breakfast, so instead, you fuel your body with a caffeinated beverage to kickstart your day.

While stuck in a traffic jam, someone pushes in, causing anger levels to rise. If there's one more red light, you might tear your hair out. The anxiety of being late to work brings about that nervous twitch you hate. You get to work late, and your boss calls you into his office. The typical feeling of dread sweeps over your entire body.

There's a large pile of new work on top of the work pile from last week. You're now sure to miss another deadline of which the anxiety is too much to deal with right now, so you go and grab your second coffee of the day which raises your adrenaline levels so much you get the shakes.

Your coworkers are as annoying as ever, and you receive a text from your other half that really annoys you. You work through lunch...again. Lack of food has you reaching for more caffeine and sugary snacks that have your hormones spiking up and down like a roller coaster. You feel out of control with your emotions and go to the bathroom to either scream or cry, whatever comes out first.

On the way home, you are stuck in yet another traffic jam which means you are late picking the kids up from after school club...again. You are wondering if the extra cost of childcare is even worth the stress of the low income that your job brings you.

You get home to a pile of bills you don't have time to look through right now. You need to get the kids ready for their karate class which you are currently running late for and on the way there some douche pulls out in front of you nearly causing an accident. Your stress levels soar.

You get home to prepare dinner. Your other half arrives home in a foul mood after his own stressful day. You forgot you were meant to visit his mother in hospital on your lunch break. You get into a heated argument.

You sit down to sort through and pay the bills even though you don't want to deal with it right now. An electricity bill is wrong, so you spend 25 minutes on the phone listening to hold music that infuriates you. You forget you have to pick the kids up from karate class and arrive half an hour late.

You get home to a burnt dinner. You ring the other half to get takeaway on the way home from visiting his sick mother in the hospital. He doesn't answer the phone the first four times of calling, which frustrates you no end. Somehow, it's your fault the dinner got burnt. Another argument ensues.

You eventually all get to eat at 8:30 pm, which stresses you as you note that you are gaining weight, shouldn't be eating takeaway and especially not at that time of night! You don't feel good in your own skin.

At 10 pm after the struggle of finally getting the kids to settle down from sugar-laden fast food, washed down with yet more sugar in the form of soda; finally, it's your time to relax.

You sit down and watch the news. Your brain fills with images of children getting blown to bits in the latest war on terror. You wonder how it would feel if that were you and your children caught up in a war, and it fills you with sadness. You watch as on home soil there is the most recent report of another school shooting.

You are filled with dread as you see the possibility of war with North Korea getting closer. You feel hopeless as you see there is no way out of the massive debt you are in as you watch a report showing fuel prices are on the rise again, and the cost of living is going up, but your wage has stayed almost exactly the same for the last three years.

You see the weather tomorrow is going to be lovely and warm, but you'll be stuck in the office filtering through the massive amount of work you have for little in return. This causes yet more anxiety.

You decide to go to bed. Once again, you are too tired to have sex. You wonder how your relationship has lasted so long with so little connection. You go to sleep stressing about the future only to dream about work and wake up the next morning feeling like you haven't slept one wink, only to do it all again...

So, what can we do about it? It is possible to limit stress, and these are a few ways to handle it;

Sunrise Alarm Clock

I use a sunrise alarm clock that is not alarming at all. It slowly wakes me up as if the sun is rising in my room, so I don't have a shocking start to my day. It allows my internal body clock to adjust slowly, without the massive release of cortisol and adrenaline that a loud alarm clock brings about.

According to researchers at Athabasca University in Canada, somewhere around 2-9% of the population of Alaska, Canada and the UK suffer from Seasonal Affective Disorder (SAD), depending on where you live, with many more suffering milder symptoms. Light therapy has long been associated with helping forms of depression, and sunrise alarm clocks have shown to be effective too.

Yoga

A great way to relieve stress and at the same time, tone and strengthen your body while becoming more flexible. Make sure to give it a chance, though. You need to do at least six classes to really 'get it' as it is very different from other forms of exercise.

The style that I like to perform to offset stress is Restorative Yoga. Each pose is held for 3-15 minutes and becomes almost like a mini-meditation. It allows you to focus on slowing your breath and to fully relax into each pose, rather than trying to keep to a more movement-based class, which has its own benefits, but for true stress relief, I do love doing a restorative session.

One pose I highly recommend doing daily, preferably either at the end of a long hard day at work when you get in the house or just before bed is the **Legs Up The Wall Pose** (Viparita Karani). The health benefits of this one simple pose, that almost anyone can do are substantial. It is a deeply relaxing pose that calms the nervous system, which, in turn, helps lower stress and anxiety. It helps improve circulation and lymphatic drainage, relieving tension and fatigue from the feet, legs and even the hips. Inverting the legs or feet has long been known as an effective therapy to help reduce swelling and pain in lower extremities. It gently stretches the hamstrings and lower back, relieving back pain. It has also been shown to improve digestion and sleep. So, give it a go! As so, below:

- Begin the pose by finding some space near a wall in a quiet room.

- Lay down on your back with your feet nearest the wall.

- Move your hips closer to the wall and bring your legs up vertically, resting your heels against the wall.

- Have your hands just away from your side, palms faced up - you can also place a pillow under your head.

- Now, try to relax every part of your body as you continue to keep your legs propped up against the wall.

- Close your eyes and breathe deeply - try to lengthen each breath as you inhale through your nose and then exhale back out through the nose.

- Stay in this posture for 5-15 minutes.

- To come out of this pose, bend your knees and push your body gently away from the wall, turning onto your side in the foetal position.

- Gently come to a seated and then a standing position, being careful not to move too quickly and causing yourself to become dizzy.

We are just about to cover meditation and breathing in more depth now, and there is much more on yoga in a later chapter.

Meditation

It really is the ultimate stress relief in today's hectic world. There are a lot of benefits to mediation. One of my favourite authors Tim Ferriss, has interviewed many famous and successful people from Jamie Foxx to Arnold Schwarzenegger to people at the top of business and world-class athletes. The one thing that more than 80% of them do is some form of daily meditation. Why? People in the know are well aware of how vital stress relief is, but the benefits go way beyond that. It will, of course, help to quiet the mind, stopping the production of stress hormones brought about by constantly thinking. But it will also bring about focus in the times you need it most as well as breakthroughs, ideas and answers to questions that you couldn't seem to recall in the busyness of your day.

The funny thing is people stress about meditating 'right'. Which really is ironic and extremely counterproductive! There is no 'right' way to meditate, so stop stressing and simply start. There are great apps out there that take you by the hand and guide you through the whole process of meditation. Use these, and you will soon get into the swing of things. Or finding a Group Meditation Class is an awesome way to learn, stay committed with a set time every week and to meet new, (generally), happy people! Meeting new, likeminded people is key to your success in becoming as healthy as possible as you'll find out in a later chapter.

Studies have proven the health benefits too. The National Center for Complementary and Integrative Health believes it can improve the quality of life for cancer patients through helping relieve anxiety, stress, fatigue, and general mood and sleep disturbances, which would apply to anybody! The Society for Integrative Oncology recommends meditation, as well as other mind-body modalities, to reduce anxiety, mood disturbance and chronic pain through evidence-based clinical practices. The American Heart Association also say there is evidence to support the use of Transcendental Meditation as part of treatment for high blood pressure.

Even more telling, for me at least, is the success researchers at the State University of New York had with women suffering from severe irritable bowel syndrome (IBS). Following up one-year after a very successful 3-month trial with subjects using Relaxation Response Meditation to treat IBS researchers noted significant additional reductions in pain and bloating, which tended to be the most distressing symptoms of IBS. Where do you usually feel stress and nervousness first? Exactly. Your guts. If you have digestive issues of any kind turning to meditation will surely help ease those symptoms.

Okay, for those of you who don't want to download an app or go to a class, try the following meditation in the safety of your own home. I call it **Meditation 101**;

- Find a quiet space where you won't be distracted.

- Sitting comfortably, spine straight. Choosing whether you are cross-legged on the floor or sitting in a chair, feet side-by-side.

- Close your eyes and simply notice your breath.

- Breathe slowly in and out through your nose.

- Notice that the air is cool as it enters your nostrils and warmer as it leaves your body.

- Feel the rise and fall of your chest.

- Follow the breath on its journey, as it enters through the nostrils, down the back of the throat, into the upper chest, and deep down into the lungs.

- Follow it on its way back up into the upper chest, through the bronchial tubes, up the back of the throat, and out through the nostrils.

- Try and slow down your breathing, taking longer breaths as you relax more, aiming to do the same length of time with your inward breath as you do on your outward breath.

- Each time you take a complete breath both in and out count down one breath at a   time from one hundred and one.

- If an external thought enters your mind, acknowledge the thought, let it go and then go back to counting starting again at 101.

- See how many slow controlled breaths you can complete without a single external thought entering your mind.

- Remember! Your mind is like a muscle, with training it will get stronger, and the exercise will get easier. *Patience* is key.

Now a key point here is that you'll likely get distracted *a lot in* the beginning. You might not even make it past 98 the first time you do the exercise! To refocus your mind, to give you the best chance of staying on track you need a mantra, that in itself is a very powerful Positive Affirmation but here we are not too focused on that. (That's for later in the book!) We are using it as a mind vehicle to get you refocused. That, by the way, is what mantra stands for, 'mind-vehicle'. Mantra is a Sanskrit word, comprised of the root words "manas" meaning mind/to-think, and "tra" meaning vehicle.

As your mind starts to wander and you think about what you are having for lunch, when you realise you are not working with an empty mind anymore you acknowledge the thought, then let it go, then repeat your mantra three times. Saying your mantra out-loud on the outward breath over the next three breaths you take. Then you start again at 101.

Here are a couple of mantras you might say. For each time you do this practice choose only one mantra you will use that day.

- **OM** - The origins of om is said to be Hindu, and started in The *Mandukya Upanishad*, an ancient Sanskrit text that is entirely devoted to om. It begins like this: "Om is the imperishable word. Om is the universe, and this is the exposition of om. The past, the present, and the future, all that was, all that is, all that will be is om. Likewise, all else that may exist beyond the bounds of time, that too is om." Sounds pretty important to me! The symbol is one of peace, tranquility and unity and reminds people to slow down and breathe. The sound, and the vibrations it makes, helps to calm the mind and the central nervous system.

  - To perform the sound, apply these simple mouth adjustments.

  - For "ahh," relax the jaw. The sound rises from the belly, lips are parted, and the tongue doesn't touch the palate.

  - In "oooh," the lips gently come together as the sound moves from the abdomen into the heart.

  - During "mmm," the tongue floats to the roof of the mouth, and the lips come together to create a buzzing in the head.

- **HAM SAH** - This mantra means 'I Am That'. In other words, *I am here now*. Which is great to get you back on track remembering that the meditation you are currently doing is so you can be in the present moment, and not thinking about the past or being anxious about the future. You can also use this as a brilliant trick to help your body relax in a stressful situation. For example, stuck in traffic and knowing you are going to be late or your child is screaming in a public place. Repeating the mantra, Ham Saw a few times reminds you that you are you. You are here right now. The situation is temporary. It is what it is...Keep calm. Your calm demeanour will also help those around you and your child!

- To perform the sound, simply perform the "Hammmmmm" while you inhale.

- Then say "Sahhhhhhhh" as you exhale.

I think we can all agree meditation is something we need to be making time for in today's hectic and crazy world. The problem is most people either don't take the time or feel like they simply don't have the time to meditate. I would sometimes fill in for teachers in a Yoga Studio in Sydney and teach their class for them if they were unable to make it. With every class came an optional 5-minute meditation at the end, to recenter and wind down the session. The hilarious thing I noticed was; the people who were constantly checking their watch throughout the class, who struggled to fully relax into their poses, the ones with places they needed to be were the ones who couldn't seemingly (in their mind at least) spare *five minutes* to meditate and left early. Of course, they were the ones who needed it the most! The ones who were breathing deeply, who weren't even wearing a watch, the ones who seemed the most relaxed, stayed behind. A little dose of irony, indeed.

And so, with that, I leave you with this awesome quote;

"You should sit in meditation for twenty minutes every day - unless you're too busy; then you should sit for an hour." - Dr Sukhraj Dhillon

Breathing

As simple as it sounds, this is a fast and very effective technique to lower stress levels. If in a stressful situation, simply walking away and taking **5-10 slow, long but shallow breaths**. This will slow the production of stress hormones and make you feel calm, again leading to better decision making. Or as mentioned you can use the mantra Ham Sah.

Beyond that, breathing is an incredibly underrated but hugely important system to health. There are breathing exercises you can do, maybe even as part of your meditation practice that can teach you how to breathe properly.

Ancient Yogis noticed that animals with a slower breathing rate lived far longer than animals that take short, shallow breaths.

Think about the lifespans and breathing rates of elephants and tortoises, versus that of a dog that pants, or cats, mice and monkeys. Tortoises take only four breaths per minute and live an average of around 150 years. When laying down, an elephant takes five breaths per minute and lives for 70 years. A whale takes six breaths per minute and has an average life expectancy of 111 years. A dog, on the other hand, takes 20-30 breaths per minute and lives for around 10-20 years. A monkey is similar, taking 32 breaths per minute and living for 18-23 years.

The reason for this is that if you slow down your breathing rate, your heart doesn't have to work as hard. Think of it as putting fewer miles on the clock of your car. Less wear and tear. A study at the Copenhagen University Hospital, Denmark showed how important your Resting Heart Rate (RHR) is. They followed 2798 men over a sixteen-year period and showed that people with an RHR of 80 beats per minute die up to five years earlier than those with an RHR of 60 beats per minute. Most people run around stressed out of their head, barely stopping to take a breath, never mind being mindful of it. Through practice, you can slowly become more aware of your breathing and then become unconsciously competent at taking control and slowing it down while going about your day to day activities.

Four Stages Of Competence

Turning to psychology for a minute to explain an important concept of learning. It's one that you need to be aware of when doing something new (and maybe even daunting to you such as yoga, meditation or breathing exercises) because as hard as something new is to learn just know that one day you will master it. That day may be sooner for some than others but stick with all the concepts in this book, and you will develop all the skills needed to live a long and healthy life regardless of whatever level you are at now. The keys are persistence and consistency. All I'm trying to say is, don't give up.

The four stages of competence are the learning model I'm just going to explain so you can get your head around doing perhaps new things to you such as meditating and practising breathing every day. In the beginning, for example, you didn't know you couldn't tie your shoelace, maybe because you didn't know what a shoelace even was! So, you were *Unconsciously Incompetent*. You didn't know what you didn't know. Then someone said, 'Hey, you don't know how to tie your shoelace.' So now you were aware of the fact you became *Consciously Incompetent*. Then you slowly learned and got better. As you were learning, you got the sequence of tying your laces but had to really think about it, so you became *Consciously Competent*. Now more than likely you can tie your shoelace without even thinking about it. The same can be said of breathing. It will take some practice, but you will eventually become so in control you don't have to even think about it. That's called *Unconsciously Competent*, and that's where we want to get to not only with breathing, but meditation, yoga and many of the other skills we will learn throughout this book.

Breathwork

To start with, let's try a simple breathing exercise I call **Natural Breath** to help you become more aware of your breath. It's actually the exact same technique I used in Meditation 101 and would likely be how you would go into most mediations, with me at least. However, because you might just want to focus on breathing right now, let's go over it again, so you get more and more comfortable with the process.

- Find a quiet space where you won't be distracted.

- Sitting comfortably, spine straight. Choosing whether you are cross-legged on the floor or sitting in a chair, feet side-by-side.

- Close your eyes and simply notice your breath.

- Breathe slowly in and out through your nose.

- Notice the air is cool as it enters your nostrils and warmer as it leaves your body.

- Feel the rise and fall of your chest.

- Follow the breath on its journey, as it enters through the nostrils, down the back of the throat, into the upper chest, and deep down into the lungs.

- Follow it on its way back up into the upper chest, through the bronchial tubes, up the back of the throat, and out through the nostrils.

- Try and slow down your breathing, taking longer breaths as you relax more, aiming to do the same length of time with your inward breath as you do on your outward breath.

- Continue focusing on your breathing for somewhere between 5-15 minutes, noticing how your body feels more and more relaxed on your outward breath and breathing becomes naturally longer and easier.

For a slightly more advanced breathing exercise, we can do **Alternate Breathing.**

- Start with 5 minutes of the exercise Natural Breath to relax and get in tune with your breathing.

- Take the index and middle finger of your right hand and place them on your forehead where your third eye is (between the eyebrows).

- Cover your right nostril with your thumb and take three natural breaths (nothing forced) exclusively through your left nostril.

- Now, uncover both nostrils. Take one breath in through your nose and out through your mouth as a resting breath.

- Now cover the left nostril using your ring finger and take three natural breaths through your right side.

- Then take a resting breath in through your nose and out through your mouth.

- You may notice it is easier to breathe through one side than the other, even struggling to complete the three breaths through one side.

- The aim here is to create balance left to right, so both sides become as strong as each other and so breathing becomes more relaxed in everyday life.

- Repeat the exercise 5 times on each side, aiming to make your breaths longer each set.

- Warning! You may get a sense of complete relaxation and even euphoria when doing this.

Meal Time

Now that we know the importance of breath, remember to take five deep breaths before you eat or drink anything. The other thing around food that we need to consider is to *slow down* in today's hectic world and take at least 20 minutes to eat a meal. We need to stop what we see as 'normal' in today's world, such as eating as we walk, eating in the car while driving or at the desk while answering emails! Stop eating in front of the TV and taking your phone to the dinner table.

Firstly, how are you going to enjoy what you are eating if your focus is not on your food? You're not going to *taste* anything while you are reading the news on your phone when you eat your beautiful organic salad. And if what you are reading or watching is triggering stress hormones to be released, alongside eating too fast, that's a double whammy of stress you could really do without.

Secondly, how are you going to know when you are full? It takes 20 minutes from the moment the food goes in your mouth until it reaches your gut and you start to feel like you've had enough. I see people eating enough food for two fully grown adults in just *ten* minutes, let alone twenty. If you're eating fast food, erm, fast you could potentially wolf down two burgers, some supersize fries and a great whopping milkshake without even knowing you were full after just one burger, a handful of fries and three sips of shake!

Go For A Walk

Instead of stressing yourself out and watching the news, in fact rather than watching any TV, go for a walk. Go for 20-60 minutes with your partner, your family, with a friend, your pet or simply by yourself. This one thing will help destress your body every day. It is easy to do, and best of all it's free! It has other noticeable health benefits as well, which we will cover in a later chapter, plus there is a social aspect if going with friends or family, which is another way to destress.

Go every day in the late afternoon, early evening (depending on where you are in the world) or early morning sun, with no sunglasses or suncream on; this will help with the natural production of Vitamin D in your body, which is a highly underrated vitamin. Our body heavily depends on getting a full spectrum of light which comes from natural sunlight. You get a massive absorption of natural sunlight through your eyes so not wearing sunglasses in the evening or early morning sun will allow your body to produce Vitamin D without the threat of damaging your eyes. The amount of organs that depend on full-spectrum light is astounding. According to researchers German Ophthalmologist Fritz Hollwich, MD and John Ott, Hon. D. Sci, 'When the eyes are exposed to natural light the pituitary gland, thyroid, adrenal glands, ovaries, testes, pancreas, liver, and kidneys all function better.'

Full-spectrum light also means ultraviolet light despite all the bad press it gets, when in fact there has never been any research showing the health benefits of blocking UV light to the eyes. But you will be hard-pressed to find any sunglasses that don't block UV light which research shows is massively counterproductive to the way our body naturally works. Beyond that, as the sunlight hits the back of your eye, it tells the body to prepare the skin for the sun and so releases higher levels of melanin which will protect you against burning. Therefore, there's no need to apply suncream in the evening or early morning sun if you are not wearing sunglasses because the body will naturally protect you. Suncream blocks sunlight from your skin and is potentially harmful in many other ways which we cover later in the book.

Going for a walk in the sunshine and looking into the distance helps the mind switch off entirely, helps produce happy hormones and Vitamin D, and is regularly used by good doctors for treatment of depression and seasonal affective disorder (SAD). If you do suffer the winter blues or any form of depression, merely taking an early morning or early evening walk as described above will most definitely be beneficial to you and a fantastic addition to anybody and everybody's day.

Journaling

One of the most amazing things I did to treat my condition eczema was journaling. After seeing a study and a fair few articles showing that people with eczema didn't express anger, I realised that that was me. Journaling is a great way to get rid of the heat and energy that builds up in the body if you don't release it physically through anger. What happens in most cases is that the energy that is not released comes out through the skin in the form of skin conditions such as eczema. So, when I learned this, I figured I'd give journaling a go.

Before bed one night, I wrote, and boy did I write, all about what had upset me in my life that I never really talked to anyone about. I wrote seven A4 pages without stopping; I then tore up the pages and threw them in the bin. What ensued was one of the most amazing but painful experiences of my life. I woke up covered in blood. My sheets, pillow and even mattress were absolutely soaked in sweat like someone had poured an entire paddling pool over me in the night. I had open wounds all over me. I then remembered the dream I had that night;

'I was Will Smith's Madame Tussaud wax model. I was stood to the back and centre of a long room. On my right was a door that was currently closed. To my left, I could see another closed door with a path out in front of me that joined the two. I was the only model that stood on a low raised platform.

The door on my right opened, and I knew it was my time to be still and silent like the wax model I was playing. Flooding in came a class of schoolchildren with a certain air of excitement about them.

They came straight over to me and started pushing pins deep into my skin. My face, my arms and my torso burned like it was on fire. I knew all I had to do was stay still and silent. As quickly as they came, they exited out of the door on the left. As soon as the door closed behind the last child, I knew I had only one minute before the next group would be coming through the door on the right.

This was my cue to scratch out and remove the pins that burned so bad. As I did, it was a feeling of ecstasy. The relief was amazingly intense, almost orgasmic. Then the door opened, and it was time to be perfectly still and silent again...'

Little did I know the damage I was doing to my body as I slept. It would be weeks before I was brave enough to journal again. You might be thinking why the hell would you do that again!? The next time was much the same;

'I was an old Chinese man whose skin had cuts of beef attached to it. I hovered; legs crossed above a cauldron full of boiling water. Much to the entertainment of tourists coming up the hill, who would stop and throw wood into the fire to make the water bubble up and cook the beef. Once they left, I would scratch until the cooked beef was gone.'

I have never worked out why I am a character with a different race to my own, but that's beside the point! Both times in the following days and weeks, my skin cleared up massive amounts. I had purged the heat and energy from my body that was the root cause of my problem, and the results were spectacular. Researchers in New Zealand also showed that journaling could physically heal older adults aged between 64 to 97 years in a paper published in 2013. In somewhat amazing results, the group that were directed to journal for 20 minutes per day for three days, had a 4-mm punch biopsy wound heal better after 11 days, and they got more sleep than the group who did not journal.

You may not have a skin condition but using me as an example is an excellent idea because I could see the physical difference in my skin, which is on the outside and visible to all.

Think of what it could do for your inner health, getting rid of any pent up anger and trapped emotions.

Think of all the times you wanted to say something but didn't. All the times you suffered in silence and never really talked to anyone. That energy could still be stored in your body, causing health issues that you can't see or feel right now, or maybe even ones that you can! Since my two experiences, I now don't journal at night. I do it in the day and then burn the paper, usually on a beach or in a park. Every time I do this, the remarks I get about my skin is truly astonishing. People are always asking what do I use on my skin? What have I been doing that's different? Then people think I'm joking when I say journaling. Beauty and health start on the inside. That much I think we can all admit to being true.

So, before you think this is way too out there, please don't think like that just yet, give it a chance and experience it. I didn't want to bring something like this into the book so early; I wanted to warm you all up with obvious changes you can make. And there's plenty of that to come very soon! But stress and the power of your mind is so powerful it can't be ignored. And for those of you who wholeheartedly agree and get what I'm saying, don't worry there's lots of funky stuff to come too! Something that I'm struggling to admit to (as I sit next to my father who is my proofreader), as having a massive impact on the health of my skin is the following;

Have A Good Cry

Fuck it. In for a penny, in for a pound. In much the same way journaling is a release of energy so is letting it go through crying. Researcher and Medical Doctor, Juan Murube showed in a 2009 paper that tears contain toxic chemicals and stress hormones, therefore crying reduces stress on the body. In a paper published in 2014 in the journal Frontiers in Psychology, researchers showed crying activates the parasympathetic nervous system (PNS), which helps people relax.

Having cried only twice in the last ten years (tough man I know!), I can honestly say the positive effect on my skin health afterwards was mindblowing. Everyone I spoke to the next day after I cried the night before, thought I had had a facial in a spa, using the fanciest products. But no, I had simply cried. Skin is a window to your inner health. So once again because I could literally see the positive effects, it was easy for me to tell the difference. You may or may not be able to either see or feel the results, but I can assure you the health benefits will be there from journalling or letting go through having a good cry.

Just as crucial as releasing negative energy is to restore it. The next chapter could have life-changing information for some of you. Most people struggle to sleep. The next chapter will have every one of you sleeping like a baby. Beyond that, I am going to show you a simple way to make you far more productive the next day (lowering stress levels and creating more time to do things like...meditating) and how to improve the time you spend with the other half in between the sheets. Before that, it is time to take action. So do the following before moving on;

Resources

Go to **www.TomBroadwell.com/resources** to see;

- The sunshine alarm clock I currently use and recommend.

- A free video showing how to perform the Legs Up The Wall pose.

- The meditation apps I use and recommend.

- Free videos on how to correctly perform the Breathwork exercises.

Action Steps

- Buy an alarm clock that will wake you up peacefully.

- Start going for a walk at the same time each day if possible, to create a new healthy habit.

- Make sure you have at least 20 uninterrupted minutes every time you sit down to eat a meal, with no phones, computers or TV's on while you eat

- Research and book a spot on a yoga class that you can get to without causing you stress. Buy a package of 6 or more lessons if possible.

- Next time you find yourself in a stressful situation, walk away and take 5-10 deep breaths or repeat the mantra Ham Sah a few times. If it's not possible to walk away because it might cost you your job, take 5-10 deep breaths as soon as you can afterwards.

- Download a meditation app and get started straight away. Or you can always look for a Group Meditation in your area which is an amazing thing to try and to meet new, (generally) happy people!

- Start journaling. Choose a subject you know has caused you grief in the past and write down everything that comes to mind. *DO NOT* reread anything that you write. Either tear up the pages and throw them away or burn them if safe to do so.

- Something I definitely need to take my own advice on and do more often is; next time you feel like crying, do it and let it go...

Chapter Three

Sweet Dreams

"A good laugh and a long sleep are the best cures in the doctor's book."– ***Irish Proverb***

I lay there.

Staring at the ceiling.

As usual.

Mind going 1 million miles per hour.

Stressing about the fact it was only 4 hours until the alarm will go off.

Thinking over what I should of said to that asshole I had an argument with earlier in the day.

Trying to get my thoughts to a more positive path.

Trying to blank my mind if at all possible.

One minute I was too hot.

Then I didn't like the fact my leg was out of the cover.

Exposed.

I tucked it in.

Only to be too hot again 2 minutes later.

Tossing.

Turning.

What to do?

As it turns out it's pretty simple.

Four Lists

That's all it takes. Write down Four Lists on a notepad with a pen. Not on your phone or a laptop but with a pen and paper. Two reasons, one is the fact when you stare at a screen just before sleeping, the light hits the back of your eye telling your brain it's daytime and it's time to wake up! The second and main reason being because of the huge amounts of movements you make with your hand when writing, compared to typing on a laptop, or worse with your thumb on a phone, activates far more areas of the brain. This leads to better memory recall, more creativity, relaxation and a far greater connection to what you write. All this is necessary especially when writing just before sleep but also when note taking in seminars and class. How will this help you sleep? This empties your mind. Allowing you to sleep peacefully.

The lists are as follows and need to be written in this particular order;

- **Contact List**: - People you need to contact. Write down everything from phoning your mother, texting your brother and emailing back that business proposal.

- **To-Do List**: - Everything you need to do. If it's the first time doing this write down short term, medium term and long term actions and goals. This will make you far more productive the next day, week and even year and will go a long way to helping you achieve your goals. Having goals will make you happier and healthier and achieving them will certainly help you sleep at night! But this is not the point, the point here is to empty your mind of thinking about what you need to do tomorrow and the next day.

- **Pissed Off List**: - Write down everything that pissed you off that day no matter how small. Get it off your chest. Get it out of your mind. Write down *everything*!

- **Gratitude List**: - Write down 20 things you are grateful for. If you are struggling, start with sight if you have it. Write this list last of all so you go to sleep with a big smile on your face and in a positive mood.

What you do with these lists will go a long way to helping you achieve goals you never thought possible. This, however, is a book on achieving your *health* goals, and so we will mainly stick to that here, although we do discuss goal setting in more depth in a later chapter. Because at the end of the day if you are achieving your life long ambitions, you're far likelier to be happier and therefore healthier. Keep your Contact List and To-Do List for the next day and use them. This will help you become more proactive instead of reactive, which in turn will lower stress levels.

Tear up your Pissed Off List and throw it in the trash. Don't reread this one. Ever.

Don't worry, this is not nearly as deep as journaling and therefore won't bring out tremendous amounts of heat or energy in the night, it will simply clear your mind allowing you to sleep better. Keep your Gratitude List, maybe in a separate notebook that you can turn into a Gratitude Journal which you can read back from time to time when you need a little motivation or a little extra happiness in your life.

To follow on from not writing your lists on your phone because of the bright lights waking you up, stopping the following will have a huge impact on your sleep.

No Screens

Don't look at any screens at least one hour before bed. That includes TV, smartphones, tablets, laptops, smart watches and any other device since brought out to the public since I wrote this sentence! Wondering why your mind is racing with thoughts when you've just read an in depth article on your tablet, got emotional about a social media post or been scared by something on TV?

This means not having a television in your bedroom.

Your bedroom should be a relaxing sanctuary without anything in there that reminds you of being awake, working, stressed or active in any way. That means get rid of all computers. Tablets and phones should never find their way into your bedroom. They are far too tempting to grab when you think you can't sleep after just five minutes! You shouldn't walk into your bedroom and see gym equipment, paperwork, or household items like vacuums that remind you of things you could or should be doing rather than sleeping.

Charging Your Phone

Charge your phone in another room, preferably downstairs if you sleep upstairs. Don't have it radiating your brain while you sleep. One study done by researchers in the USA and Sweden found that radiation from mobile phones adversely affected sleep. They looked at the difference between giving people the same radiation as a mobile phone before sleep, and another group sham radiation (meaning no radiation) and the difference was significant.

The studies of what phones are doing to our brains (and our balls) are extensive. So much so we have an entire chapter dedicated to it later in the book. But for now, to keep the mood light, I have a little (true) story. Someone once showed me a video a little while back of a group of phones ringing and turning corn kernels into popcorn. They thought it was, 'Well cool!'. I said, imagine what they are doing to your brain when you sleep with it next to your head. They didn't think it was that cool anymore.

If you live in a one room apartment or a cabin like I have for long periods of my life, put it onto airplane mode. Some people say, 'Oh no I can't what if someone needs to reach me in an emergency.' I ask them how many emergencies have they raced out to solve in the middle of the night in their entire life? The answer is usually zero. It's obviously up to you, but I think the longterm damage on your health is not worth the off chance of being called to an emergency for the first time in your life. Talking of TV's in bedrooms and balls this next subject should excite you more than any other. You should only ever use your bed for two things...

S&S

Sleeping and...sex. That's it. Nothing else. Not for watching TV. Not scrolling through your smartphone. And not for reading 50 Shades of Grey. I mean how messed up is it that most women are more excited about a fictional character than the very man laid next to her (who is probably reading about the latest going on in his favourite sport, meaning he's spending time reading about muscular men getting sweaty rather than getting down n dirty with his own wife!). C'mon people stop with all the bullshit distractions and start making love or continue to do so if you already are. Tip of the hat to you if you are! When you lay down in bed, if it is only used for the above two things, then your mind is already preparing to sleep. Don't confuse it by laying down to watch 12 episodes of your favourite series or to read a book. If you like reading in bed to relax, no problem, but do it *sat up*.

This was proven in a massive study of 4 million people in 80 countries. When the study was performed in 2010, it was found that simply *owning* a TV (anywhere in the house!) would have a 6% reduction in the likelihood of couples having sex. Never mind having one in the bedroom. In the updated paper, the researchers say that because the survey was done before the widespread use of smartphones, the real sex-life killer today will be more than likely just that. The study shows a rather worrying trend of replacing human companionship with that of an electronic device.

Food Before Bedtime

Much more on food coming up, but when it comes to sleep; let's not have simple sugars rushing around your bloodstream or be taxing the digestive system with heavy meals containing starch and meat. Let's have your (or your child's!) last sugary treat *at least* 4 hours before bed, if not *sooner*. Let's have your last large meal around the same timeframe. In a pivotal study published in the Journal of Clinical Sleep Medicine, researchers found that people with a diet of low fibre and high sugar foods spend significantly less time experiencing deep, slow-wave sleep. This type of sleep is essential for restoration, and the healing of the body, mind and soul.

When was your last coffee or soda?

Before 3 pm hopefully...In another paper published in the Journal of Clinical Sleep Medicine in 2013 found that even a moderate intake of caffeine 6 hours before bed severely affected both the quality and length of sleep someone can expect. In another paper published in the journal Science Translational Medicine, caffeine was shown to delay your circadian clock, which puts you completely out of metabolic rhythm with the world around you.

And if you're dead set against sugar or wondering why a heavy meal would ever be a good idea don't worry I have you covered later in the book! However, this may be news for some people. Which is fine, you don't know what you don't know. So, let's start with small, achievable, realistic goals for all. And if you are worried, you'll have to give up sugar completely, or thinking you'll be *starving* after a long day at work and need a big meal, don't worry I have you covered too! Let's start striving for progress and not perfection...Last but not least (with much more physical reasons you might not be able to sleep covered in a later chapter) let's look at something that is almost never discussed when it comes to sleep.

Mouth Breathing

If you have broken sleep through feeling the need to pee in the night, breathing through your mouth and not your nose might well be the reason why. See, I was told by my Holistic Dentist in Sydney (Dr Charlotte de Courcey-Bayley, more to come from her in a later chapter), that if you breathe through your nose at night your body relaxes as it allows you to take longer, deeper breaths which in turn produces hormones responsible for telling you to fill your bladder. If you breathe through your mouth this doesn't happen, as you take shallow, shorts breaths that that trigger the fight or flight response, causing an increase in the production of those pesky stress hormones, which in turn causes a terrible night's sleep and your bladder is not told to fill up.

Studies show nasal breathing lowers adrenaline levels, blood pressure and relaxes the body. That's why it is practiced in Yoga. Dr Charlotte showed me a most sadistic way of correcting mouth breathing, but it works! And it helps your teeth and gums through not exposing them to the constant attack of the elements throughout the night. You have to tape your mouth shut while you sleep. With a special tape usually called 'sleep strips' or 'mouth strips', not just any old duct tape! Start for a few nights by still having the corner of your mouth free. Then go for the full mouth after 4-7 nights. Don't say I didn't say it would get funky. But would you rather have good teeth and a great night's sleep? Of course, you would. So, get it done.

Now obviously there's a ton of other physical things you can do to sleep better, which are all covered in this book. Start with the specific Action Steps from this chapter and you will feel a huge difference and then, as you go through all of the steps in this book, you'll see your sleep getting better and better.

In the next chapter, we will look at one specific subject that is very high up on the list of the most important things for your health, and that thing is *water*. You definitely need it to survive, but I will show you just how important the *type* of water you choose is for your health. You're going to learn how to increase your metabolism with one simple trick, and I'll give you the details on how to avoid potentially the greatest scam of the 21st century. Beyond all that I'll show you how to save lots of money by showing you precisely what bottled water you should be choosing, and which ones are as good for your health as the water, you get for free out of your tap. Before that, we must take some Action Steps to keep you on the path to optimal health.

Resources

Go to **www.TomBroadwell.com/resources** to see;

- The tape I used to become a nasal breather.

Action Steps

- Tonight, before sleeping write the down Four Lists using a pen or pencil, then continue this every night until it becomes routine.

- Remove the TV from your bedroom (DO IT!).

- Make your room a relaxing sanctuary removing everything that reminds you of work, chores or being active - also not allowing devices such as phones and tablets into your sleep space.

- Tonight, charge your phone in a separate room from your bedroom and/or put it on airplane mode.

- Tonight, make love to your partner if you have one. Or at least start with a kiss and a cuddle to reconnect. Start showing them you're interested if it's been a while.

- Limit the times you eat sugar, starch or red meat after 6pm. This could depend on your bedtime which could well be daytime if you're on night shift (your bedtime now might also change due to not giving yourself pure energy just before bed!).

- Don't have caffeine in any form after 3pm.

- Make sure to buy your tape if you are a mouth breather.

Chapter Four
Life Begins With Water

"When you drink the water, remember the spring." – ***Chinese Proverb***

I asked my brother;

"Why do you use the most expensive fuel for your car?"

"Because it gets much better performance out of the engine. I can feel the difference when I drive," he replied.

"Why do you drink tap water?" I asked.

"Because it's free. Why the hell would I pay for water!?!" he questioned.

Hmm...

We see this type of inverted values all the time in today's day and age. People prefer to spend time and money on their cars, their houses and not their own body. Yet, our body is made up of approximately 60% water. Our brain and heart are around 75% water. If you are replacing this with poor quality water, then don't expect to be in good health a lot of the time! Okay let's get an often asked question out of the way first.

How Much Water?

Everyone tells me it's eight glasses a day, but why are you drinking the same as a 250 lbs guy? If you are thinking 'because Tom, I am a 250 lbs guy'. Fair enough, but why are you drinking the same as a 120 lbs woman? We are all different. The lowest volume of water you should drink per day is half of your body weight measured in pounds, in fluid ounces. That's if you are sedentary...Breaking that down for my peeps in different parts of the world;

Weight	Fluid Ounces	Litres	Glasses
250 lbs / 113.4kg / 17.8 stones	125	3.7	15.5
200 lbs / 90.7kg / 14.3 stones	100	3	12.5
150 lbs / 68kg / 10.7 stones	75	2.2	9.5
100 lbs / 45.4kg / 7.1 stones	50	1.5	6.25

Now for something simple to kickstart your metabolism and start losing unwanted fat:

Drink two glasses of water immediately upon waking.

This gets your body moving and metabolism going for the day, helping your body to function and to burn fat. If you are still thinking that drinking more water is a bad idea because the thoughts, "I will need to pee all the time" are running through your head, please consider this is precisely why you should do it! You should be peeing to rid your body of the build-up of toxins (more on that in a later chapter). Other than that, it was found by researchers at Berlin's Franz-Volhard Clinical Research Center in Germany that after drinking 17 oz of water, their subjects metabolic rates increased by 30%. They estimate that over one year, a person who increases their water consumption by 1.5 litres a day would experience a weight loss of approximately five pounds. How about that for motivation! Want to lose weight? Drink more water. Now, let's look at what is even more key to your health.

The Type Of Water

Filtered Water

I've avoided tap water for the last ten years. I will always buy bottled water in restaurants. Why? Firstly, tap water contains the chemicals chlorine and in some parts of the world fluoride. As far as chlorine goes, I used to dose a swimming pool in a large Health Club in Leeds and to do that job; you first have to complete a short safety training course. To handle chlorine, you have to wear a full bodysuit, wellingtons, gloves and a gas mask with two filters! Meaning in its purest form chlorine is a highly toxic chemical. For example, if you swim in a pool that has too much chlorine, your eyes burn. Jump into one that is freshly dosed and your skin burns. This means you are having an acute reaction (one that is happening right now). So surely; bathing, and swimming in and then drinking the diluted form every day could cause chronic illness, no?

According to the US Council Of Environmental Quality, there is 'significant evidence' of increased cancer risks among people who drink chlorinated water versus those who don't. They put the risk of some forms of cancer among people drinking chlorinated water at 93% higher than among those whose water does not contain chlorine. *Ninety-three per cent!* A statement that the Chlorine Institute in New York said appeared to reinforce other studies on the effects of chlorine in the water. They said, 'I guess we can't dispute it at this point.' These findings were way back in 1980, from which nothing has changed...

The other chemical added to our water supply is *sodium fluoride* which is highly toxic to both the environment and the human body. Many studies are backing up this claim. Researchers at the University of Kent and London School of Hygiene and Tropical Medicine came to the conclusion that fluoride can cause *significant* human health problems while having only *modest* effects on dental health. They believe the act of adding fluoride to the water supply artificially should be rethought on a global level, and laws should be tightened because of the devastating effects on the environment.

Put it this way, there is one active ingredient in your toothpaste (sodium fluoride, good guess) and it says on the label; 'If swallowed seek immediate medical attention'. So why the fuck is it in your *drinking* water!?! It's in there because of one of the largest cons of all time. It's in there because huge aluminium companies needed somewhere to dump the toxic by-product when making aluminium, namely fluoride. The dumping of it in rivers was poisoning crops and making livestock sick and was costing millions of dollars in fines. So, they needed to convince the American public that it was a good idea to dump it in the water supply, for profit, nonetheless. The research to support the dumping of fluoride in the water supply was underwritten by the Aluminium Industry, Steel Industry, Dupont, and National Institute of Dental Research.

Enter Edward Bernays, who was also known as 'The Father of Spin' and the nephew of Sigmund Freud. He was also the author of many books, one conveniently called *Propaganda*. He was hired by the aforementioned companies to convince the general public that they needed fluoride in their water supply. It went from costing companies millions to the multibillion-dollar industry that we see today.

There is mounting evidence fluoride damages the thyroid gland. In the study of the largest population ever recorded in regard to adverse effects of elevated fluoride exposure, it was found that the city of Birmingham in the UK, which fluoridates water, compared with Manchester, UK which does not, has twice as many reports of hypothyroidism. This was after controlling for factors such as sex and age (women are more likely than men to have the condition, and the elderly more likely than the young). Because water consumption is widely considered to be the bulk of a person's fluoride intake, and the sheer size of the study (it covered 99% of England!) you'd think it would be seen as pretty comprehensive. But no, as you'll see throughout this book, there's always (for some reason rather angry) science bloggers who personally attack the authors who don't tread the mainstream line of thought, and then doctors who always seem to have a vested interest to disagree... You'll meet plenty of them as we go through the book.

Now beyond all that, is fluoride even good for your teeth? That question *will* be answered in a later chapter, and I have to tell you right now, the outcome is *comprehensive* and absolutely *jaw-dropping*. That is two chemicals that almost everyone knows about. However, there are many more chemicals that contaminate our drinking supply most would never expect to find in their nice refreshing glass of water. A 2019 report by the non-profit Environmental Working Group and Northeastern University showed an estimated 19 million people are exposed to water contaminated with

PFAS chemicals. The Centers for Disease Control and Prevention (CDC) states these chemicals have been linked to health issues that include birth defects, cancers and infertility.

David Andrews, a senior scientist for the Environmental Working Group, said; "This should be frightening to all Americans in many ways. These chemicals don't break down in our body, and they don't break down in our environment, and they actually stick to our blood. So, levels tend to increase over time."

If you are going to drink tap water, filter it.

There are some great filter jugs out there that get rid of almost everything, including fluoride. These can be a cheaper option if a filtration system for your entire house is too expensive right now. Be aware, because some of the larger brands actually state on the packaging that they keep the fluoride in for your health... 'facepalm'.

There are also very affordable filters for your shower head without having to get your whole system filtered. And let me tell you as a person who suffers from eczema that they work! When drinking filtered tap water, it is easy to see the difference; the taste is worlds apart. However, telling the difference when showering is a little more difficult unless you have very sensitive skin like me. In the big cities where I have lived, like London and Sydney, I've noticed the water is extremely harsh. This is because they are supplying millions of people when compared to the countryside and smaller towns. When my suffering was at its worst with eczema, the harsher water used to have me itching uncontrollably for a good 10-20 minutes after a shower. But when the water was filtered, I had no problem at all...

Bottled Water

In restaurants, I always order water sold in a glass bottle. Ever wondered why there's a sell-by date on bottled water? Well, water doesn't go off, so what is going on!? That's the date the plastic will break down so much there will be plastic leaching into your bloodstream. Next time you take a sip of bottled water that has sat in the sun too long, and it tastes nasty, that's not because the water is warm as one friend of mine claimed. I inquired, "So the water you use in your tea tastes terrible, does it?" No, it's the plastic that has broken down contaminating the water.

So, if are buying bottled water in a plastic bottle you need to remember two things. Only use plastic bottles once. The number in a triangle on the bottom of the bottle relates to the type of plastic. If it is the number 1 only use it once and then recycle it. That's why you'll never see me using the reusable plastic sports bottles in the gym. They are often made of poor quality plastic - maybe not number 1 on the triangle system but not much better. They will not usually last the amount of time you are considering using them for and more often than not contain carcinogenic compounds such as BPA. And even when they don't contain BPA, researchers in Austin, Texas found that the replacement plastics still cause estrogenic activity which we are trying to avoid. Once the plastic starts breaking down, then these chemicals will then enter your bloodstream. Lovely.

The quality of the water is only as good as the bottle it is in.

So, do yourself and the environment a favour and try to buy water in glass bottles as much as possible. The next thing to know when buying bottled water is only ever to buy water that is; **Bottled at the Source**. If not, you are paying for tap water. Talking of crazy, paying for tap water is crazy! It is tap water no matter what, even if it says, 'Natural Spring Water' and has pictures of birds, trees and mountains on the label. It's tap water. What will really make you happy is the fact that the best water is 100% free. It is truly bottled at the source. By YOU!

Spring Water

The absolute best tasting, freshest, cleanest and healthiest water I have ever found was from a spring in the Yorkshire Dales that I bottled at the source *myself*. If you can find a spring, you have literally hit gold and found the Fountain of Youth. The best place to start is **www.findaspring.com**. This is an amazing free website on which people submit the location of springs they have found. This means people all over the world can have access to the freshest, cleanest, freest water available.

We can't talk about water without talking about food. This will be discussed in the next chapter and boy it is an epic one! If you've learned something new already be ready to be taken to school in the next chapter! Just make sure you're sitting down and have some protective headgear on...because I am going to blow your mind...Take the next Action Steps first, before going on to the next chapter.

Resources

Go to **www.TomBroadwell.com/resources** to see;

- The filter jug I use and recommend.

- The shower filter I use and recommend.

- A clickable link to www.findaspring.com.

Action Steps

- Go to www.findaspring.com and see if there is a spring near you! If not, start asking around at your local yoga class, alternative health events, organic food markets etc.

- Buy a filter that filters *everything* toxic.

- Work out how much water you need and start planning on drinking that much every day, beginning with two glasses as soon as you wake up in the morning. A good way to reach this quota is to always have a bottle or glass of water with you, as you'll automatically sip from it throughout the day.

- Read the label of the bottled water you have been buying and figure out which brands are good or not so good. Remembering it must say Bottled at the Source.

Chapter Five
You Are What You Eat...

*"The food you eat can be either the safest and most powerful form of medicine or the slowest form of poison." - **Ann Wigmore***

As the goalkeeper cleared the sweat from his eyes, he looked out from the edge of his penalty area to see who he could pass to among his 8-year-old teammates.

"Fatty pass me the ball!"

"Pass me the ball Fatty."

Cries rang out from all over the football field.

Little did this affect his ability as it might in today's day and age of political correctness but allowed him to throw the ball more accurately as he answered to his nickname.

For he was the only overweight child on the pitch in 1993...

Yet today it would cause great confusion if you were to call, "Fatty pass me the ball." As most children would go to pass you a ball that wasn't even in their possession. Sad. But true. You purchased a book that described itself as the 'The *No Bullshit* Guide...' so here you have it. Have a look at what you are feeding not only yourself but your children. After what I show you in this chapter, hopefully, you are thinking, 'What the actual fuck am I doing!?!' If you do not think that, then I am sorry, it may be too late. I can't help you, so please stop reading and head back to Weight Watchers and Walmart. Sorry to not beat around the bush, but I need to prepare you for what you are going to read.

Processed Food

Okay, so a small survey to start; 'Who agrees that food has changed dramatically over the last 50-100 years?' Okay good, glad to have most of you still here. Over the past 50 years, the health of Americans has gotten worse. Now 71% of Americans are overweight or obese—not 66%, which was reported just five years ago.

A staggering 100 million men, women and children in America are obese.

However, I am not just pointing the finger at America. I have spent long periods of time in Australia, Britain and Canada over the last few years and I have to say that these countries are all quickly catching up to America in terms of the amount of processed food people eat.

This is highlighted in an amazingly enlightening paper by medical doctor Joel Fuhrman, published in The American Journal of Lifestyle Medicine in which he goes through the hidden dangers of fast and processed food. He describes the standard American diet (SAD), showing that over 55% of the SAD's calories are processed foods, and about 33% of calories come from animal products.

The consumption of fresh produce (fruits and vegetables) is at 10%, but in actuality, it is less than 5%, because it includes French fries and ketchup!

A proper nutritarian diet is rich in micronutrients such as phytochemicals and antioxidants. It is mainly vegetable-based, utilising a wide assortment of colourful vegetables, root vegetables, green vegetables, peas, beans, nuts, seeds, and some intact whole grains. In comparison, the SAD is almost the opposite of a nutritarian diet. Not only the SAD but most traditional diets are grain-based and therefore lack sufficient amounts of antioxidants and phytochemicals which have anti-cancer effects. As well as being high glycemic foods, which means sugar release in the blood is very fast and therefore can lead to weight gain and diseases such as type 2 diabetes and heart disease.

Processed foods such as bread, pasta, boxed cereals, breakfast bars, ketchup, mayonnaise, doughnuts, cookies, chips, soda, and popcorn do not contain a significant micronutrient benefit. A piece of meat is like a piece of toast because they are both rich sources of macronutrients (calories), but neither one contains the necessary amounts of micronutrients, especially the antioxidants and phytochemicals only found in plants.

One problem with the SAD is that it is pushed on people from a very young age. This, in a country that has children eating its daily recommended amount of fruits and vegetables per day, but classifies pizza, fries and ketchup as vegetables! Once those sugary, high carb options have gone down the hatch, the children then need to add other high carb grains to reach a 'balanced' diet. It's madness! So, what's in our food that wasn't in it one hundred and twenty years ago? The best place to start is;

Refined Sugar

This subject could have a chapter of its own, but I'll keep it short and sweet. Excuse the pun. Put it this way...Again, for some real stark truth. Time and again, people I come across say that their disease or even weight gain, 'runs in the family'. It's genetics, they say. As you will soon learn in a later chapter that is far from the truth. However, when I speak to clients, they genuinely think their genetics have blighted them. Though no fault of their own. Doctors often say, "It runs in your family." So, does that mean you have to have that disease? Or does it mean that maybe, just maybe you have the same lifestyle as your family members past and present? Think about this fact for one moment.

In 1700, the average person consumed approximately 4.9 grams each day of sugar (4 pounds of sugar each year). This then rose to around 22.4 grams each day (18 pounds of sugar each year) up until 1840. Then sugar consumption exploded, and as of 2009, 50% of Americans consumed approximately 227 grams (1/2 pound) of sugar each day - equating to 180 pounds each year. Half a fucking pound per day!

The average person consumes 70 grams of fructose each day – 300% above the recommended amount. Fructose in its purest form, as part of naturally occurring fruit is somewhat healthy (we will cover why not 100% healthy in a later chapter), but when added to processed food, it is stripped of all of its fibre and nutrients and will lead to serious health problems when consumed in the amounts discussed. Studies show that large amounts of sugar can lead to severe metabolic problems, including insulin resistance, metabolic syndrome, elevated cholesterol and triglycerides. Added sugar is one of the main drivers of diseases like obesity, type 2 diabetes, heart disease and cancer.

With the massive rise in sugar consumption, we have also seen an enormous increase in diseases related directly to sugar, such as type 2 diabetes. At the turn of the 20th-century, diabetes affected *one-tenth of 1%* of the population. According to the Centers for Disease Control and Prevention (CDC), in 1958, diabetes affected less than 1% of the population.

Today around 10% of people in America are diagnosed as having diabetes, and even more shocking than that, new cases doubled every year from 1990-2010.

Looking back, not so surprising considering it was just a few short years after Coca-Cola and Pepsi Co went from using refined sugar to the even more dangerous High Fructose Corn Syrup in their soda drinks. Today, more than *100 million* US adults are now living with diabetes or prediabetes.

Rather sadly and shockingly 31% of adults and 13% of children suffer from non-alcoholic fatty liver disease (also called NAFLD). This is a fatty liver that is not caused by drinking too much alcohol, but usually by consuming too much processed food that is high in sugar. NAFLD is characterised by excess fat that builds up in the liver. That is a massive number of children suffering from a disease purely caused by bad food choices. And so again I ask you, do you think the above examples of considerable increases in specific health issues are caused by it 'running in the family' or with the changes in our food? Answer that honestly and then start to make the changes, not only for yourself but your children as well.

Beyond the obvious health problems sugar can bring, there is also the fact it is highly addictive. In a paper published in the British Journal of Sports Medicine researchers show that sugar may be more addictive than *cocaine* in humans. Their studies showed animals get more addicted to refined sugar than the other white powder. Sugar is the most consumed addictive substance in the world. I have seen first hand what sugar can do to a child who, prior to trying a sugary snake sweet, had never consumed refined sugar once in his four short years on this world. His mother, a health advocate and Yogi had made sure his diet was pure and contained no processed foods. That was before I witnessed the child's uncle offering all the children at the family gathering sugary sweets. His father, who was always confused as to why his mother was so strict with their child's diet, told the uncle that it was, "all good, it's only a little bit of sugar, let's see what happens".

Even to me, the results were *shocking*, to say the least. The usually well behaved, balanced little boy, ate the sugary sweet and then proceeded to act like he was high on cocaine. He ran around like a madman, screaming at the top of his voice, clearly loving the sugar high. At one point he even ran full pelt into the side of a solid wooden table, was taken clean off of his feet as his forehead smashed into it, then proceeded to jump to his feet laughing out loud and carried on running. Amazing. From then I vowed any children I have would not eat processed food until they were able to make the informed decision themselves because children who can barely talk don't need sugary foods. As much as mothers, fathers, aunties, uncles, grandparents and the like think they are being nice to small children by buying them 'treats', they are not. You could be causing unnecessary addiction to sugar and food and uncalled for health problems. If not now, then later in life. The child could have to deal with weight problems, obesity, diabetes, heart issues, self-esteem issues and much more. All of this was caused during their early childhood when they didn't have a voice.

This next statement really shouldn't be shocking to anyone, but amazingly people are still suckered in by low-fat food choices...

Fat does *not* make you fat, sugar does!

Fats in food being the same word as fat in your body has confused people for decades, but it is such old science that fat makes you fat it is incredible to see how many people still think this way. I see qualified Personal Trainers cutting the fat off of chicken breast in the hope their body fat will lower. It's madness. Fat is essential to the human body. If I were to suck all the fat out of your body in one go, you would instantly drop dead. Yes, there are good fats and bad fats which we will cover soon. But none of them make you fat. Sugar does! Essential fats are so-called because they are...well, essential.

Sugar makes you fat through releasing the carrier hormone insulin. Insulin takes the sugar and stores it in your fat cells, which makes the fat cells grow larger. It does this to lower your blood sugar levels, which spike to dangerous highs when you eat too much sugar. Refined sugar spikes it faster than other forms of sugar. Refined sugar is in pretty much all processed foods. Please, please take control of your own health and your own weight and *stop eating processed food* (or at the very least limit it at this point in our journey). Not only for limiting the amount of refined sugar but for the following;

Americans each eat an average of around 6-9 pounds of chemical additives per person, per year.

That my friends is absolutely fucking mental, what's even crazier is that statistic is from 1978! How much do you think the average person now consumes? Food in America has changed dramatically since the Food and Drug Administration (FDA) took control of what chemicals are deemed fit for human consumption in 1958. Since then thousands of chemicals have flooded the food that people consume on a daily basis. This is an example of a very common problem you'll see throughout this book, of a government agency maybe not having your best interests at heart. Do you think your body was designed to deal with this chemical *shitstorm*? I don't think so either ...let's now take a look at the synthetic chemicals processed food contains.

Preservatives

Did you hear of the story of the Icelandic man called Hjörtur Smárason who bought the country's last McDonald's cheeseburger and fries in 2009? He had it in his garage in a plastic bag for three years and noticed it had not changed. No mould. No nothing. So, he decided to donate the meal to the National Museum of Iceland. After deciding they don't deal with food, they gave it back to him. It is now in its new home the Snotra House, a hostel in southern Iceland. They have a live stream of the burger and fries on their website that gets around 400,000 hits daily. To this day, eleven years later, it still looks the same! Just wow!

Think about the health implications of putting that inside of your body. Does this break down in your intestines? Probably not since it's obviously got enough synthetic chemicals in it to be designed not to break down for years at a time. Think about the small intestines for a moment; it's very warm at around 99°F (37°C), it's very long at around 20ft, it's dark, and it's moist. This is a perfect and quite disgusting place for bacteria and a lot of other nasty things to grow from the food that is stuck in your gut, which can then have devastating effects on your health. The big question is, does heavily preserved food naturally exit your body? Probably not. Again...More to come in a later chapter.

If you're thinking this asshole keeps trying to make me read his book, you're right. It's good for your health to continue reading. Well, sitting on your ass reading will not help your health, but at least you can make more informed decisions going forward! Oh, and by the way, two things to take from the above story. One is obviously that fast food is terrible. Two is that Iceland banned McDonald's. There is also no Starbucks and no army. It is also the only country in the world that jailed all the corrupt bankers after the 2008 world financial crisis. What a country! What else is in processed food that causes us major health concerns?

Additives

Ever wondered why you have never, ever craved an organic cabbage? Because synthetic chemical additives are put in food to make you addicted to that food. Once You Pop, You Can't Stop! Know that slogan? Never a truer statement said. Ever tried eating through a whole mixing sized bowl of raw broccoli? I love raw broccoli, but even I would find eating an entire mixing bowl of the stuff near impossible. A massive bowl of chips? Never failed, E-A-S-Y!

Processed food is much like nicotine in cigarettes. It changes the chemistry of your brain, making you need that food to keep the new chemistry in balance. Massive food companies are constantly in a race to find the latest, most addictive additive they can add to your food to increase their profits through you craving their food over others. Researchers at University Street, Montreal, Canada and Yale University amazingly showed that the exact same areas lit up in the brain when someone craved processed food and smoking.

You read that right; food today is as addictive as smoking.

In 2011 researchers from Yale University went one further and showed that food addiction is similar to drug abuse when looking at brain patterns. They found that similar patterns of neural activation are implicated in addictive-like eating behaviour and substance dependence. Many people reading this would be horrified by the thought of taking any illegal drugs. However, you have to realise that today's processed food would not be recognisable as food to your great-grandparents. It has the same addictive, controlling grip as illegal drugs and is actually responsible for far more deaths in the Western world. Now, I'm not saying illegal drugs are good, but when looking at the evidence, we cannot ignore that problems with food are at epidemic levels, and processed food is showing the same addictive qualities as drugs.

Thinking about that, don't get angry at your children when they kick and scream wanting, no, *needing* their bright neon-blue frozen beverage or their caramel chocolate cookie ice-cream *right now*! Or how they behave after the rush of getting their fix. That there, ladies and gentlemen is an *addiction* caused by food. Just remember that when you are fed up of how needy and hyperactive the kids are today.

I don't want to overwhelm you with too much scientific language right now by listing out a whole list of synthetic additives with long-ass scientific names, and exactly how they are destroying your health. I'm saving that for a later chapter when you're all warmed up. Still, to come in this very chapter, there are some specific, key ingredients you might want to avoid, then the rest will come later. However, the takeaway from all of this really is to stop eating processed food to curb food cravings and overcome addiction, lose weight, clear up your skin, solve your digestive issues and almost every other ailment you have. Easier said than done, I know, but I will show you how never to crave food again. In a later chapter (sorry...not really). What other wonders do they put in your food?

Artificial Sweeteners

Again, this subject could easily have its own chapter, if not its own book! These abominations are in over 10'000 products today. Where to start...I just thought that to myself as I stared out of the aeroplane window. That's not writer's block. That's a case of too much information to tell I don't know where to start! So, buckle up for the story of how messed up your food is and how screwed up the people in charge of it are.

Aspartame is possibly the most (in)famous sweetener. It took the FDA 16 years to pass aspartame fit for human consumption. That could be because there was a huge trend of it causing brain tumours to grow in many of the lab animals that it was tested on. It then made it into your food, because the politician who was in charge of the FDA at the time, a Mr Arthur Hull Hayes Jr. went against an FDA Board of Inquiry. The board had unanimously voted against aspartame ever been put in human food. Mr Hayes then put it in food just one year later in 1981 as one of his first acts as the new FDA commissioner.

The reason he became commissioner was largely down to the fact he was handpicked by the newly elected Ronald Reagan's transition team. The team included none other than Donald Rumsfeld, who was CEO of G.D. Searle, a chemical company that held the patent to aspartame. Aha! Yeah, go figure. In 1983 Mr Hayes passed aspartame for use in carbonated beverages. Soon after that, he quit his job on the FDA amid accusations that he was accepting corporate gifts for political favours and then started working for...G.D. Searle. Yes, again. Go figure.

Just two years after aspartame was put in diet soft drinks, rates of brain cancer went up by 10% and in people over the age of 65, an alarming 60%.

Aspartame is the food additive with the most complaints in the FDA's history. In 1995 under the Freedom of Information Act, the FDA had to make a list of symptoms thought to be caused by aspartame as brought about by more than 10'000 complaints. Here is a list of diseases it is thought to trigger or exacerbate; depression, birth defects, Alzheimer's, Parkinson's, epilepsy, mental retardation, brain tumours and chronic fatigue. They even listed death, which is a pretty severe symptom. The problem is not only money, but it's also the fact the huge companies that produce these chemicals have so much influence that they pay for their own studies to prove these chemicals are safe. However, 83 independent studies and counting, done over decades showed there were many adverse side effects to aspartame being put in your food.

Other artificial sweeteners such as **acesulfame-K** have been shown to cause leukaemia, tumours and respiratory diseases. **Sucralose** (which I think might be conveniently named to look a lot like the naturally occurring sucrose), has a very similar history to aspartame. It has had a marketing plan that seemingly tries to pull the wool over consumer's eyes, pretending it's natural when in fact it's far from so. Rather worryingly artificial sweeteners, including sucralose, are regulated as food additives and so the screening overall is less stringent than that required for drugs. Remembering these foods have zero edible calories and are made up of mainly synthetic chemicals, and so should not really be classed as food.

Researchers at North Carolina State University found sucralose to be mutagenic at elevated concentrations. They also found that it may alter glucose and insulin levels. This means that sucralose is toxic and if you have enough of it, remembering that it's in thousands of products today, it can cause mutation of cells. Meaning it can lead to diseases such as cancer. It also means that sucralose and every other artificial sweetener can still make you fat. This can happen even though they have zero calories, which amazes some people. Your tastebuds do not know the difference between sweeteners and sugar, and so the same hormones such as insulin elevate when you eat them, meaning you still gain weight. Remember that the whole calories in, calories out concept is bullshit. Weight gain is far more complicated than cutting back on calories, which is proven once again in the prior study on zero-calorie sweeteners and many more studies like it.

The oldest artificial sweetener of them all is **saccharin** which has had the same dodgy political past as most of the manmade foods in this chapter. Way back in 1977, the FDA proposed saccharin be banned for use in food because it was shown to cause cancer in studies using animals, which is fair as mice and humans share virtually the same set of genes. Almost every single gene so far that is found in one has been found in the other. This is one of the reasons rodents are used so often for use in laboratory tests. Congress, however, said it was not to be, and that saccharin should be allowed as long as the food carried a warning label. Since then in May 2000, the US Department of Health and Human Services removed saccharin from its list of cancer-causing chemicals after pressure from the diet-food industry. Later that year congress removed the warning labels. So, as I always say, take your health into your own hands and read the labels, as I will prove throughout the book that some powerful people within governments all around the world seldom have your best interests at heart.

We then have the amazing history of stevia, which *is* a naturally occurring sweetener from a plant native to South America, that has been used as a sweetener for hundreds of years. Astonishingly this is the only one mentioned to get banned in the US for being unsafe.

When in fact stevia has been shown to be safe in more than 200 studies, and indeed no experiments have ever proven it to be unsafe at all.

It was banned when an 'unnamed company' complained about it in 1994, with rumours circling it was the manufacturers of aspartame. Hmmm. Even when the FDA passed it again to be used in products, they stated that no one company in the US could say it is a sweetener on the label, despite being 300 times sweeter than sugar and containing no calories...I'll let you make your own mind up on that one!

I also have to warn you that you have to read the labels when it comes down to choosing your stevia. Ten years ago, there were very few stevia products, and all were pretty darn good. However, as people are becoming more aware of the dangers of synthetic chemical sweeteners, they are now looking for more natural alternatives. And so as with any chance to increase profits with the latest trend, the big corporations came out with their version of stevia, which a little bit of stevia mixed in with a whole lot of junk. Only buy 100% pure stevia and nothing else!

Trans Fats

These are man-made fats. Once again if something is touched by the hand of man, it appears that it will be a hazard to your health! Why did man start making his own Frankenfats? Because they declared war on saturated fats found in things like butter, cream and meat. It was claimed that these were clogging up your arteries and causing high cholesterol. Which they do contribute to in a small way. Maybe. However, your body can process naturally occurring saturated fats and get rid of them. However, trans fats are not so easy for your body to get rid of. Regardless of this, through clever marketing, the world went mad for trans fats.

The result; Today, trans fats are found in 40% of the products on your supermarket shelves. Where are they found? Processed foods. The problem? They have a much worse effect on clogging up your arteries and increasing your LDL cholesterol (the bad stuff) and decreasing your HDL cholesterol (the good stuff) than saturated fats. Great work! It has been shown that saturated fat is not actually associated with coronary heart disease, stroke or type 2 diabetes. Researchers at McMaster University in Canada proved this in their paper published in the British Medical Journal in which they found that trans fats are associated with all-cause mortality. The main concern here is that trans fats were advertised for years as a healthy alternative. What was this healthy alternative that was (and amazingly in some circles still is) raved about? *Margarine.*

But new findings are coming to light from the groundbreaking Nurse's Health Study, a study of 121,700 women at the time of its initiation in 1976. Participants are required to fill out follow up surveys every two to four years on a range of lifestyle topics. In the very successful study, the response rate is at 90% in most follow-ups. Results showed women who consumed the highest amount of trans fats in their diet had a 53% higher risk of heart attack compared to women who consumed the least. The time of highest consumption was between the 1950s and 1980s when trans fats were pushed as the healthier alternative.

Researchers at Slovak Medical University have linked trans fats to a lot more than just heart health issues. They found the greatest danger from trans fat lies in its capacity to distort the cell membranes and it having an adverse effect on the brain and nervous system. Trans fat from the diet is incorporated into brain cell membranes and alters the ability of neurons to communicate. This was then linked to low mental performance, depression and showed there was growing evidence for a possible role of trans fat in the development of Alzheimer's disease and cognitive decline with age.

Fear not, there are ways to reverse the damage of such things. Keep reading, and all will become clear. One thing you can do is immediately is to stop consuming trans fats. Replace them with the much healthier **polyunsaturated** and **monounsaturated** fats. You'll find these in nuts, seeds, avocados and oils such as olive, coconut, and avocado oil. It is thought that the body will replace the trans fats held in your cell membranes with these healthier fats over time. This is another time when you need to know how to read labels as trans fats can still be hidden in your food under different names. Avoid the following if, for some reason, you are still going to eat processed foods. If you do, making sure your cookies, ice cream, bread etc. are organic is the best way to avoid most of the nasty ingredients listed in this chapter. However, we will cover that in much more detail in a later chapter. Trans fats can be hidden in labels as the following;

- hydrogenated

- partially hydrogenated (such as 'partially hydrogenated soybean oil')

- shortening

- margarine

- monoglycerides

- diglycerides

Sugar Sweetened Drinks

One area of nutrition I originally felt I didn't even need to cover because I thought it's fairly obvious to most people how bad soda pop is. However, looking at the money made by companies that produce these products and how many people I see walking around with a can of the sweet stuff, it appears I still need to give an education on the subject! That fact is driven home when you realise soda is the number one source of additional sugar in America. Often drinks sold in America have more sugar in them than the exact same product in another country, especially across Europe where health organisations have more influence to implement their ideas. Graham MacGregor, a professor of cardiovascular medicine at Queen Mary, University of London is head of 'Action on Sugar', a group that conducted a product analysis to show this. They made a strong connection between sugary drinks and the obesity epidemic sweeping much of the world. They say soda manufacturers should lower the amount of sugar in their drinks, as 88% of the products tested had more sugar in just one standard 330ml (12oz) can, than someone's entire daily recommended amount.

In response to this claim, the American Beverage Association who is also representative of the industry's stance in Canada and the UK said rather *hilariously*: "Soda doesn't make you gain weight, calories do." Oh, my word that is literally piss your pants funny! There are so many ways to dissect that and tear it apart I'm not going to even bother...Anyway, let's look at the evidence as to why this is a *ridiculous* statement of epic proportions. Firstly, the obvious was proven in a paper published in the journal Circulation in 2019, that the consumption of sugar-sweetened beverages is directly linked to mortality. It was shown that the more you drink, the higher the risk of you dying is, mainly from coronary heart disease.

In 2011 The New York City Health Department launched a campaign to show the American people how much sugar they were consuming without even knowing it most of the time.

They show that drinking just one soda per day is equivalent to 50 lbs of sugar per year!

Put another way, that's a full suitcase worth of sugar going into your body *every single year* when you state, "Yeah I drink soda, but only about one per day" or something I've heard too many times, "No I don't really drink soda, maybe one a day (I give them a confused look)...at most!"

At more than four additional pounds per month, that is going to hit your health and the scales, *hard*! In a paper published in 2016 in the journal Behavioural Brain Research, researchers from Sydney found that only short term exposure to liquid sugar caused inflammation and memory deficits in rats after only one week! Having them flickers of memory loss might have you reaching for another can since it was shown in 2011 by researchers from Harvard that liquid sugar does not make you feel as full as having the same amount of sugar as in solid foods. Doesn't sound too surprising, but that's a dangerous game to be playing when your mind's telling you no, but your body is telling you yes. Don't go forgetting that two sodas per day and we are talking 100lbs of additional sugar per year, which is two full suitcases. Have you ever tried to lift two suitcases? That's a lot of *additional* sugar.

And it's not just us that is affected by this. Our children, who are not old enough to form their own opinions, let alone speak them are almost force-fed sugar without even knowing about it. Almost every school meal throughout the US comes with a beverage of choice. By innocently choosing a bottle of milk, which comes in all the fun flavours such as strawberry and chocolate, a child is consuming far more than its daily allowance of added sugar in just *one* drink. Jamie Oliver, who is a chef and health advocate in the UK, came over to try and influence some change to help with the obesity epidemic sweeping America's children. He was met with a lot of resistance from not only schools but politicians and even the children clueless parents. In one stunt he showed how much sugar the children of The Los Angeles Unified School District consumed in one week from just their flavoured milk. He filled a broken-down school bus with 57 tonnes of white sand to represent the children drowning in sugar. And we wonder why our children can't focus in school and why they are fatter and sicker than ever?

Worse than that though, the larger soda manufacturers went from using sugar to high fructose corn syrup (HFCS) in America in 1984. Again, it sounds like I'm picking on America here, but the research really points to different laws and attitudes in the US versus much of the rest of the world. These laws and attitudes are truly killing Americans at a quicker rate, as their waistbands expand and health deteriorates faster than the rest of the modern world, with the case of HFCS being a perfect example of this. In many countries around the world, the soda manufacturers were never allowed to switch from using sugar to HFCS, or they have been made to switch back. Not so in the US.

Longtime researcher into the subject of HFCS, Michael Goran states; 'fructose is much more harmful than glucose. Glucose is used for energy in the body. Fructose is taken up much more readily by the liver, where it is used as fat. That conversion causes a lot of metabolic problems. We now know that fructose has more negative effects. The $6 billion a year corn refining industry repeats the mantra that sugar is sugar." Remembering the fact that so many children in the US have Non-Alcoholic Fatty Liver Disease, now we can see one of the major reasons why. And once you start messing with the liver and it's more than 500 functions, it can be a downward spiral for your health and one of the hardest things to recover from. This is where we must become very aware of what our children are consuming as sodas in the US and some other countries are far more complex than just a sugary treat that they maybe once were, a long time ago. I mean, cola goes into the body black in colour and comes out of you clear, where do all those artificial colourings and flavours go?

Cola is so acidic it is used as a pesticide in India as it is cheaper than traditional products and will kill the bugs and slugs in your garden if you leave a bowl of it out.

It can also be used to clean rust and stains off of metal and clean a car battery. Now, is that polishing the inside of your body or stripping the calcium from your bones? Well, we will cover that in much more depth in a later chapter, but the answer was the latter as shown by researchers in a paper published in The American Journal of Clinical Nutrition in 2006. They showed consumption of cola, in particular, gives ladies a lower bone mineral density which then leads to a higher risk of osteoporosis and other bone-related diseases. People often ask me, what can I do to help my osteoporosis or osteopenia? Well, if you are drinking soda which is shown to block calcium absorption, there is an easy fix. Stop. Replace it with stevia lemonade, which is a fanatically refreshing, healthy alternative and sugar-free to boot!

Tom's Spicy Stevia Lemonade

Ingredients:

- 3-4 Organic Lemons

- 1 Litre of either Sparkling Mineral Water or Still Mineral Water (depending on if you want it fizzy and would like to drink then, or for it to last in the fridge for a few days)

- Organic Pure Stevia Extract (check your brand of stevia conversion rate and use equivalent to 1/4-3/4 cup of sugar depending on your taste)

- Optional: A thumb of ginger

Method:

1. To get the most juice out of your lemons, using a juicer is best. This also means you can leave on the peel, which has tons of nutrients in it.

2. The next best option to a juicer is a wooden reamer. This will allow you to easily get more juice than merely squeezing your lemons.

3. The final option is to roll your lemons thoroughly (which is a good idea anyway). Then rather than cutting the lemon in half, cut it lengthways just off centre, leaving four pieces and the core. When the lemon is in two pieces, it is so strong it is difficult for even the toughest man to get much juice out! Five separate pieces is a much easier squeeze, leaving you with loads of juice.

4. Pour the lemon juice into a pitcher.

5. Stir the stevia into the lemon juice and continue stirring until the stevia has completely dissolved into the liquid.

6. If you have a juicer (which is highly recommended for many reasons discussed a little later in the book), juice the ginger and add to the pitcher while stirring it in.

7. Add the water.

8. Stir thoroughly.

9. Serve over a glass with ice and a garnish of lemon.

Sugar-Free Drinks

Talking of sugar-free, let's talk about diet soda, zero sugar, or sugar-free, whichever name they've decided to call their product. We already mentioned the shocking statistic of the increase in brain cancer when it hit the market. In a study of 452,000 people in 10 European countries, published in the Journal of the American Medical Association in 2019, it was shown that both regular and diet soda was responsible for all-cause mortality. Sugary drinks were responsible for more deaths due to digestive diseases, and sugar-free soda was responsible for more deaths associated with circulatory diseases. Both increase the risk of death from Parkinson's disease.

In a study published in the journal Stroke in 2017, sugar-free drinks were shown to be directly linked to an increased risk of both stroke and dementia, which included Alzheimer's. In contrast, sugar-sweetened drinks were not associated with an increased risk of either disease. More shocking than that, researchers in Japan published a paper in The European Journal of Nutrition in 2013, showed that consumption of *diet* soda was significantly associated with an increased risk for *diabetes*! This was proven again by researchers in Israel in 2014, who showed that diet soda induces glucose intolerance by altering the gut microbiota. The gut is essential to your overall health and will be discussed at length in this chapter. This shows that diet sodas are good for no one, even diabetics. Get into stevia lemonade if you need a refreshing change from water! People also flavour their water to make it more interesting, but the packaged products nearly always contain artificial sweeteners and flavourings. So flavour it yourself, but with fresh fruits and herbs. It's very easy to make a large pitcher on a morning filled with filtered water and fresh fruits and simply let it infuse all on its own. I love fresh mint and lime. Cucumber is another nice flavour that goes with mint, or it's delicious on its own.

As mentioned, there is *a lot* to take into account when we look at why people gain weight rather than simply calories in versus calories out. Zero-calorie drinks are often linked to the rise in obesity, and researchers at San Diego University went out to show one of the reasons why. They showed that diet soda drinkers have greater activation in the area of the brain that releases dopamine when they consume something with a sweet taste. The more someone drinks diet soda, the greater the activation. This shows why diet sodas are so addictive, but also shows that addiction can spread across a wide variety of sweet-tasting foods, therefore, leading to weight gain and obesity.

Energy Drinks

And then we *have* to talk about energy drinks. The biggest brand of energy drinks sold a whopping 7.5 billion cans in 2019. And here I was thinking just how ridiculous these concoctions were was obvious and so I wouldn't need to talk about it! Before getting into some science, just going to go on a quick rant here but it's a rare something that actually gets me quite pissed off.

The other day my friend was showing me YouTube videos of one of his favourite surfers who was sponsored by an energy drink. In every video, he was holding a can of the pure poison, but as I pointed out, never drank from the flipping thing! My friend said this was a common comment from subscribers and so showed me a video where 'he proved everyone wrong'. The video came up and basically showed him taking a swig of an open can as he walked down to the surf. "An open can?" I asked. "He could have anything in there."

My point is, I understand why a top athlete would never want to put anything like an energy drink in his body. But why promote the stuff? The celebrities who promote sodas, fast food, energy drinks and other poison would never put that into their own bodies, and I guarantee they wouldn't feed that shit to their kids. But they promote it to their fans (who they dearly love and appreciate...barf) who the most susceptible of are children and teenagers. Don't they have enough money without getting paid to promote products that are going to make people fat and sick? Why would they ruin kids' lives to make another buck? It's a fucking disgrace, to be honest. One of the better things about this pandemic we are currently going through in 2020 (I told you this section about soda was literally a last-minute addition as I am currently editing the already finished book) is that we've (hopefully) realised people who grow, make and sell food, who give you electricity and clean running water, healthcare professionals and others who provide things that are key to life are far more important to us than celebrities and sports stars.

Okay, rant over. The first thing about energy drinks that we should know is, they have found a loophole in the law which allows them to classify themselves as food supplements. This means they are not governed under the same laws as other drinks such as soda and coffee, which are not allowed to contain too much caffeine; otherwise, they cause heart problems...see where this is going? So now we have these super caffeinated beverages that are also mixed in with taurine and other stimulants and then a boat-load of sugar, even more than most sodas in many cases - unless you get the sugar-free version - please don't...*just don't*.

Companies can put in as much caffeine as they like due to been regulated under a different set of rules to food and drinks, and so you have over 800 energy drinks on the market today competing to grab your attention, and one of those ways is to give you the biggest buzz. You have some brands today with more than 300mg of caffeine in a small 236ml (8 fl oz) can. The daily recommend amount for anyone of any size is 400mg per day (which I personally think is a little crazy by being too high) and no more than 200mg in a single go. 300mg is comfortably more than 3 cups of coffee in one small can.

Then for some reason, at one point in time, they started bringing out larger cans. When I first moved to Australia, I had to do a double-take at people walking down the street at 8 am with what I thought was a can of beer. But no, I found out it was an energy drink. I was *dumbfounded*. Was one small can not enough caffeine, sugar, stimulants and synthetic additives in one go? These cans often contain over 80 grams of sugar plus the caffeine, plus the other stimulants and additives. Talk about either not giving a shit about your health, being severely misinformed, or being an absolute sucker for your favourite sports star or celebrity. Who by the way, more than likely treats their body like a temple, but doesn't mind you screwing up yours for some extra cash in the bank account. Sickening.

The amount of people who visit the emergency room because of consuming energy drinks keeps on increasing. From 2007 to 2011 the number doubled, by 2016 there were 20'000 visits in America alone. In a paper published in the Journal of the American Heart Association, researchers showed the massive difference between drinking an energy drink and another caffeinated beverage with the same amount of caffeine but none of the other ingredients. Researchers measured the participants' blood pressure and used an electrocardiogram (ECG) to measure heart electrical activity for 24 hours after the subjects consumed the drinks. Energy drinks significantly prolonged their QTc intervals, which is the time it takes for the ventricles of the heart to contract and relax. Their blood pressure increased by 5 points compared to less than one point when consuming the plain caffeinated beverage and continued to be raised for 6 hours afterwards. The problem is there is not a lot of studies out there regarding energy drinks, and so they hide behind their clever marketing and tell everyone there is no difference between energy drinks and coffee when clearly there is. My advice as always is, don't be the guinea pig when it comes to drinking this stuff.

One final thing when it comes to discussing energy drinks and health - many people complain about headaches, poor sleep and having an irritable mood and so wonder what to do about it. Following all the Action Steps in this book is a great place to start, however, let's hone in on and potentially eliminate one particular contributor to a lot of people's health issues both young and old. In a study conducted in Finland on a group of more than 9000 13-year-olds, it was found that consumers of energy drinks had a 4.6 times greater odds of headaches, 3.6 times greater odds of sleeping problems, and 4.1 times greater odds of having an irritable mood compared to non-consumers.

If any young people you know are struggling with any of these problems, now could be a good time to ask them about their consumption of energy drinks. This was all nicely summed up by Dr Josiemer Mattei, Assistant Professor of Nutrition based at the Harvard T.H. Chan School of Public Health, Boston, USA, who published a study in Frontiers in Public Health. He said, "We summarise the consequences of energy drink consumption, which include heart, kidney, and dental problems, as well as risk-seeking behaviour and poor mental health." He goes on to say, "The evidence suggests they are harmful to health and should be limited through more stringent regulation by restricting their sales to children and adolescents, as well as setting an evidence-based upper limit on the amount of caffeine."

Marketing Marvels

What has history taught us? There is one rule I tell all clients. One rule that if you follow it will make a world of difference to your health. That rule is;

Always eat as close to as nature intended.

When it comes down to a choice, if faced with choosing between butter and margarine - choose butter. If offered the choice of a regular soda or a diet soda - choose regular. If offered full-fat milk or skimmed milk

- choose full-fat. This is shocking to most people, but time and again, the 'healthier' alternative has proven to be the *unhealthiest* option. Just trust in mother nature and forget about buying from large companies who profit from you being addicted to their foods. Trust in nature rather than the very companies who profit from you being fat and sick. Now I'm not saying that regular soda, milk or butter are good for you, far from it. But they are way better for your health than the 'diet' alternatives.

Never, ever eat food that uses the words diet, light, lite, low-fat, 1 or 2% fat, fat-free, slimline, sugar-free, zero sugar, etc.

I can guarantee the fat has been replaced with refined sugar, or even worse the sugar has been replaced with synthetic chemicals. All this talk about eating as close to as nature intended and avoiding processed food points to one thing...

Prepare Your Own Food

Everyone knows cooking your own food is always going to be better than takeaways, fast food and ready meals. But let us look at why to really drive home the real consequences of eating this stuff. First off whoever snuck the 's' in fast food is a genius! We've already heard of the story of the Icelandic gentleman. If that didn't put you off of all fast food that really is quite astonishing. By the way, it's all the same, don't let clever marketing from one company positioning themselves as the healthy alternative kid you.

But let us go further. When I lived in Sydney, a good friend of mine worked for a local organic supermarket which also did catering for business meetings. She told me, whenever all the top executives of a certain, prevalent fast-food chain had business meetings, they would order organic food. They never ate fast food. They didn't even eat regular supermarket food. But only *organic* food. Now, what does that tell you? This is far from the only time I've heard of this kind of thing. I've had clients who are doctors who prescribe medication but never take it. Top people in food, supplement, and pharmaceutical companies would rarely ever consume their own products.

Microwaves

Now for a personal story because I see people who consider themselves to work long hours making claims all they have the time or energy to prepare when they get home is a microwave meal. Yuck. I have worked from 5:30 am-9:30 pm as a Personal Trainer, Monday-Thursday and still managed to make my own food without even owning a microwave. I also worked 'half days' 6 am-2 pm on Friday and Saturday before you say anything! Anyway, that's beside the point. I will show you very soon how always to eat a home-cooked meal no matter what the hours you work.

Before that, we need to look at the dangers; Yes, the *dangers* of microwaves. There are a few things to consider when looking at microwaving your food. The major problem is how a microwave cooks your food. It vibrates the water molecules within the food at 2.5 billion times per second. This causes the cells of the food to deform, so your body has a difficult time recognising it for the food it once was. You see, when I was first working in the fitness industry, I knew nothing of what I do now. Working shifts in the gym meant I would sometimes get home between 8-10:30 pm. Reheating the mostly healthy home-cooked dinner, my mum had made me was commonplace. Of course, I used the microwave as most people would do. The problem was, from the age of 17 years old when I was trying my best to bulk up and add muscle, but I could not finish a meal for the life of me. My mother, who stands at a towering 5' 3" could eat three times as much food as me in one sitting.

A standard sized meal would take me three sittings over about 3 hours to finish. I didn't know what was going on; neither did the doctors. I was prescribed all sorts of drugs. I had cameras shoved down my throat to see what was going on. And...nothing. Nothing changed. The doctor said, "We don't have a clue what's going on, but you're a big strong lad who is otherwise healthy, so we will leave it there." I'm like, "Da, fuck?" Well, obviously, I didn't say that at the time because the doctor is always right. 'Trust me; I'm a doctor.' Correct?

Well, little did I know that would be the start of developing me into the person who I am today — the person writing this book. So, I went forward thinking that was it, I would never be able to eat a full meal never mind like the aspiring bodybuilder I once was. That was until I first worked on cruise ships at the age of 23 years old. On a cruise ship, nothing is microwaved. Everything is fresh. Within two weeks, I was eating like a person my size should be able to. I didn't know what was going on. I didn't realise it was the microwaves to blame until I read about them in a book. Then it dawned on me. Ahh...The only thing that had changed since living on there was, I didn't eat microwaved food anymore. Wow.

Since then, I have been able to eat normally. The only time I can't finish a meal is when there is something microwaved, which I would never do myself. I don't own one and threw my parent's microwave out as soon as I got back home after learning what I had learned. Before working on cruise ships, I couldn't finish any meal. Now it just seems to be microwaved food. The reason I know this is, soon after my first contract on cruise ships had come to an end, I was at a friend's house, and I ate literally one bite of steak, and I felt full. I sat there thinking; 'Hang on. I've just seen them barbecuing all the meat. What is going on?' So, I turned to my friend and asked, "Out of interest, has any of this food been microwaved?" My friend said, "Yes, I didn't have time to defrost the meat, so I did it in the microwave." Huh. Wow.

Besides my personal experience, research published by the Atlantis Rising Educational Center in Oregon shows very similar findings. The Soviets originally conducted the research showing carcinogens form in nearly all types of food during microwaving. This amazingly led them to ban microwaves nationwide way back in 1976. They showed that *every* type of food changes into carcinogenic compounds. Even thawing frozen fruit in your microwave will cause the glucosides and galactosides to convert into carcinogenic compounds. The same is for plant foods, in which alkaloids turn into carcinogens and hazardous free radicals.

Not only do microwaves change the molecular structure, but they also nuke the food so much that most of the nutrition is lost. A study done in 2003 by The Journal of the Science of Food and Agriculture found that microwaved broccoli lost 97% of its antioxidants. Compare that to only 11% when steamed. And 0% raw.

So far, we have microwaved food, causing cancer and losing most of its nutrition. The next thing to consider is what does most microwave food come in? Packaging containing plastic. In a paper published in Environmental Health Perspectives, researchers analysed 455 common plastic products which included BPA-free ones. They found that 70% tested positive for estrogenic activity; that number went up to 95% when the plastics were microwaved, which can cause anything from an increased chance of mental health issues to leukaemia, and almost everything in between. We will be discussing endocrine disruptors in far more detail in an upcoming chapter.

Bulk Food Preparation

So how do you always eat home-cooked food? If pressed for time as most of us are today, prepare food in bulk rather than cooking one meal at a time. I would always choose Sunday and Wednesday evenings to prepare lunches that would last for a few days. I use a **slow cooker** to bulk cook meals that can easily be kept in the fridge and then reheated *using a pan* (not a microwave) for dinners. If I'm at home making dinner, I will always make enough food for two or three meals which I will then eat for lunch or dinner for the next couple of days.

Think about the time saved, and it's easily achievable for everyone. One meal might ordinarily take an average of 60 minutes to prepare. Preparing meals, one meal at a time could *easily* take fourteen or more hours per week just for lunch and dinner each day. Whereas, when preparing in bulk twice per week, it will take around 3-4 hours in total. You've just saved at least 10 hours and eaten healthy and felt great all week! I've not even added in the increase in energy and improvement of sleep, which will add to productivity, creating even more spare time to play with! If you enjoy cooking like I do, and you have the spare time then do it every day if you please. However, if you know you'll be pushed for time the next day plan ahead and make enough food to last a couple of extra meals, so you don't go reaching for the phone to order a not so healthy takeaway.

Now, let's look at the quantity of food. Because that is all that is ever focused on in the mainstream media, right? Calories in vs calories out. We've already obviously covered what bullshit this is in Chapter 1 and already earlier in this chapter, but one thing we didn't cover in any detail is when we take this concept to the extreme.

Fad Diets

Ladies and gentlemen big news just in...Diets don't work!! No seriously. Even the latest diet, the one that came out just last week. I know, I know. It's heart-wrenching news that there is no short cut to optimal health and permanent weight loss. But the good news is you don't have to starve yourself anymore. Yay! By diet, I mean a way of eating that has a beginning and an end date. With an end date it is basically showing us that, it is not sustainable, and therefore it's *not healthy*. Let's just look at the facts, shall we? We have religiously been eating less and exercising more since the 1950s. Is it working? There are more gyms and diets than ever before, but more people are struggling with their weight than at any other point in history.

Let's do a small survey, shall we? Answer honestly. Have you been on a diet before? Have you been on more than one diet? Do not count any that you are *currently* on (as they all work to some degree when you are on them, the failure happens afterwards), but did *any* of them work for you on a permanent basis...For 99% of people, the answer to the final question will be a very big no! Why is this? Why do diets not work?

Well, firstly, diets usually have you consuming fewer calories than you need even to function properly. Even a smaller woman will have a basal metabolic rate (BMR) of around 1200 calories or more, which is the number of calories per day that you need to function at rest. Most diets will have you consuming around 500-1000 cal per day. Think about that as a male who needs 1800-2200 calories on average just to function. As a survival mechanism, your body then goes into what we call starvation mode. Your body was designed for hunting and foraging, and not for a time like today. A time where you can get your hands on any amount of prepackaged food at any time of day if you are living in the Western world. And so, when you are not consuming enough fuel, your body feels the need to store fat as part of that survival mechanism. It is not sure where the next meal is coming from and so stores fuel for future hard times ahead. However, your body still needs to function. Since it's not getting enough energy from food and is storing fat instead of burning it, your body needs a new energy source. Muscle now becomes your primary energy source. And so, on a typical diet, you will gain fat and lose muscle. Since muscle weighs more than fat, you'll be getting lighter on the scales. You will then win awards at your local diet club, of which there are many brands. Slimmer of the Week! Well done! But not really, since you are getting weaker and slowly killing your metabolism. If you are a yoyo dieter who goes back to your diet club whenever you have a holiday or wedding come up, you might start to develop health complications. And worse than any of that, you actually start to look worse without your clothes on! (Joking about not looking good naked being as important as your health...I think). What do I mean by killing your metabolism you may ask? Well, the clue has always been in the word;

Take the 't' off of diet, and what do you get?

The less muscle you have, the fewer calories you burn at rest and so the slower your metabolism, which is why dieting kills your metabolism. Besides getting slowly fatter the more diets you go on, when did a yoyo dieter ever feel (or look) healthy? Lethargy, food cravings, constipation, thyroid complications, premature ageing and dark circles around the eyes are just a few of the very common ailments dealt with by yoyo dieters. And so, you are also killing yourself! So, stop. Stop doing the same thing over and over and expecting a different result - that my friends, is the definition of insanity. So, let's *stop* focusing on the quantity of food. Let's look more at what is far more important than quantity; let 's look at the *quality* of food.

As mentioned, it's a subject that the mainstream media rarely covers, but it's far more important than the quantity of food. The quality of today's food is by far and away the biggest reason why so many people are currently overweight. It is the number one reason why more people are suffering from lifestyle diseases such as heart disease and diabetes than at any other point in history.

Researchers at The Center for Science in the Public Interest found that poor nutrition is the leading cause of disease in America. It caused 19.1% of disease in 2016 (with High BMI making up another 13.9% which is surely caused by...never mind). Think about the following for a moment; when I take a sick dog to a veterinarian, the first question I'm asked is, 'What has he been eating?' When was the last time your doctor asked you that? And why is it that the division of the government who are entrusted to battle the major obesity problem in the United States, had funding of only $47.6 million? On the flip side, The Hershey's Company spent more than 12 times that on advertising at a whopping $562 million! Or put it another way, there are more obese Americans than there were for each dollar spent to battle the problem that year. More than 78 million Americans being classified as obese in 2016. Are people in government really taking this problem seriously when you look at almost laughable statistics like that?

Do you entrust these people with your health, or is it time to take it into your own hands?

What else do we have to consider when it comes to the quality of food? In a later chapter, we will look into fresh produce such as fruits, vegetables, nuts, seeds, oils and proteins such as fish, eggs and meat in more depth. So far these may seem like great choices (and they are for now!), but more factors still have to be considered.

Gut Health

There are currently over 10'000 papers written linking your gut health to overall wellbeing. It appears Hippocrates wasn't too far off when he said his now-famous saying...

"All Disease Begins in The Gut." - Hippocrates

Okay, maybe not all. But it's now being proven time and again that Hippocrates wasn't too far off with his suggestions. In a paper published in Therapeutic Advances in Gastroenterology in 2013, researchers in Cork, Ireland found that the gut influences human physiology, metabolism, nutrition and immune function. They also found that if there is an imbalance in the bacteria found within its walls, this can then cause chronic gastrointestinal diseases. We'll talk more about what to add to your routine to create a better bacterial balance in a later chapter, but we first have to look at taking away what's causing damage and imbalances within the digestive system because it's this damage which can then lead to almost all diseases starting in the gut.

Gluten

You've probably heard a thousand times to avoid gluten, but why? Here's the scientific lowdown. Gluten is a protein that is found in wheat, rye, and barley. Grains contain proteins called lectins which are not broken down in the normal digestive process. Gluten contains the worst of the lectins although oats and rice contain a similar protein which is not as bad for your gut health, but it's still pretty close! Protease is an enzyme which is released to help break down protein; however, in a one, two punch to the guts, grains contain protease *inhibitors*. As does dairy, which is pretty bad news all round for various reasons we will cover later, but for now, we will focus on gluten.

These large, intact lectins now enter through your intestinal wall causing major damage to the lining. Your immune system now responds, thinking the lectins are a foreign invader. Antibodies are made to attach to the lectins to neutralise their toxic effects. Unfortunately, lectins look a lot like other proteins in our body. If your immune system starts attacking the proteins in your pancreas where insulin is made, the tissue is damaged, and you develop type 1 diabetes. If the protein is in your thyroid gland, you develop Hashimoto's thyroiditis or Grave's disease. If tissue is attacked in the protective myelin sheath surrounding nerves in the central nervous system, you develop multiple sclerosis (MS).

Proteins are throughout your entire body and within every organ. Not only do we have literally hundreds of diseases that now link back to lectins, but we also have the damaged intestinal wall to think about. As it develops holes along the lining, your gut can now empty its entire contents into your system. This is why almost every disease starts in the guts. Its contents can now make their way into you! Everything from bacteria and viruses that were held in there, to rotten putrified food and toxic synthetic chemicals make their way into your bloodstream, that feeds every cell in your body. Wherever you are genetically weak, you may start to develop a disease.

As food is dumped into your duodenum by the stomach, the gall bladder is supposed to be releasing bile to help the breakdown of fats and proteins. However, the signal for it to release bile is blocked when the intestinal wall is damaged, therefore leading to cholesterol crystals to form in the gall bladder, which leads to gall stones. Around half a million surgeries to remove the gall bladder are performed per year in the United States alone! Of course, as with almost all surgeries, you are treating a *symptom* when removing the gall bladder and not getting to the route cause, which is the damage of the intestinal wall caused mainly through poor nutrition.

Grains also contain phytates which are known as anti-nutrients, which is something that blocks nutrient absorption. Phytates bind to calcium, magnesium, zinc, and iron, which then are not absorbed by the body. Are you popping calcium supplements with your toast, cereal and glass of milk on a morning and wondering why your osteoporosis is only seemingly getting worse? Don't worry, by the end of the book; you'll have all your answers and health back on track.

So, there we have the wonders of not only gluten-containing grains, but all grains bar a couple, as they all have a similar makeup that we want to avoid for the most part. Now let us continue on our health journey and look at how you should be combining food.

Food Combining

We know now how vital good digestion is, so what foods should you be eating together to aid that process? That's a question rarely asked but is extremely important. In fact, food combining principles first appeared in the Ayurvedic medicine of ancient India and was popularised around the year 1890 under the name trophology, which means, 'the science of food combining.' All that time, yet strangely it seems hidden from the public eye in today's world. What you've got to understand when it comes down to digestion is the pH Scale.

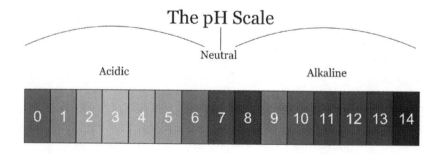

The 'pH' in the pH Scale originally stood for the power of Hydrogen. Or as we British now like to say potential Hydrogen. Either way, it's all the same thing. The more acidic a water-soluble substance is, the closer it is to zero on the scale. The more alkaline a water-soluble substance is, the closer it is to fourteen. In the middle (#7) is neutral, which is where water sits. We are going into the ph Scale and just how important it is for your health in a chapter very soon. For now, we are just looking at it in terms of digestion which is also pretty darn important.

Different food groups digest at different speeds and need different enzymes to do so properly. To do its best work, an enzyme needs certain conditions, such as an alkaline or an acidic environment. Amylases break down starch into simple sugars and need an alkaline environment in the duodenum (first part of the small intestine after the stomach) to function fully. Pepsins are the enzymes that break down proteins in the stomach and work best in an acidic environment. Both are pretty much rendered inactive in the opposite environment to what it needs. As starch and sugar travel through the stomach, they can impede the proper breakdown of proteins into usable amino acids. When the proteins are not broken down properly, they enter into the system as a macromolecule, and as we saw with gluten, the body starts to attack itself, leading to autoimmune disorders. Improperly digested protein becomes a toxic burden on the body.

Fats enter into the duodenum and are emulsified by bile releasing fatty acids. If this happens while carbohydrates are in there, the alkaline environment is neutralised. The undigested carbohydrates are left and start to ferment, producing gas. Fermentation creates inflammation which is a leading cause of disease and will be discussed at length later in the book.

If food needs opposing digestive conditions to each other, then eating them together is going to affect the body's ability to break down food. This leads to poor absorption of all nutrients, including essential vitamins and minerals, therefore leading to malnutrition and disease. We then have poorly digested food left in the intestines, remembering it's a very long, dark, warm, moist place which becomes a perfect environment for food like meat to rot, creating unwanted bacteria. This becomes heavily toxic in the body. Of course, undigested, rotting, fermenting, putrid food can cause gas, bloating and damage the intestinal wall - leading to leaky gut syndrome, irritable bowel syndrome, colitis, diverticulitis and different forms of cancer.

Let's look at the different food groups and what they best pair with;

- **Non-Starchy Vegetables** are considered neutral and contain their own digestive enzymes and so can be paired with anything.

- **Starch** such as potato, rice, pasta, bread and cereal needs an alkaline environment to digest.

- **Protein** is the opposite of starch and needs an acidic environment. This means avoid eating meat with starch, because in chemistry if you mix acid and alkaline, then you cause a neutral environment. However, if you have a little think about it, what is everyone's favourite food combination?...That's right! Meat and potatoes, burger in a bun, salami sandwich, spaghetti bolognese, chicken and rice, chicken and pasta, sausages and hash browns...I could go on.

- **Fruit** should only be eaten on its own due to its rapid absorption rate. Eating it with anything else slows down digestion and could lead to gas and bloating. It can be eaten as a starter 30 minutes before your main meal or as a dessert 1-2 hours after finishing.

- **Liquids** should not be consumed too close to or during a meal as they water down the digestive enzymes. Drink freely 30 minutes before or 1 hour after a meal. During a meal limit the amount of liquid you drink. For now, have a small glass of wine or warm water with dinner or a coffee with breakfast if it makes you happy, but avoid cold water, beer and other drinks.

The main crux of this is that we shouldn't be eating what are the most popular meals across the world. The digestive system is so important that it can and will affect the health of the rest of the body. So, we need to start taking much better care of it through pairing naturally occurring foods we are designed to eat together in better ways. By 'designed to eat' I mean limiting the bread, pasta and cereals that we didn't eat when we were hunting and foraging for food. More to come on that in...THIS chapter! See, I wasn't an asshole this time; you only have to read a few more paragraphs for that information!

Some perfect meals to get you started with food combining and losing weight would be as follows;

- Wild caught salmon + broccoli + green beans

- Organic chicken + sautéed kale + cauliflower mash

- Organic grass-fed beef strips + asparagus + spinach + capsicum + onions

- Organic scrambled eggs + onions + capsicum + spinach

- Tofu + spinach curry + cauliflower rice

- Quinoa + black beans + veggies

- Lentil soup with vegetable broth + mixed veggies

If you like the look of these, I'll be sending you recipes and tons of other valuable stuff so be sure to check your inbox for emails from me. Hey! That is not a shameless plug! If you have so far got value out of the book, then it will be well worth your time to learn more of where this information came from right!? And c'mon, if you're saying you haven't got any value so far, we all know that's a lie because you wouldn't still be reading! Anyway, swiftly moving on to that little nugget, I promised a few paragraphs back.

Wheat

"Government-sponsored guides to healthy eating, such as the USDA's food pyramid, which advocates six to eleven servings of grains daily for everyone, lag far behind current research and continue to preach dangerously old-fashioned ideas. Popular beliefs and politically motivated promotion, not science, continue to dictate dietary recommendations, leading to debilitating and deadly diseases that are wholly or partly preventable." - Ron Hoggan

If you are a little overwhelmed or calling bullshit on what I am saying, do yourself a favour and do just this next one thing for the next 30 days. Give up *wheat*. By wheat, I mean all bread, pasta, crackers, pizza, cereal, cakes and anything else containing wheat. You should lose weight if you are struggling by making this one little change. Obviously, if you want permanent change, then you will need to implement other things from this book afterwards. But for now, try that. I know even this one thing is going to be damned difficult, as grains, particularly the gluten-containing grains, contain molecules that fit into the opiate receptors in our brain. This makes them incredibly addictive as they are the same receptors that work with heroin. It doesn't matter if it's whole grain, it's all pretty much the same thing. When giving up wheat, you need to give it *all* up.

You will feel better. If you suffer from gas, bloating, IBS and the like then the symptoms will at least subside if not go away altogether. You will have more energy. You will be more regular. You will sleep better. Then you will know...that Tom is always right. Ha. Jokes. But at least you will have the motivation to implement the rest of what I am saying. If you have more motivation than that, then start taking the other Action Steps straight away. Don't wait. This just for my peeps who are overwhelmed. Which I completely understand. This is why it is a step-by-step guide. Small steps. Progress, not perfection. It is also for the naysayers. Of which I can guarantee you, there are many! And if you are thinking well, Tom, you said it yourself; "They won't have read this far." Maybe you can help someone you love who needs help but won't make the necessary changes by saying, "I bet you can't give bread up for just one month." Some might accept the challenge. After a few days ask how they feel. After a week point out how good they are looking. Then maybe they might start doing something beyond just giving up bread, which is positive for their health too. And before you know it, you just might have changed someone's life forever.

Now. If you are feeling flat. Lethargic. If you have difficulty moving. Then the next chapter is for you. We are going to get the vehicle that is your body moving like a well-oiled machine. Yes, exercise is that one thing that is difficult to start. It takes effort. But it's never too late. Guys and gals if you don't use it, you...lose it. And I'm not going to be asking you to train like an exercise freak. I'm going to show you how just 20 minutes three times per week can have a huge impact on the way you look, the way you feel and your health. Can you manage 20 minutes, three times per week? I'll show you many different ways to exercise, and you can pick and choose between low impact and more vigorous forms of exercise. Variety is the spice of life! What I cover will show you that there is truly something for everybody and every body when it comes to exercise.

First, time to take some Action Steps. If you're feeling a little overwhelmed, remember that you can revisit this chapter and any other chapter as and when you need it. This book is so full of information and Action Steps that you might just need to read it 3 or 4 times to do everything. That's okay, though. You've saved time because you now don't need to read the latest diet book your fat friend just recommended you. Everything you need is right here...

Resources

Go to **www.TomBroadwell.com/resources** to see;

- The Stevia product I use and recommend.

- A free video of me making Tom's Spicy Stevia Lemonade

- The slow cooker I use and recommend.

Action Steps

- Give up wheat for the next 30 days.

- Cut the plug off the microwave and dispose of it safely.

- Buy a slow cooker to replace the microwave.

- Vouch to never go on a diet again.

- Either cut out or cut down on sugary or sugar-free drinks.

- Limit the amount of processed food you consume, aiming for that magical 80% good and 20% treat yourself number.

- Eat fruit in limited amounts and only on its own.

- Limit the volume of liquids you drink with your meals.

- Make healthier meal choices in the correct food combinations when eating out.

- Cook and prepare food at home, choose two nights a week where you can bulk cook or prepare meals in the correct food combinations and take them to work for lunch.

- If pressed for time, prepare meal options in bulk for dinner too and eat the same thing 2-3 days in a row.

- If not time poor, commit to cooking at home for at least 4-5 evening meals per week.

Chapter Six
Move It Or Lose It

*"We do not stop exercising because we grow old - we grow old because we stop exercising."– **Kenneth Cooper***

You could almost smell the money as the elderly couple approached.

The lady extended a jewellery laden hand as a greeting.

Her wrist was draped in beautiful bracelets.

Diamond encrusted everything.

She seemed to run the show here.

The weary gentleman nodded his head and followed her as I encouraged them to follow me to my office.

Both struggled as they lowered themselves into their chairs.

She was a larger set lady, holding the excess weight in the usual areas of her upper arms, tummy region, hips and thighs.

He seemed to be a shadow of his former self.

I could see a fire in his eyes that once burned brightly.

I guessed that fire seemed to be fading as his health did the same thing.

He was very slim with a potbelly.

As I went through their health forms, I was shocked to see that they were only in their early sixties.

I would have guessed at least 75 if not older.

"Why do you want to do Personal Training?" I asked.

The lady answered, "We discussed it was time to do something since we are both now retired and want to fully enjoy the travelling that we plan to do."

"What do you mean by enjoy?" I replied.

"Well, we want to see places other than Florida. We both love walking but didn't have the time until now. We want to find it easy to get around, because right now we find it a struggle to walk for more than 5 minutes and stairs are somewhat impossible."

"Okay excellent, you like walking. When was the last time you both did walking regularly as exercise?"

"Well, before the birth of our first child, we were very active...We just celebrated his 40th birthday."

The saddest thing for me is to see someone who has just retired. Put everything into a career or raising their family. Or both, putting everyone and everything else first. They have all the money in the world, and they can't get out of a freaking chair...I have seen the above example in my consultation room hundreds of times. People who are trying to buy their health back. If they had simply done something regularly through the last 40 years, they would be far more likely to be able to enjoy retirement to the fullest.

Something we will discuss at length in the next chapter is how genetics has *very little* to do with the outcome of your health or longevity. One study on exercise that proves this was performed in Finland on 15'902 identical twins. Over 20 years, 1,253 participants died. Even after accounting for other risk factors, exercise proved strongly protective. Twins who exercised regularly were 56% less likely to die than their sedentary siblings, and even twins who exercised only occasionally (less than six times per month) had a 34% lower death rate than their sedentary identical twins. That in itself should be motivation to at least move your body most days.

People often ask me, "What is the best form of exercise?" My answer is always, "It doesn't matter."

If you like walking, walk. If you like yoga, do yoga. If you like swimming, lifting weights, cycling, horse riding...Whatever it is. Do it. Consistently.

If you like whatever it is you are doing, then you are much more likely to do it. The best thing to do would be a combination of all forms of exercise. And choosing whatever you feel like doing on that day. I regularly do yoga, walking, swimming, resistance training, pilates and cycling. I choose whatever takes my fancy that day.

For clients, I constantly mix it up. No client of mine ever does the same workout twice when paying for a Personal Training session. That is unless there is a point to them repeating the workout which could be any of the following reasons;

- They were trying to beat their best score in a challenge.

- If they were unable to complete the workout to the fullest of their ability the last time out, for whatever reason.

- If we wanted to check progress and make sure they were getting stronger and fitter by repeating either some exercises or the entire workout.

- If they simply loved it and so requested to do it again.

There really is no other reason for someone to repeat a workout, with the same exercises with the same weights for the same amount of repetitions. I'd always have a general plan for a client, but if they walk in looking absolutely shattered, I might do yoga instead. Sometimes I've had clients who were depressed or under an ungodly amount of stress and so I would put them through a guided meditation instead of causing their body more stress through exercise.

My point is, listen to your mind and body, and perform whatever exercise feels right to you that day. That is why my website www.tombroadwell.com is chocked full of different styles of workouts. From breathwork to stretching to yoga to pilates to resistance training to high-intensity cardio. You can pick and choose the workout that you want to do that day. Often I hear people saying they don't have time to exercise. I ask them what they feel like is a reasonable amount of time to workout? They talk about needing to do at least 1 hour in the gym. Some even say they heard that they need to do 45 minutes of cardio and then 1 hour of weights. Taking into account the time to get to the gym, take a shower after their workout and then the time to get home, I'm not surprised most people feel they don't have time!

I'm here to tell you right now that you don't need that amount of time to exercise! My Personal Training sessions were only 30 minutes. Some of that was warming up and cooling down, the real meat of the workout was always around 20 minutes, and the results were as good, if not better than other trainers who do 1-hour sessions. When comparing it to when I used to do 1-hour sessions, I have to say the results were far better. The shorter sessions are way more fun for both the client and me. People are more focused and engaged, which leads to more intense workouts with far greater results.

All the workouts on my website are around 20 minutes long. They all use minimal or no equipment. Meaning they can be done at home or at work. There is something on there for everyone, at any level of fitness. So, whether you are travelling and don't have access to a gym, or you simply don't want to join a gym, now you don't have to. You can have a great workout anywhere at any time. Boom! There goes the excuse of no time. Boom! There goes the excuse of no gym. The workouts all vary in difficulty. If you fancy a slower less intense workout one day because you're feeling burned out after a long day, it is right there at the click of a button. Boom! There goes the excuse of no energy.

Within the workouts are special challenges that you can repeat and therefore see that you are progressing. My style of Personal Training on land meant me having a whole mirror to myself in the gym on which I write upon with special window pens. I would host different competitions. For example, I hosted my own Olympic Games, which celebrated all forms of fitness, from cardio to strength, flexibility to balance and more. All this while the Olympics were on and all of my client's names, nationalities and scores would be written on the mirror, and it would become a competition, but a fun one! It truly was a World Championship too as I had more than 50 active clients in a city as diverse as Sydney, and so every continent in the world was represented! At one point, seven different ladies lead the seven different events as my heptathlon (the workout) allowed everyone, regardless of age or fitness level, to be competitive and good at something. Not to blow my own whistle (again) but please go and find me a Personal Trainer who would go to such lengths and show so much creativity to make everyone feel so good about themselves and to have such fun but results-driven workouts.

My website is also based on the same friendly competition. You can either compete against yourself or others that have already joined The Tribe. Boom! There goes the excuse of no motivation. Having goals and challenges creates motivation. However, I admit it; you don't need my website to succeed. It is simply there as a tool. On it, you will be guided by an expert. Hopefully, at this point, someone you can trust. Boom! There goes the excuse of, 'I don't know what I'm doing'.

You will have the motivation to do something, most days — not every day. No one is asking you to become an exercise freak. Amazing results can be achieved with much less effort and way less time than most people think they need to put into exercise. As far as types of exercise go, here is an in-depth list of what you need to be doing for a good mix of health improvements, weight loss, flexibility, strength gains and to look better naked. Each one starts with the main benefits you can expect from doing the exercise consistently (arguments could be made for other benefits not listed) and I go on to show you how I would implement it for maximum results.

Walking

- Cardiovascular health

- Lower body muscular endurance

- Stress relief

- Mental health

If you can put aside 1 hour a day for walking, that would be one of the most amazing things to do for your health. Preferably outside, not on a treadmill. Unless the treadmill is your only choice right now due to a whole host of reasons, such as but not limited to; feeling safer indoors, using it to zone out for stress relief (rather than walking around objects, people and dogs), you are currently quarantined due to a global pandemic, or that it is simply what you enjoy more. However, as we will discuss in a later chapter, getting outside in nature will hold far more benefits than walking or running inside on a treadmill.

If you don't have time or the physical capabilities to walk for 1 hour, do what you can, when you can. Easy habits to implement into your current lifestyle is parking the car a couple of blocks from work and walking the rest. Get off the bus 1 or 2 stops early. Walk the kids to school rather than jumping in the car (helps them create good habits too, the number of people I see taking their kids to school in the car when it's a 5-10-minute walk is unbelievable!). Take the stairs, not the elevator. Simple things everyone knows, but you will actually start to implement. Today. Or tomorrow if you are reading this sat up at night. But don't wait any longer! Start now...Research has proven how good walking is for your health in dramatic fashion over the years. The Harvard Alumni Study is an ongoing study of over 12'500 men who studied at Harvard University between 1916 and 1950 that was initiated in 1962.

It found that men who found that men who just walk 1.3 miles per day had a 22% lower death rate than sedentary men!

If you need me to give you a good reason to take the stairs, in the study, those who average at least eight flights a day enjoy a 33% lower mortality rate than men who are sedentary - a third lower chance of dying, just for taking the stairs!

As mentioned already, the best habit you can start is to turn off the TV and go for an walk in the evening sun. Twenty minutes minimum if you can currently go that long, building up to an hour. Enjoy it. Walk in nature. Stare into the distance. Appreciate the trees and plants around you. Absorb the sunlight in through your eyes and skin. Go with the family or your partner for the social aspect. Or your pet. Or yourself. But go. Every day...

Resistance Training

- Whole-body muscular strength

- Whole-body muscular endurance

- Core strength

- Increased muscle tone

- Increased muscle size (if you want it, but don't fear there are ways to make sure your muscles don't grow - ladies I'm looking at you)

- Fat burning

- Increased Basal Metabolic Rate

- Improved posture

- Relieve pain

- Cardiovascular health and fitness

- Mental health

- Improved self-esteem

People sometimes seem confused when I talk about burning fat when lifting weights. Even if you are doing a slow strength training program, where you are sat resting in-between sets, researchers published a paper in 2002 in the European Journal of Applied Physiology showing you will continue to burn fat for up to 38 hours after your workout! This is something that has never been reported with cardio. A slow strength training program, by the way, is not something I will never prescribe you on a regular basis, as you are likely not a bodybuilder and I doubt you want to look like one. If you are one or want to build huge amounts of muscle, then we would need to look at what to do in the gym differently, and I could most certainly prescribe you a killer workout regime!

However, for most people, there are far more efficient and healthier ways to train than doing three sets of 10 repetitions of the heaviest weight possible. But once again, variety is the spice of life and these types of training methods can be prescribed as part of a complete workout regime for everybody to get some benefits from. The majority of your workouts, however, should be made up of a resistance training type circuit. Of which there are many training methods to implement, which are all covered on my website. This time-saver will give you all the benefits of cardiovascular work and weight training at once in a fraction of the time! On a fat-burning note, you also have to realise, the more muscle you add, the higher you Basal Metabolic Rate (BMR) will go. So, you'll burn more energy at rest, for the other 23 hours of the day you are not exercising! This has been proven many a time, with a paper published in the journal Medicine & Science in Sports & Exercise showing men increased their BMR 9% and females 4% using resistance training, over 24 weeks. The reason I chose this study was they disproved an age-old myth that you can't build muscle after 40 years old when this paper showed age has *nothing* to do with the rise in the resting metabolic rate and therefore the amount of muscle gained.

The other thing to consider when talking about resistance training is *how* do you lift the weights. I regularly talk to people of a certain age who go to the gym consistently 3-5 times per week, and they still struggle to get out of a chair or lift their hand luggage into the overhead compartment on an aeroplane. I ask them what strength training do they do in the gym? It's pretty much always the same answer of, "I do a circuit of the weights machines."

So, what's the problem you may ask? They are working out consistently like I asked, right? Firstly, I said do what you *love* or at least like. Has anyone in the history of mankind ever loved doing the same monotonous circuit of the weights machines in the gym? Day after day, week after week, month after month, year after year. Just writing that has depressed me a little bit. Never mind actually doing it!

Secondly, it is simply not how the human body is designed to move or how you actually move in real life. When have you ever sat in a chair and lifted weights that are in a fixed plane of motion?

Most people sit down too much as it is and then they go to the gym and sit in a chair to exercise!

It doesn't make any sense. The problem people mainly have is stabilising themselves as they move their body or lift something. When the weight you are lifting is *fixed* in a singular plane of motion, you don't recruit any of the stabilising muscles, so you remain weak. Hence, when you try to go from seated to standing or pick something off of the ground, it's a real struggle. Or when trying to lift something overhead, you just don't seem to have the strength.

A shoulder press machine is nothing like lifting a fairly heavy object over your head in real life, regardless of the weight it says you are lifting on the machine itself because it is fixed. Even if someone throws some free weight exercises into the mix, it's not quite enough to become strong in real life. A bicep curl mainly works the muscles in the arm and not much besides. The problem is, you never lift anything from the ground just using your arm. A whole chain of muscles come into play in a certain order, working in unison to lift even the lightest object from the ground, such as a pencil. You'll find yourself recruiting everything from muscles in your feet to your lower legs, all the way up through the upper legs and glutes, to the lower back muscles through to upper back and shoulders. At the same time this is happening, the muscles in your hands are working with the muscles in your arms and again up to the shoulders. If you are not strong in this kinetic chain and through these kinds of movements, then you are not going to be very strong in real life.

I've seen guys in the gym who train exclusively on machines and use single muscle free weight exercises such as bicep curls, and the next thing you hear is that they are injured. How? One particularly muscular guy put his back out, picking up a CD from the ground! No joke. The way you should train is moving your body the same way it is designed and using a collection of muscle groups together in a kinetic chain. Now I am not saying doing bicep curls, or a lat pulldown is no good at all. These movements can be used in a complete training regime. However, the majority of your workout should be made up of movements that consist of using the body the way it was designed. Mixed in there can be movements that are designed predominantly to make your body look better naked. And there is nothing wrong with that! Mix the two, however, and it's damn near perfection.

Rather than filling the rest of this book with pictures of exercises and tons of written notes on how to perform them perfectly, which would be a great waste of paper as in today's day and age when a video would convey the message far, far better. I am instead going to show you one exercise that works every single muscle in your body. This exercise will get your heart rate up, burn fat, make you fitter, build strength throughout the entire body *and* make you look better naked. It also turns boys into men...What more could you ask for? (Don't sweat ladies it's not just for the men, it's simply in the name...The Man Maker which I've since renamed The [Wo]man Maker).

It is one of the most testing exercises for even the most advanced athlete; however, it can be toned down (regressed) to a level of which I have seen more than 99% of people I've trained being able to perform it. If you are already working out, this is an amazing exercise to learn so you can put it in your own workouts and reap the benefits. If you are just starting out or just getting back into it, then this is a great place to kickstart your journey.

As mentioned to get the form *perfect*, I am not going to write it in this book. Having observed over many years people in gyms struggling, trying to follow written programs, who end up using the most horrendous exercise form, I quickly realised this is not the way to do it. In fact, I've read many books on exercise and even with my extensive qualifications, years of training and in-depth knowledge I still struggle to follow along with how to perform exercises perfectly when it is written in books or on sheets of paper. Even with great explanations and high-quality photographs, it's difficult to know that you are performing it absolutely perfectly. To perform an exercise perfectly, you have so much to focus on most wouldn't believe it! You have to;

- Engage the correct muscles.

- Push or pull through the correct part of your body (e.g. pushing through your toes rather than your heel on certain movements can be dangerous for the knees).

- Disengage other muscles that shouldn't be working but will try and take over the movement because of your current muscle imbalances.

- Make sure you're using the correct plane of motion.

- Use a full range of movement.

- Have your posture in the perfect position.

- Use the correct movement speed in both the positive and negative phase.

- Know when and how to breathe.

- Know which muscles to contract, for how long and when is the correct time to do so in the movement.

- Which muscles to stretch and how to do without hyperextending the joints.

- Assure your body is in the correct alignment.

- Know when you are starting to use the imperfect form so you can either correct it or stop the exercise altogether.

If I struggle to gain all that insight with exercises written on paper and a couple of photographs, I guess you do too. So, to save you from having to take this book to the gym and look down at the pictures every 2 seconds with a weight above your head (a surefire way to injure yourself). Or to save you from leaving the book at home and then trying to remember everything I wrote, which will more than likely lead to crappy form, possible injury and terrible results. Instead, what I've done is recorded a free video of me performing the exercise with perfect form, teaching you step-by-step, the correct movements. They say a picture speaks a thousand words; a video, however, must speak 10'000 more. Most people have a device they can take to the gym with them and watch the video online. But as with anything I show you, you don't even need a gym. You can easily perform this at home, at work, or even on vacation. All you need is two dumbbells. Simply head to the Resources section, and it's right there waiting for you.

Yoga

- Flexibility

- Stress relief

- Improved breathing

- Cardiovascular health

- Whole-body muscular strength

- Whole-body muscular endurance

- Increased muscle tone

- Improved posture

- Relieve pain

- Detoxification

As mentioned before, you have to give yoga a proper go. Coming from a traditional gym education, it took me six lessons to 'get it' and a lot more to really understand and feel it. Now I love it. Anytime I go for longer than a few weeks without doing yoga, my back or hips start to hurt. When I pick it back up again, the pain goes away. Beyond the benefits of flexibility, yoga should have a massive part in everyone's life as a form of stress relief. Quieting the mind in today's hectic world is a must. Yoga is a great way to do that. Research done at The University of Mississippi showed that yoga improved muscular strength, flexibility and respiratory and cardiovascular function. It promoted recovery from addiction, reduced stress, anxiety, depression, and chronic pain, improved sleep patterns, and enhanced overall well-being and quality of life.

Beyond even all of that, if you get into a class with a teacher that will push you, yoga suddenly becomes a tough workout! Muscles will burn and sweat will pour. You'll start to use muscles you didn't even know existed in ways that the gym will never fully replicate. Static holds are commonplace in yoga and will build a different type of strength to most resistance training. The reason I have written detoxification down as a benefit is that there are yoga poses that will detoxify certain organs of the body. If you get a well trained and highly knowledgeable yoga instructor to teach you, the workouts go way beyond building a strong, flexible body on the outside. It really is a different world once you go deep into practising yoga. And beyond all of that, there really is nothing quite like a yoga bum...

Swimming, Cycling And Running

- Cardiovascular health and fitness

- Whole-body muscular endurance (Swimming)

- Lower body muscular endurance (Cycling and Running)

- Fat burning

- Injury rehabilitation (Swimming and Cycling)

- Stress relief

- Mental health

All three of these are great ways to work your heart and lungs. However, you can work out the cardiovascular system far quicker and more efficiently doing a good weights circuit if that is your main goal. You will also burn more fat lifting weights in the correct way than you would be doing any of these activities. Yes, I know this might be news to some of you, but I have friends who have stayed overweight after training for and running a marathon. Others who have kept their beer belly after training for and cycling the Tour De France mountain stage!

The fitness required for each of those is of epic proportions, however, doing the same movement over and over such as running or cycling doesn't keep the body guessing long enough to burn maximal amounts of fat. As mentioned earlier in the Resistance Training section, a creative weights circuit that can be changed every time you do it shocks the body each time, leading to superior fat loss in far less time. Researchers at McMaster University, Canada showed that using a low-volume High-Intensity Interval Training with a commitment of fewer than 30 minutes (including warm-up and cool down!), three times per week had great results in a matter of a few weeks. It showed effective in both healthy individuals and people with cardiometabolic disorders, so please don't worry if you don't feel particularly fit right now or you think you are too old. It's not the case!

Having said all that, running, cycling and swimming are fantastic ways to stay healthy, both physically and mentally. Getting lost in your mind on a long swim, cycle or run is incredibly good for your mental health. The release of endorphins and a sense of achievement will only add to that.

Doing any of these activities outside will only add to the benefits. Running and cycling outside gives you the elements of fresh air and sunshine to increase health benefits massively when compared to running on a treadmill or on an exercise bike in the gym. When done in groups, you also have the social aspect which will only improve health and increase happiness. The best place in which to swim is the ocean, of which we will cover the health benefits of later in the book.

Pilates

- Core strength

- Flexibility

- Improved posture

- Relieve pain

- Injury rehabilitation

- Improved breathing

- Whole-body muscular endurance

- Increased muscle tone

Just like yoga, you have to dedicate some time to really understand and feel pilates the way you need to, to get the most benefit out of it. Pilates will connect you to the deep core muscles as very few gym routines can. It is all about focus and using the correct muscles rather than just allowing strong, overworked muscles take over movements. If you have a good teacher, you will work muscles you didn't even know existed even after years of exercise experience working out in gyms. If you are an experienced weight-lifter, you'll find it difficult in the beginning to grasp the breathing technique as it is the complete opposite to the when working out in the gym but stick with it as the benefits are substantial.

You will start working out all the muscles that you are missing in your gym workouts, which is absolutely key in a complete workout regime because if the muscles remain unworked, it can lead to muscle imbalances and therefore, injuries. Pilates will go a long way to preventing injury, and if you have any underlying problems, it can help you fix them too. Many men and some women look at pilates as an easy workout when watching from the outside, but it can cause so much working (good) pain you'll see grown men literally rolling around on the floor in agony. Fun times...

Suspension Training

- Whole-body muscular strength

- Whole-body muscular endurance

- Core strength

- Increased muscle tone

- Fat burning

- Increased Basal Metabolic Rate

- Injury rehabilitation

- Improved posture

- Relieve pain

- Cardiovascular health and fitness

- Mental health

- Improved self-esteem

This is technically a form of resistance training, but I gave it its own category because it is so diverse, there are so many benefits and because so many of my clients and I love it so much. A Suspension Trainer usually compromises of a couple of straps made out of something very strong and durable like parachute material, with some handles which you can hold or place your feet into. You can attach it anywhere that is strong enough to hold your weight, like the top of a door (without any glass in), a solid tree branch or a wall mount you can put up just for that purpose.

It entails using your own body weight as resistance while holding the Suspension Trainer or having your feet strapped in there. Sounds a little scary at first but absolutely everyone I've ever trained has been able to do the basics at the very least. This can not only make exercises more advanced than just using your own body weight, but it can also make some exercises far more comfortable for people who feel pain or pressure in their joints or who are rehabbing an injury. For example, I find it works amazingly well for people who can't normally perform a lunge or a squat due to bad knees. It can also make core work, such as planks far more challenging and fun because of its unstable nature.

As well as all the benefits, they are amazingly diverse. More than 300 exercises can be performed on my favourite Suspension Trainer, working every muscle in your body. I've used it everywhere; I've hung it from a hook in the garage, suspended it in my living room door and the door of a hotel room (it's really lightweight and compact, easy to travel with), and hung it from a sturdy tree branch in my garden and the local park. It is literally like having your own fully equipped gym in a bag that you can hold in one hand.

With that we round out the Foundations of your Health House. Making sure you have implemented most (if not all) of the Action Steps from this and the previous five chapters is key to your overall health and wellbeing and will most certainly give you the best chance of losing weight permanently. As funny as it sounds, the next chapter is really what the entire concept of this book is about, and so is the most important chapter to understand. Why are we only looking at it in Chapter 7 you may ask? Well, this is what we've been warming up to, this is where things start to get a little funky and way less mainstream. Before we move on, let's look at taking some Action Steps and a couple of Resources that can make life easier.

Resources

Go to **www.TomBroadwell.com/resources** to see;

- A video on how to perform The [Wo]Man Maker exercise.

- The Suspension Trainer that I use in my workouts and with my clients.

Action Steps

- Get up and go for a walk (unless you're in bed reading..sat up!...go for one in the morning or park further away from work etc.).

- Buy a pair of dumbbells you can use at home. If just starting out, a pair of 4 to 6 lbs dumbbells are usually suitable for a female and around 8 to 10 lbs is often is ideal for a male. If experienced, go with a weight that you can perform a Shoulder Press for 15-20 repetitions to failure.

- Go to my Resources page and aim to do 10x [Wo]Man Makers in a row to start with, once it's too easy up the weights or start to mix up your training with a PT you trust or with me over at my website.

- If you didn't start already and think yoga might be something you want to do regularly, search out a yoga class in your local area and commit to at least six sessions. If it's something you want to try at home, my website offers some yoga lessons to get you started.

- Do the same with pilates. Find a trusted teacher in your area and start classes. Even better than that, if your budget allows both yoga and pilates are best done one-on-one or in small intimate groups with a teacher who can fully focus on you. Your choice but start either way! Again, my website offers some pilates videos to get you on your way.

- If you've always wanted to run a marathon, swim in the ocean or cycle a 100km, then start to do your chosen activity. It doesn't matter how far you go or how fast, all it takes is that first step. There may be running or cycling or even swimming groups in your area. Search them out if you don't want to go alone and add in the social wellness factor.

- Buy a Suspension Trainer. Trust me, it's worth it!

Section Two

The Walls of Your
Health House

*"Even paradise could become a prison if one had enough time to take notice of the walls." – **Morgan Rhodes***

Chapter Seven

The perfectHealth Scale

"Cancerous tissues are acidic, whereas healthy tissues are alkaline."–
Dr. Otto Warburg

The doctor beamed with pride as he went to collect his prize.

He had finally done it, what every young scientist dreamed of.

He had practised his speech in the mirror a thousand times over.

He was on his way to collect the biggest prize of them all.

A Nobel Prize Award.

What it was for would be the greatest discovery in history, that he was certain.

His research had found what caused cancer.

It was 1931, so cancer wasn't yet a huge worry, but the numbers didn't lie.

It was on the rise and fast.

It would be an epidemic by the end of the century is what the numbers were saying.

But Otto Warburg had put a stop to all that.

He had shown the world that cancer could not live in an alkaline body.

He had shown that if people simply kept their body in an alkaline state, then they would never get cancer.

Pure fantasy?

Dr Otto Warburg

No. In fact, this is all written in the chronicles of history. In 1931, a German doctor by the name of Otto Warburg did win the Nobel Prize Award in Physiology for his "discovery of the nature and mode of action of the respiratory enzyme". Basically put, he won the Nobel Prize for discovering the cause of cancer. He investigated the metabolism of tumours and the respiration of cells. He demonstrated that all forms of cancer are characterised by two basic conditions; acidosis and hypoxia (lack of oxygen). These two conditions are one in the same, as you are about to discover for yourself. Where you have hypoxia, you will find acidosis.

Dr Otto Warburg was a German physiologist, medical doctor, and Nobel laureate. In total, he was nominated for the award 47 *times* throughout his career. Three scientists who worked in Warburg's lab, went on to win the Nobel Prize in future years. He was often awarded honorary doctorates from universities around the world. However, in his own words, he was obsessed with his work, and he would ask officials to mail him medals so as to avoid a ceremony that would separate him from his laboratory. Warburg pursued his research until the age of 86. He is highly regarded for his outstanding achievements and has what is regarded as the highest award in Germany for biochemists and molecular biologists named after him. The Otto Warburg Medal has been awarded annually since 1963 by the German Society for Biochemistry and Molecular Biology.

Utterly convinced and quite rightly so of the accuracy of his conclusions, Warburg expressed dismay at the "continual discovery of cancer agents and cancer viruses" that he expected to "hinder necessary preventive measures and thereby become responsible for cancer cases". Today cancer is widely considered a genetic disease involving nuclear mutations in oncogenes and tumour suppressor genes.

However, once again, extremely strong emerging evidence suggests that cancer is a mitochondrial metabolic disease, as was the original theory of Dr Otto Warburg.

In a paper published in the journal Frontiers in Cell and Developmental Biology in 2015 researchers state, "real progress in cancer management and prevention will emerge once the cancer field abandons the somatic mutation theory and comes to recognize the role of the mitochondria in the origin, management, and prevention of the disease."

In 1966, Dr Otto Warburg delivered a lecture at an annual meeting of Nobelist's in Lindau, Germany. In his speech, he described the cause of cancer as the following: "The prime cause of cancer is the replacement of the respiration of oxygen in normal body cells by a fermentation of sugar. All normal body cells meet their energy needs by respiration of oxygen, whereas cancer cells meet their energy needs in great part by fermentation. All normal body cells are thus obligate aerobes, whereas all cancer cells are partial anaerobes. From the standpoint of the physics and chemistry of life, this difference between normal and cancer cells is so great that one can scarcely picture a greater difference. Oxygen gas, the donor of energy in plants and animals is dethroned in the cancer cells and replaced by an energy yielding reaction of the lowest living forms. Namely, a fermentation of glucose."

The idea that a cancer cell has a lack of oxygen and the entire concept that cancerous tissues are acidic, whereas healthy tissues are alkaline is backed up in more recent research too. What is known as The Warburg Effect has been documented for over 90 years but extensively studied far more in recent times, as over the past 13 years, *thousands* of papers have reported on it. One such paper was published in The British Journal of Nutrition. Researchers at Bastyr University, Seattle found that diet-induced acidosis is a very real thing and has a significant impact on peoples longterm health. They believe it can be neutralised through nutrition.

In 2017 researchers at The VP Research Institute, Sao Paulo evaluated the many studies published over the last ten years. They concluded that excessive consumption of acid precursor foods while eating less alkaline-forming foods can lead to reduced bone density and muscle mass while leading to an increased risk of type 2 diabetes, hypertension and non-alcoholic liver disease.

Stick with me here, because there's a little bit of scientific and medical language to get through. I need to back up what I'm stating so that everyone is on board with what I'm saying, even the more scientific-minded of you! When I present health seminars around the world, most (*not all!*) doctors agree with pretty much everything I say. They quickly become my biggest fans because they understand what I am saying from a scientific and medical standpoint. *It just makes sense.* To do that, I cite a lot of medical research, which I need to do here. Don't worry if you have no prior training in any field related to health. Or indeed any understanding of this at all, as I'll simplify everything (as I always do). Then we can all be on the same page.

Genes

Beyond what Warburg stated, more and more people are coming to the realisation that disease is far more about choice than it is about genes. Pioneer, award-winning genomic researcher Craig Venter who deciphered essentially all the genes in human DNA, states; "Human biology is actually far more complicated than we imagine. Everybody talks about the genes that they received from their mother and father, for this trait or the other. But in reality, those genes have very little impact on life outcomes. Our biology is way too complicated for that and deals with hundreds of thousands of independent factors.

Genes are absolutely *not* our fate.

They can give us useful information about the increased risk of disease. But in most cases, they will not determine the actual cause of the disease or the actual incidence of somebody getting it. Most biology will come from the complex interaction of all the proteins and cells working with environmental factors, not driven directly by the genetic code."

One of the scarier diseases to most people is Alzheimer's and the thought of losing one's mind. According to the Alzheimer's Association, 'only a small percentage of people with Alzheimer's disease (less than 1 per cent) have an early-onset type associated with genetic mutations." So more than 99% is preventable through healthy lifestyle choices. Eight researchers at The University of Texas in their paper titled; 'Cancer is a Preventable Disease that Requires Major Lifestyle

Changes' concluded that only 5–10% of all cancer cases can be attributed to genetic defects, whereas the remaining 90–95% have their roots in the environment and lifestyle.

That means that somewhere around 90-99% of disease comes down to *choice*.

This is backed up time and again by studies done on identical twins. One such study of 1811 pairs of female twins was performed at the University of Southern California, Los Angeles. Researchers found that the incidence of breast cancer in both identical twins was found only about a quarter of the time, with diagnosis years apart. Remembering that twins will usually have the same *lifestyle* and so would increase the likelihood of both getting the same disease. Just putting it out there, but women are maiming their own body by opting for elective bilateral mastectomy because their mother had breast cancer. When, in fact, genes have little to do with it. Or...they are following whatever agenda the mainstream is pushing and doing the same thing as their favourite celebrity, which is even sadder.

All of the previous research is brought together perfectly by researchers from the National Institute of Environmental Health Sciences. They used data from 49,731 Sister Study participants (women whose sister had, had breast cancer). They concluded that women eating more acid-forming foods had; 'greater acid-forming potential, was associated with increased risk of overall and invasive breast cancer'. That is a massive study that drives home the point that I'm trying to make; it's the lifestyle choices you make that impact your health most of the time. This is, in fact, the Foundation of everything in our Health House.

Everything discussed in this book is basically leading to a lifestyle that keeps your body effortlessly functioning in an alkaline state.

Just in case you were thinking, why I put it in as the first *Wall* of Your Health House instead of the Foundation is because I had to warm you up to this first. Otherwise, cynical people may have shut the book in the first chapter! And I want to help as many people reach their goals as possible (cynical or not). I believe that starting with subjects such as food, water and exercise was a good way to get people into alignment with what I was saying, before bringing out the information that *no one* talks about (at least in the mainstream) and so might lead people to be cynical and not believe and therefore not do.

So, I'm hoping I still have most of you with me. And if you stay, the evidence I will now build will be very hard to dismiss even for the most cynical of minds. Whatever your current mindset, the most awesome thing for you to realise from all this is one thing;

You are in complete control of your health.

If you choose to lead an acidic lifestyle, then you are choosing poor health — time for some straight-up *truth*. If you have high blood pressure, high cholesterol, diabetes or any other lifestyle disease, you *chose* it. Sounds *harsh*, but *it's true*. And the sooner you realise that, the sooner you take responsibility for it, the sooner you can get your health back on track. Don't worry; I'm as harsh on myself as I am on you guys. I *chose* to have the condition eczema for the longest time. I know that and I fully admit it.

My Story

What I mean by this is today in 2020, while living on land I don't have the condition eczema. However, in 2008, my condition was so bad every morning when I woke up, I would have to change my sheets because they were covered in puss and blood. *Covered.* It would take me over an hour each morning to become brave enough to shower because water touching my skin felt like I was on fire. To be honest, I sometimes thought it would be nicer to be dead than to live like I was.

Today, after a journey of epic proportions, which lead me to write this book. I got rid of eczema in the most part by practising everything in this book (around 80% of the time) and then controlling any flare-ups severity through lifestyle choices such as, but not limited to, not eating much wheat and dairy. If I do consume these products over a prolonged period of time, I've noticed my skin flares up. I'm so in tune with my body; I know exactly what causes the condition that I have. That's where I want you to be by the end of our journey together. If you are living with a disease or pain every day, I know what you are going through. I've been there, I've felt your pain, I am here to help.

You have to however, first help yourself by taking full responsibility for the disease or condition that you have.

Yes, I know that nobody probably told you about all of this before you found me, so how can you take responsibility if you didn't know? It's okay. You know now. So, let's not dwell on the past, but look to a brighter, healthier and happier future.

You now have the choice; you can choose to be sick or decide to be healthy.

Now, you may have a couple of questions about what you've just read, namely, what do I mean "I chose eczema"? And what do I mean by "while living on land", we all do don't we? What I mean is, I currently spend 9-10 months of the year living and working on cruise ships. I love it. I love the lifestyle, the travel, working with people from all over the world, public speaking about all this stuff and working one on one with fresh clients every week. I love everything about it...almost. I hate the false air, the harsh lighting, showering in water that is so concentrated in chlorine you can smell it on your skin after a shower. I also don't like not having access to fresh organic food. And I put me having eczema while living on a ship down to living in air conditioning almost 24/7 and the water that I shower in. It changes the pH of my skin and so the condition eczema flares up.

So, when working on ships, I choose to have eczema for around nine months of the year. Why? Because I chose to work and live on cruise ships. Waking up in a different country every morning is well worth a little bit of eczema in my book. And it is my book so there! However, I choose to control the severity of eczema by controlling what I put in my mouth. You see today, my eczema is barely noticeable and completely under control whether I'm living on ships or on land. It flares up a little bit while working on a cruise ship, but nothing compared to 9 or 10 years ago, or even 6-7 years ago while living exclusively on land! The difference today, compared to when I started my health journey is incomprehensible. I practice this self-control every day, whether on land or on board a ship, without becoming *obsessed* about it. If I choose to eat pizza every night while living on land, I'd be choosing the condition eczema, due to the amount of wheat and dairy that I'd be consuming. But I also wouldn't turn down pizza if that is what everyone else was ordering at a social gathering. Get my drift? It's *all* a choice.

The Acid vs Alkaline Balance

Remembering our pH scale from Chapter 5: You Are What You Eat..., your blood is right there on the scale at a finely balanced 7.35-7.45. Slightly *alkaline*. Your body will do anything it can to stay there. The body's buffer systems will rapidly control any change in blood pH. It wants to avoid acidosis (pH lower than 7.35) at all costs. Or even alkalosis (pH higher than 7.45). However, just note, if it drops to 7.2, that is when it all ends, my friend — human death.

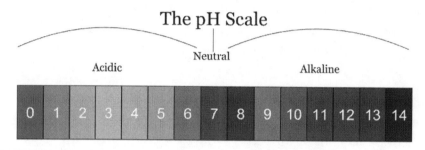

The pH Scale

*7.35-7.45 (Human Blood pH)

Just to make myself clear, from now on, if I speak about a certain food or product being acid or alkaline, I'm *not* talking about its pH Level as it would appear on the scale, if we tested it in the outside world. I'm always talking about it being acid-forming or alkaline-forming *in the body*. There's a huge difference. As you will see, lemons and limes are some of the most alkaline-forming foods, which confuses a lot of people as they are generally thought of as acidic. What's really important is where the food is at on the pH Scale once it has gone through the digestive system.

Many arguments I see going against the alkaline theory is that eating alkaline foods won't make you more alkaline, because your blood is always alkaline. To which I agree, and I would never argue against that. But that's not the point I'm making. This approach is not about making your body more alkaline; your body is amazing at doing that by itself. However, to constantly consume acidic foods is detrimental to your health, because your body keeps itself in an alkaline state by using your natural buffer systems. It's when these buffer systems kick in that the health problems arise.

When your body starts to use water from within cells, to neutralise the acid, it is called chronic inflammation. We all know this as a bad thing in the fact inflammation links back to most diseases. Another buffering system is when we start to leach calcium from our bones. This is because calcium is alkaline. And this is when we start to see diseases such as osteopenia, osteoporosis and certain types of arthritis.

Other buffer systems are, but not limited to plasma bicarbonate which is a form of carbon dioxide in your blood. A low level of bicarbonate in your blood can cause too much acid in the body. This can be caused by kidney disease and liver failure, both of which are linked back to having too many toxins (acid) in the body. Other systems are haemoglobin from the red blood cells causing anaemia and magnesium being used from the muscle, causing muscle wasting. High levels of cholesterol are used to bind acids and patch up lesions in the arteries, leading to stroke and heart attack.

This is why when we look at the research, diet-induced acidosis (however slight the acidosis is), is linked to all types of health problems. It can cause everything from obesity, back pain, loss of muscle mass, and lower bone density leading to diseases such as osteoporosis, brittle bone disease, arthritis, type 2 diabetes, hypertension, liver disease and cancer. Yes, you read that right, eating alkaline can help back pain according to Researchers at The University of Alberta. As well as, 'maybe benefiting bone health, reducing muscle wasting, as well as mitigating other chronic diseases such as hypertension and strokes, even improving memory and cognition.'

Oh, and please note most of the scientific and medical research I've read say 'may' or 'maybe' a lot! And I mean, a lot. Even the breast cancer study from before was done on nearly 50'000 people over seven years said 'may', a lot. Even though when I looked at the statistics, I found it extremely comprehensive. It's almost like researchers who are studying concepts that are not seen as mainstream are afraid of being ridiculed. This is fair enough because they rely on a lot of their funding coming from huge corporations, which in turn would rather keep certain information from becoming mainstream. So, you, as the reader need to read between the lines and as with the prior example say, "Well fuck yeah, most of the women getting breast cancer were eating lots of acid-forming foods. And most of the ones who weren't were not!"

When we eat alkalising foods and expose ourselves to less stress and toxins, we begin to get to the root cause of most people's health problems. Rather than just treating a symptom, we begin to give the body what it needs to heal itself and prevent the disease from happening in the first place. Put it this way; there are only three things that cause disease in the body.

- **Genetics** - We can't do much about when a disease is caused purely by genetics, but that is rare compared to what most people believe. You may be genetically weaker in one area of your body, or more predisposed to get a disease than the next person. But it doesn't mean you *have* to develop that disease.

- **Toxins** - All toxins are acidic on the body and come from a massive variety of places. In a later chapter (and in fact, throughout the entire book), we will go through toxins and find out what might be causing your disease. They can also lead to weight gain, especially around the abdominal region, hips, thighs and upper arms. We will discover what may cause you health issues or undesirable weight gain in the future.

- **Malnutrition** - As mentioned food is fuel and is necessary for our body. The right amount of certain nutrients is essential to keeping the body balanced, healthy and functioning in an optimal way. The nutrients are also used to protect us against toxins that enter our body on a daily basis.

Acid vs Alkaline Foods

In this chapter, we will keep it simple. We will focus on alkaline-forming *foods* you should eat more of, and acid-forming *foods* you should be eating less of. Then as we continue on our journey together, we will look at other lifestyle choices that will help keep your body functioning effortlessly in an alkaline state. This equates to a state of optimal health, and you becoming more and more like the fat burning machine we all are born to be. We have already covered some of the lifestyle choices in earlier chapters.

Emotions, stress and a lack of exercise all contribute to this. Emotions and stress can directly affect our blood and have affected our health twice as much as any food can! Which is why the made up our very first Foundations, with Chapter 1 being called Mindset Mastery Matters Most, and Chapter 2 was called Stress Less. Hopefully, the techniques and information I provided helped to get those two highly essential factors into check at least a little bit! If not yet, keep working on it! Exercise was covered in Chapter 6: Move It Or Lose It because it is crucial. It pumps our blood and lymphatic system, which removes waste and helps to deliver more oxygen to cells. This is entirely in alignment with Dr Otto Warburg's research.

Some might say; "Whoa! I'm in my 50's Tom; my metabolism has slowed down. It's harder to lose weight now. Blah, blah, blah." To which I say; "Have you ever seen an animal in the wild, who eats what it was designed to eat and moves the way it was meant to move, get halfway through its life and suddenly develop a middle-aged spread? Or have you ever seen a cave painting of an overweight caveman?" The answer is *no*. We were never meant to be fat. So, you now need to decide to get out of your own way and back into your natural state of optimal health with a banging body to boot!

A lot of naysayers in the scientific community who attack the alkaline approach base everything solely on measuring the potential renal acid load (PRAL) and its influence on urine pH. Which is not as accurate as measuring the blood itself, but unfortunately is what most (around 90%) of the food charts you'll find online are based on. Rather than looking at PRAL, we will base our food chart mainly on the work of one of the original and major researchers into the alkaline lifestyle, Robert O. Young. It is based upon the results from blood work, of which he has analysed over 40,000 blood tests. Blood work is almost always more accurate than urine when it comes to measuring things in the body.

What you'll see next is a table of Acidifying vs Alkalising foods choices. The aim to get as close to 80% alkaline choices as you can with 20% coming from the acid side of the table. This is not saying you need 20% acidifying foods to be healthy. However, life is for enjoyment, so if you want some wine and cheese, don't stress, enjoy it and then move on, fair do's?

Acidifying vs Alkalising Foods

Highly Acidic	Moderately Acidic	Mildly Acidic	Mildly Alkaline	Moderately Alkaline	Highly Alkaline
Alcohol	Apple	Bottled Water	Almonds	Beetroot	Alkaline Water
Artificial Sweetener	Banana	Apple Cider Vinegar	Almond Milk	Brussel Sprouts	Algae
Balsamic Vinegar	Blueberries	Brazil Nuts	Amaranth	Capsicum Pepper	Arugula / Rocket
Beef	Butter	Brown Rice	Artichoke	Cabbage	Avocado
Boxed Cereal	Cranberries	Cashew Nuts	Asparagus	Butter Beans	Basil
Black Tea	Grapes	Cherry	Avocado Oil	Carrots	Broccoli
Cheese	Freshly Squeezed Fruit Juice	Dark Chocolate (>80%)	Bottled Water (Bottled At The Source)	Chia Seeds	Grasses (e.g. Wheatgrass, Barley Grass)
Chicken	Goat's Cheese	Gluten Free Bread	Brussel Sprouts	Chickpeas	Coriander / Cilantro
Coffee	Mango	Ghee	Buckwheat	Chillies	Cucumber
Condiments	Orange	Gluten Free Cereal	Cauliflower	Chives	Fresh Veggie Juice
Cow's Milk	Peach	Gluten Free Pasta	Courgette / Zucchini	Coconut	Flaxseed
Dried Fruit	Pineapple	Green Tea	Filtered Water	Coconut Milk	Flaxseed Oil
Egg	Raspberries	Hazelnuts	Grapefruit	Coconut Oil	Celery
Farmed Fish	Red Wine	Melon	Herbal Tea	Fresh Coconut Water	Himalayan Pink Salt
Fruit Juice	Strawberries	Millet	Herbs (Other)	Garlic	Kale
Jam	Raw Honey	Nectarine	Leek	Ginger	Kelp
Lamb	Raw Sugar	Oats	Pomegranate	Green Beans	Lettuce
Malt Vinegar	Soy Milk	Pecans	Olive Oil	Hemp Seeds	Parsley
Milk Chocolate	Vegetable Oils	Plum	New Baby Potatoes	Homemade Hummus	Silverbeet / Chard
Mushrooms	Walnuts	Potato	Raw Cacao	Kidney Beans	Seaweed
Peanuts	Wholemeal Bread	Rice Milk	Raw Vegan Sprouted Protein	Lemon	Sprouts (Alfalfa, Bean, Pea etc.)
Pork	White Rice	Stevia	Sauerkraut	Lettuce	Spinach
Processed Foods	Wholemeal Pasta	Sunflower Seeds	Sea Salt	Lentils	Watercress
Shellfish		Wild Fish	Sesame Seeds	Lime	
Soda			Sesame Oil	Onion	
Syrup			Spices (Other)	Quinoa	
Tap Water			Squash	Peas	
White Bread			Swede	Radish	

Okay, so there you have it. Hopefully, you have a fair few foods that you enjoy on the Alkaline side of the chart. As we continue on our journey together, you will find it easier and easier to give up the foods you may well be addicted to on the Acid side. Trust me; once this journey is complete, you will crave not one piece of processed junk. That doesn't mean you can't eat it, but you will be in complete control of whether you do or not!

PRAL vs Blood Analysis

I also need to point out a couple of mistakes I've made in the past when advising clients regarding acid versus alkaline foods. Rest assured as my knowledge grows; I will own up to mistakes and adapt my approach, for the benefit of both you and I! Some of you might be confused at seeing fruit, raw honey and apple cider vinegar in the Acid side of the table. When researching in the past, I've only ever come across the PRAL method of measuring pH in urine, which puts all of the above on the Alkaline side of the chart. However, looking at Blood Analysis and the work of Robert Young, which I see as more accurate, I now find it far more logical to consider these foods acidic.

Apple cider vinegar, for example, is fermented, which is exactly what we need to be avoiding according to Dr Warburg! And thus, fermentation makes it more towards the acid-forming side. It is far more alkaline than other kinds of vinegar, and that's where some of the confusion lays. It certainly does have health benefits, including helping me kickstart the process of healing my skin. But for these purposes and going forward, I have to hold my hands up and say it is acid-forming in the body.

Raw honey does have many health benefits, but because of its high sugar content this makes it acidic in the body. Knowing that sugar ferments and again looking at Dr Warburg's extensive, award-winning research, the difference between a healthy cell and a cancerous cell is one takes in oxygen, and the other the oxygen is replaced as a form of fermentation.

Which brings us nicely onto fruit, well most fruits anyway. Looking at the list we can see pomegranates, lemons, limes, grapefruit and rhubarb are amazing for you and melon ain't too bad either. But because of the high sugar content of most fruits, this leads to the exact same problem as with honey and so should be eaten in moderation. They are far better than reaching for a chocolate bar or some cake, but as mentioned earlier in the book, eat them on their own and in small quantities.

Making Life Easier

Now, let's go through some ways to make this whole process easier, so you can get somewhere close to your 80% with as little stress or brainpower being used as possible. First, we have to understand that all meat and the five most common carbohydrates that make up most people's meals in today's modern world; bread, pasta, potatoes, rice and cereal are all acidic. As mentioned we should not be eating these carbs and meat together anyway, so hopefully, we've already cut down on the heavy carb intake. Not only meat but all animal products are heavily acidic. To tackle this problem, consider the following Action Steps;

- **Cut down on meat intake.** Albert Einstein once said, "Nothing will benefit health or increase chances of survival on Earth as the evolution to a vegetarian diet." Now, I am not vegetarian or vegan, and neither was Einstein for most of his life, but there is something very true in his words. All animal proteins break down into acid. Also, consider as meat travels round your very long, and very warm colon, it will begin to rot. Fish will digest quicker and easier than a piece of steak or chicken, but in the end, the blood will end up pulling in rotten carcasses which it then feeds to every cell in your body. You don't need an 16oz (1lb or 450g) steak or two chicken breasts! You are likely not a bodybuilder and will build muscle with far less protein than you think. Forget about the popular diets right now, which focus far too much on protein, they in time will be proven wrong as all popular diets always are...

- **Cut out the starchy carbs.** There are a lot of alternatives to the staples of this world, bread, pasta, rice, potatoes and cereal. Even when you go for the brown, wholewheat, or wholemeal, these are not considered good choices for your health and especially not if you are trying to lose weight. The better alternatives are naturally gluten-free grains such as **quinoa,**

buckwheat, millet and **amaranth.** You can do some amazing things with **cauliflower** such as rice, mash and even popcorn! Purchasing a **spiralizer** and making your own **vegetable pasta** is a fantastic way to go. I often have the still starchy but far kinder **chickpeas, kidney beans** or **lentils** with salads, stir-fries and chilli (while not having any animal protein) which makes my belly feel full while avoiding bread and rice. Then we have still starchy but far more complex vegetables, which are full of nutrients so far better for you than their white counterparts; **sweet potato, squash** and **swede.** And if, if you are really craving pasta or bread, there are healthier options available, however, as with anything you need to read the label. Some are full of synthetic chemicals. The best ones (but still read the label!) are found in health food stores where you can find such items as **quinoa pasta** and **sprouted grain bread.**

- **Cut down on dairy.** The dairy we consume today is a long way removed from the raw milk, butter, yoghurt and cheese that was produced worldwide in times gone by. Raw dairy is now banned in some states of America, but still sold in vending machines in some countries of Europe! This shows it is safe, as long as the cows are grass-fed, and the farms are well maintained. On the large scale commercial farms, we see across America today, that practice confined animal feeding operations (CAFOs), the milk must be pasteurised to kill the bacteria and then it is homogenised to extend its shelf life. Unfortunately, pasteurisation destroys nutrients such as Vitamins B-12, B-6, C, A, the beneficial bacteria naturally found in milk, as well as denatures delicate milk proteins and vital enzymes.

Robert Cohen, Executive Director of the Dairy Education Board, wrote in his 2007 article "Homogenized Milk: Rocket Fuel for Cancer," that homogenisation is, 'the worst thing dairymen have done to milk.' Raw dairy is still acidic, but far, far healthier than the mass-produced dairy we see today. However, a little bit of cheese here and there won't kill anyone, but gulping down pints of milk never was and never will be healthy. If mass-produced even peoples go-to healthy snack, Greek yoghurt is *not* healthy. All dairy products cause inflammation throughout the body.

Researchers at Channing Laboratory, Boston found no correlation between a higher dairy consumption lowering the risk of fractures. In fact, if we look at it with fresh eyes, dairy doesn't help with bone health, it instead robs your bones of their calcium because it is highly acidic. After all, as mentioned animal proteins always break down into acid, and calcium is an excellent acid-neutraliser.

If you have teenagers, please be aware that multiple studies have shown dairy causes acne and being something, I had to endure in my time as a teen, it's something I wish someone had told me about earlier in life! To look at this from an angle of common sense, I turn to an awesome quote from Dr Michael A. Klaper, 'the purpose of cow's milk is to turn a 65-pound calf into a 400-pound cow as rapidly as possible. Cow's milk is baby-calf growth fluid.' And so, if you don't want to be a 400-pound cow, don't drink loads of cow's milk! Even when raw, this quote applies, but as mentioned a little bit of raw dairy won't kill you either. The best alternatives are **almond** and **coconut milk**, and a taste sensation is **coconut yoghurt**. Use it to replace your beloved Greek or natural yoghurt. Now, I'm not saying the following is alkaline, but it's far healthier than ice cream made from cows' milk, and you can call it a healthy treat if you like, but you've got to try **organic coconut ice cream**. My word it's amazing! **Soy milk** is still one up for debate and in some circles increases the risk for breast cancer in both males and females. For me, right now, I'd prefer to stick with the safer alternatives I've mentioned.

- *All* **herbs** and **spices** are alkaline in their purest form and have amazing disease-fighting qualities. In a paper published in the Journal of AOAC International, researcher Jiang T. Alan found that spices and herbs have antioxidant, anti-inflammatory, anti-tumorigenic, and anti-carcinogenic properties. Plus, glucose and cholesterol-lowering activities. So, add them to everything! Add **cinnamon** to your breakfast and smoothies, add fresh **garlic** and **Himalayan pink salt** (HPS) to almost any meal along with **ginger** and **turmeric** if it goes! Throw in fresh **basil**, **coriander** or **parsley** (depending on what you're making) to any soup, stew, stir fry or curry. And please don't go mistaking table salt with HPS or sea salt. Table salt is stripped of every nutrient, and so you load up your arteries with sodium, and that's about it, whereas HPS has 84 different minerals and trace elements and as we'll soon learn sea salt has incredible healing properties.

- **Warm lemon water** and **HPS** in the morning. After downing your first two glasses of water first thing, another great addition to your morning routine is warm lemon water. You can always sip a small cup of this with breakfast and if you feel the need to have some form of liquid when you eat, a small serving of warm lemon water is the best choice to have with any meal. Before eating anything on a morning, make a small, shootable cup of 1 teaspoon of HPS with the juice of half a lemon in warm water.

- **Spinach** is very alkaline and can be added to almost anything, whether it's raw or cooked. It's a great addition when raw to smoothies and juices. When cooked it reduces down to almost nothing, meaning it will fit in pretty much any recipe and doesn't have a strong taste, so throw it in there. It's great to feed the kids if they currently have a problem eating vegetables!

- *Give up* **vegetable oils** and start cooking with either **avocado oil** or **coconut oil**. Both have a high burn rate which means they don't become toxic when you cook with it. **Olive oil** is fantastic but should only be used as a dressing but should never be cooked with because of its low burn rate, which turns it into a cancerogenic as shown by research done in Austria in 1993 and then again in New York in 2011.

- **Coconut** is awesomely alkaline, so start consuming as much coconut as possible. Whether its coconut water, oil, milk, yoghurt, cream, or the flesh. Preferably fresh coconut and don't worry about consuming it every day! I say this because some of you will still be programmed by mainstream media and will worry about the amount of fat it contains. So just to remind you, good fats are essential and help you rid the trans fats out of your cells. Remember also that fat *doesn't* make you fat, sugar does. Just to put it to bed once and for all, good fats are essential for the health of your brain, heart, joints, blood, eyes, hair, nails, skin...I could go on. But they sound pretty important to me!

- **Vegetable juices** are the absolute bomb when it comes to being alkaline. It should be something you're adding into your daily routine; preferably every morning make a vegetable juice as part of your breakfast. It will flood your system with phytochemicals and antioxidants and all the good stuff it needs to fight disease and give you a huge, but gradual energy boost in the morning, or indeed any time of the day. However, I know that in the beginning, your tastebuds might still need some training. So if you follow my recipe below for a still alkaline but sweeter juice, this is a great place to start, and then you can switch in or out as many alkaline ingredients as you like, preferably switching out any fruit (that isn't lemon or lime) to vegetables, herbs and spices.

Super Sweet Alkaline Juice

Ingredients:

- 1/3 a Honeydew Melon

- 2 Beetroots

- 200g French Beans

- 200g Spinach

- 1 Lemon

- One thumb of Ginger

- One thumb of Turmeric

Method:

1. Wash all vegetables and spices thoroughly.

2. Peel beetroot and melon then cut into small pieces.

3. Peel the lemon and cut into small pieces.

4. Leave the skin on ginger and turmeric, cut into small pieces.

5. Top and tail french beans, then chop in half.

6. Chop spinach into small manageable pieces.

7. Juice ginger and turmeric first.

8. Follow with rest of ingredients.

Look at the Resources at the end of the chapter for a link to a video of me making this juice, which is a far more fun and time-efficient way to follow a recipe. Get the kids involved, as I do in most of my juice videos. Juicing can be healthy fun had by all. Don't worry, with a bit of adult supervision kids can readily use knives and the like, you just need to trust the little buggers!

- **Grasses** such as **wheatgrass** and **barley grass** are the most alkaline food types, and if you can get fresh (or grow your own), they should be added to juices. If you struggle to find fresh, you can buy 'Super Greens' type powders to add to your juices and smoothies. Hang tight for Chapter 9: SupplementNation to see how to read labels and know you are getting the best bang for your buck.

- **Sprouts** such as **alfalfa, bean** and **pea sprouts** as well as **watercress** are all super alkaline and should be added to every salad and stir fry that you make.

- You may have noticed **anything green** is awesomely alkaline. Using a lot of **spinach, kale, lettuce, chard, cucumber, broccoli** and the like at every meal is a surefire way to help your body stay effortlessly alkaline. How to do this? Have a **side salad** with every meal, whether you are eating in or eating out. When eating at home, add raw broccoli which is full of flavour, but most people kill it by cooking it. And of course, you can add any of these greens to your **daily green juice**...

- The most obvious thing to do is to **avoid processed food** as much as possible. That means being organised. Preparing and taking your own food to work, on road trips and on flights. If forced to eat something processed, go organic as much as possible as will be discussed in more detail later in a chapter that will kill any of your theories on why organic is not worth it. Avoid food that is mass-produced by huge corporations.

There you have it. Some simple, easy to do things that can get you pretty darn close if not more than the 80/20 we are looking for, in favour of alkaline food. In the next chapter, we will learn what are comfortably the most acidic products that people put into their body on a sometimes daily basis. This time it's not the food that people are consuming, but in some cases, it seems just as necessary to survive. We will learn what industry the highest profiting companies in the world belong to. One that has positioned itself through billions of dollars spent on fancy marketing, to be as necessary as the air that you breathe. However, we will question whether it is true or not. Do we really need synthetic drugs to survive, or in most cases, can we succeed to be healthy through changes to our lifestyle?

If we can improve our health through lifestyle so that the body can heal itself without the need for Big Pharma's pills and potions, how would that sound to you? Keep on taking the Action Steps in each chapter, and you will give yourself the biggest chance of not relying on medication to keep your body in a state of homeostasis. As you will see, it is totally possible to most people, no matter where you are on your journey through life, as crazy as that might sound to some of you who have been on different drugs for decades. Once you've done the following Action Steps, I'll see you in the very next chapter...

Resources

Go to **www.TomBroadwell.com/resources** to see;

- The juicer I use and recommend if you don't have one already.

- The fun video for Super Sweet Alkaline Juice.

- A free video on how to make Cauliflower Rice.

- The 'Super Greens' powder I use and recommend when fresh is not available.

Action Steps

- Buy different herbs and spices (preferably fresh and organic) to add to your cooking from now on. Even better is to plant them. You need minimal gardening skills as they are far easier to grow than most plants and vegetables, so give it a go! (You can the kids involved in this too).

- Buy some extra virgin coconut oil and if you can find it, some organic avocado oil to cook with.

- Cut down on your animal produce intake.

- Cut down rice, pasta, bread, white potatoes and cereal to an absolute minimum.

- Buy a juicer, head over to the Resources page, and you can have one heading to you in a matter of minutes. Don't put this off! Do it now. Although not cheap, it is easily one of the best investments you can make for you and your families health.

- Either plant some wheat grass or buy some green powder to add to juices and smoothies.

- Make it a habit to order a side salad every time you eat out.

- Make it a habit to buy ingredients such as spinach, alfalfa sprouts and watercress every time you shop and add them to every salad you make from now on.

- Use coconut as an alternative when it comes to dairy.

- If you haven't already, decide now is the time you will start preparing more of your own food and taking it with you for lunch and snacks. Use the time-saving techniques found in Chapter 5: You Are What You Eat... to make this process as painless as possible.

Chapter Eight
Trust Me, I'm *Not* A Doctor
"The best doctor gives the least medicines."– **Benjamin Franklin**

There was once a client of mine who took aspirin for the headache...

that was caused by the antihistamine he took for the hives,

that he got from the loperamide he used for the upset stomach,

that was caused by the sildenafil he used for erectile dysfunction,

which was brought about from the finasteride he used for hair loss,

which happened when he used the isotretinoin for the acne,

caused by the barbiturate he took for a sleeping disorder,

that he developed from taking fluoxetine for the depression,

caused by the laxatives, he relied on for his constipation,

brought about from the sertraline he used for anxiety,

created by the statin, he was using for his high cholesterol,

brought on by the use of warfarin to thin his blood,

as a result of a blood clot,

caused by the synthetic fat burning pill he took to combat his out of control weight gain...

Recognise this picture? You might well do since this is a regular occurrence looking at my working with the American public onboard cruise ships. A fact that most people can agree with is that Big Pharma is all about profits. At the end of the day, that is their promise to their shareholders - to make a profit. My question to you is, do they profit from sick people or healthy people? That's right. Sick people.

It's not actually Healthcare; it's Sickcare.

Obscene Profit

The profit is so great that in 2002, the Top Ten pharmaceutical companies in America made more profit than the other 490, Fortune 500 companies put together, that my friends, is fucking mental. The following quote is from Dr Marcia Angell, the former Editor in Chief of the prestigious New England Journal of Medicine, "The combined profits for the ten drug companies in the Fortune 500 ($35.9 billion) were more than the profits for all the other 490 businesses put together ($33.7 billion) [in 2002]. Over the past two decades, the pharmaceutical industry has moved very far from its original high purpose of discovering and producing useful new drugs. Now primarily a marketing machine to sell drugs of dubious benefit, this industry uses its wealth and power to co-opt every institution that might stand in its way, including the US Congress, the FDA, academic medical centers, and the medical profession itself."

It's gone from bad to worse, just 16 years later in 2018 the Top Three pharmaceutical companies in America brought a combined profit of $45 Billion and spent more on Sales & Marketing then they did on Research & Development. That speaks *volumes* about what I am trying to say here. Most drugs today are minor variations of highly profitable pharmaceutical drugs already on the market. For example, from 1998 through 2003, 487 drugs were approved by the US Food and Drug Administration. Only 14% of them were actually new compounds considered likely to be improvements over older drugs.

If you are thinking it's not all about the money, just look at the drug Harvoni for the treatment of hepatitis C, which was designed by Gilead Sciences. It was a drug that was said to cure hepatitis C in 12 weeks. When Harvoni was introduced, a 12-week course in the US cost $94,500. In India, the same 12-week course of treatment cost only $900. Not only the massive price difference but curing diseases is clearly bad for business, as reported in a Goldman Sachs article when they asked, "Is curing patients a sustainable business model?" after lamenting that Harvoni's profits went down from a peak of $12.5 billion in 2015 to *only* $4 billion in 2018.

The reporter says, "The potential to deliver 'one shot cures' is one of the most attractive aspects of gene therapy, genetically-engineered cell therapy and gene editing. However, such treatments offer a very different outlook with regard to recurring revenue versus chronic therapies... While this proposition carries tremendous value for patients and society, it could represent a challenge for genome medicine developers looking for sustained cash flow."

Making the whole thing even more sickening, the reporter goes on to say, "[Gilead]'s rapid rise and fall of its hepatitis C franchise highlights one of the dynamics of an effective drug that permanently cures a disease, resulting in a gradual exhaustion of the prevalent pool of patients".

The report noted that diseases such as common cancers—where the "incident pool remains stable"— are less risky for business.

So, I put to you, do you really think with all the billions that are donated each year to cancer research, that they are actually looking for a cure? Spending on cancer medicines totalled $107 billion worldwide in 2015 and was projected to exceed $150 billion by 2020. In America, even the cheapest cancer treatments top $100'000 per year. A rather sad study published in the Journal of Clinical Oncology in 2018 shows that almost half of patients who have to pay more than $2,000 out of their own pocket for pills to treat cancer have to abandon that treatment altogether.

Medical bills are the renowned number one cause of bankruptcy in America.

A company called Spark Therapeutics developed a drug called Luxturna, which was widely described by the media in 2018 as a curative treatment that 'restores vision' and was priced at $850k! However, as a paper published in 2019 in the journal Drug Discovery Today showed, FDA documents later revealed that the drug is not expected to restore normal vision. Only about half of treated patients met the FDA's threshold for minimally meaningful improvement, and that improvement might not persist long-term. This amongst the fact that two people experienced permanent vision loss. Lovely.

Financially Motivated Research

The evidence is clear that financial relationships between pharmaceutical manufacturers and researchers, doctors, and scientists create certain research outcomes. The paper "Taking Financial Relationships into Account When Assessing Research" that was published in the journal Accountability in Research in 2013 goes into fantastic detail of this subject. One study published in 1998 in The New England Journal of Medicine found that a shocking 96% of authors publishing studies reporting outcomes that favoured the use of calcium channel blockers had financial relationships with the companies sponsoring the research. In a paper published in JAMA in 1999 researchers found that *only 5%* of articles with industry funding reported negative results for cancer treatments, which increased to a far larger 38% of articles not sponsored by the industry.

In a paper published in 2003 in The BMJ that was a systematic review of 30 studies found that those with industry funding were more likely to report results that favoured the company's products than studies with independent sources of funding. Another paper published in JAMA this time in 2003 reviewed 11 previous studies and found that industry-funded biomedical research was almost *four times* more likely to yield results favourable to industry than independently funded research. Researchers concluded that 'Financial relationships among industry, scientific investigators, and academic institutions are widespread. Conflicts of interest arising from these ties can influence biomedical research in important ways.' In a systematic review of 19 articles done in 2008, that examined the relationship between industry funding and research outcomes in clinical research found that 17 articles reported a strong positive correlation, whereas only *two* did not.

Corporate Corruption

Knowing there are financial implications for research done in the medical field doesn't create too much confidence, but then what shatters it is when we take a quick look at the corruption which bubbles to the surface now and then. Even though it only rears its ugly head intermittently, it seems that it is always there and there is a vast amount of money invested, so it doesn't become common knowledge to folks like you and me. We will look at just one drug here, but as we have just seen, please understand this sort of practice is not limited to the one company in question, however across the entire pharmaceutical industry.

This particular evidence came to light after researchers got to review documents that became available during litigation related to rofecoxib (Vioxx), a drug manufactured by the pharmaceutical company Merck. It was to be used for the treatment of acute and chronic symptoms of osteoarthritis, rheumatoid arthritis, acute pain and menstrual pain. Then low and behold, some incredibly underhand practices came to light. At the time of approval, the company's trials indicated there was not an increased risk of cardiovascular events with rofecoxib compared with placebo or other NSAIDs. Merck pulled the drug from the market in 2004 amid a chorus of praise from doctors. The lead researcher of the Vioxx Gastrointestinal Outcomes Research said withdrawing the drug was "pretty honourable and gutsy of [Merck]." She was part of an advisory group to the company, of which many members recommended the drug *not* be withdrawn because patients need various drug options, even though during the study, 79 of the 4,000 patients taking Vioxx suffered serious heart problems or died.

This is all after Merck executives had become aware of potential cardiovascular risks associated with the drug as early as May 2000; however, maybe it was a little too painful to pull its second-biggest money maker. It was shown how this whole event happened in two separate papers published in 2008 in JAMA; the first paper showed the problem was as we have already mentioned. Many publications concerning Merck's rofecoxib that were attributed primarily or solely to academic investigators were actually written by Merck employees or medical publishing companies hired by Merck! The other paper showed that the company manipulated the data analysis in 2 clinical trials to minimise the increased mortality associated with the drug.

The Lancet reported in 2004 that as many as 88,000 people suffered heart attacks after taking Vioxx, and an estimated 38,000 died. While some of the individuals had a prior history of heart problems, others did not. Merck has so far settled Vioxx Cases for upwards of $4.85 Billion. They agreed to pay another $950 million to the United States Department of Justice in 2011 to resolve criminal charges and civil claims related to its alleged illegal promotion and marketing of Vioxx. The main point here is large companies that you trust with your health will seemingly lie and risk people's lives for profit.

A Rose Between Many Thorns

However, even amongst all of this damning evidence, I admit it! In some (fairly rare) cases, Western medicine is absolutely necessary. Western medicine has accomplished and continues to accomplish many incredible advancements, especially when it comes to life-threatening events. Life-saving methods, medical equipment, and critical care procedures are some of the most amazing examples of this. Hospitals can repair broken bones, save lives, and stabilise serious life-threatening situations. Unfortunately, however, the facts speak for themselves. When it comes to pharmaceutical drugs, most of the time, they are not the safest option and simply not necessary if some lifestyle changes are implemented. Besides that, there are some worrying things about the whole industry that need addressing.

"We won't ever have a cure for diseases until we first have a cure for greed." - Dr Sachin Patel

Firstly, almost every synthetic drug ever made has not cured a single disease and the ones that claim to do usually end up being dodgy claims, as we just witnessed with the apparent cure for blindness. Western medicine treats the symptom, not the root cause. Why cure a disease when you can make astronomical profits having people take a pill every day for the rest of their lives? Secondly, every single pharmaceutical drug comes with a list of side effects. This, above all else, leads to greater profits. Take one drug regularly for long enough, and the next drug you start taking might well be a side effect from the first one. People rarely link the two.

Most people also take pills without ever really questioning why they are taking them and researching what they can do to heal themselves naturally. The notion 'Trust me I'm a doctor' is put forth the world over, and people believe it. This belief really is killing people.

Over 100,000 Americans die every year from taking their *prescribed* amount of medication.

America consumes around 50% of the world's medication. The same amount as the rest of the population of the entire world! That is 300 million people taking the same amount of pharmaceutical drugs as over 7 billion other people. It would be okay if America was the picture of health and topped the life expectancy list. But it doesn't. According to the CIA's World Factbook, America ranks as 43rd on the life expectancy list of people born in 2017. That is way down the list if 'healthcare' actually worked. The US spends about twice what other high-income nations do on health care. But it has the lowest life expectancy and the highest infant mortality rates, a 2018 study by the London School of Economics and the Harvard T.H. Chan School of Public Health in Boston has shown.

Vaccines

Let's take a look at one form of medicine which is seen as the holy grail of Western medicine. I'm unsure if I could have chosen a more controversial subject to write about! If anything, this subject does have the ability to completely polarise my audience. However, before you freak out and shut the book up without giving me a chance to explain myself, please give me a chance! Firstly, I included 'The No Bullshit Guide' in the subtitle for a reason. I don't beat around the bush as a person and I most certainly won't when I figure people's health is on the line! Secondly, I'm just going to present some facts and figures and let you make up your own mind, so don't worry you shouldn't start hating me too much (or at least you shouldn't hate anybody for having a different opinion to you on such things, that's not healthy).

Now, please understand that I could have skipped over this subject, as I see most people in the Alternative Health arena do, for fear of either ridicule or losing income in one way or another. However, I won't allow myself to be one of those people when I have hard facts staring at me in the face. I'm here to tell you the truth, and nothing but the truth, as I understand it at this very moment. If it means facing hate, ridicule or losing income that's okay with me as long as I can stand in my truth, knowing I did my best to help people on their health journey. Until presented with convincing enough evidence to sway my opinion, I will keep the information coming. But of course, as I keep reiterating, this is only my opinion, and you should always do your own research.

The subject of vaccines ranks up there with religion, politics and cancer in terms of how taboo it is to discuss it. I've covered most of those subjects in this very book because I believe no subject should be off the table, especially when the very future of mankind is at stake! I truly think these are taboo subjects that should 'never be discussed' because if people do start talking about them, they might just find out the truth. People at the top of politics and pharmaceutical companies don't want the general public realising they've been lied to by having in-depth discussions about anything other than what they've seen on the TV.

What I am saying is I am not covering this subject for my own good, it's for each and every one of you. All I ask is for you to enter with an open mind. I'm writing about vaccinations because large groups of people seem to blindly believe that vaccines are safe. I believe this to be the case because vaccines are heavily pushed in the media by doctors, governments and organisations such as the WHO to be safe and effective. Why is it pushed hard? One reason is that it is the profit is in the *billions* and keeps growing year on year. People who question their safety are often thought of as either batshit crazy, a 'fringe' group or even conspiracy theorists. Numbers are actually way higher than the mainstream media lead you to believe. In a 2011 National Public Radio (NPR) nationwide poll of 3,000 parents, a little more than a quarter of households had concerns about the safety or value of vaccines. The talk then turns to the research that is done that shows vaccines can be dangerous, and it is said that they are 'fringe' studies. Nope, they are in the most prestigious journals, much of which are cited throughout this book.

And when you talk to people who question vaccines, they are often well-read and have done a large amount of research. In my line of work, I have also personally spoken to parents whose child was perfectly fine, healthy, bright and cognisant before their vaccination and then developed severe autism afterwards. Looking at a report published in Generation Rescue, Inc. in 2009, 'The United States has the highest number of mandated vaccines for children under 5 in the world (36, double the Western world average of 18), and the highest autism rate in the world (1 in 150 children, 10 times or more the rate of some other Western countries).' This is up from 1 in 10'000 children suffering from autism in 1970. Or to put it another way, an increase of more than 6000%. The vaccine schedule has grown considerably since 1990 with 25 additional vaccines. According to the CDC data, it shows just how much rates of autism have increased from 2000-2014. It shows an increase of 1 in 150 to 1 in 59 over that period of time, a 254 per cent increase. That works out to an extremely worrying annual average of 18 per cent.

Of course, people who believe in vaccines ridicule people who research anything. They claim how crazy it is that you have researched something on the internet for a few hours and think you are an expert when doctors go through years of medical school—asking how a doctor could possibly be wrong? And again, some doctors will blindly believe what they got taught, which is fine for them, but they can and have been wrong *many* times before. Telling people that it was healthy to smoke over the course of *three* decades and getting paid for it is the *perfect* example of this.

An article published in the Journal of Public Safety in September 2013 shows just how many mistakes healthcare professionals make each and every year. Researchers found that a minimum of 210,000 preventable deaths per year occurs in the US and that the number may actually exceed 400,000 because of the limitations of the search tools they used. Incredibly, they also determined that serious harm to patients in hospitals may be 10-20 times greater than that horrific lethal number of 400,000!

That potentially means between 4 million and 8 million people are seriously harmed in hospitals annually in America alone.

As far as vaccines safety goes, go and type "vaccine adverse effects" on PubMed (the National Institutes of Health Database of scientific and medical literature) and it returns more than 100'000 different studies for you to mull over! If they truly were safe, why would so many studies have been documented? I love how people ridicule those who do research and call them crazy, yet the internet provides us with an entire database of scientific studies to develop a deep understanding of many subjects regarding your health and the health of those around you. People who ridicule think parents who don't get their children vaccinated are sat watching YouTube videos with a tinfoil hat on. No, there is a lot of *evidence* out there, if you chose to turn off the TV and go and look for yourself. And this is not to bash anyone. If you have ridiculed others in the past for opting out of vaccinating their children, it's okay. I understand the power of the media and the government. But now is your chance to break *free* of that grip and see for yourself. I'm not asking you to blindly believe me, go see for yourself...

Now, please consider that in America alone, $4.3 Billion has been paid out since 1988 via the National Vaccine Injury Compensation Program. This is a program that was established after there were so many lawsuits against vaccine manufacturers and healthcare providers for causing serious injury that it threatened to cause vaccine shortages and reduce vaccination rates, which is obviously bad for business.

The US childhood immunisation schedule requires 26 vaccine doses for infants aged less than one year, which is the most in the world. Yet the US has the highest infant mortality rate of any developed nation. Mississippi has the highest rate of vaccination in the US and the highest infant mortality rate. In a paper published in 2011 in the journal Human & Experimental Toxicology, researchers found that nations that require more vaccine doses tend to have higher infant mortality rates. They found significant differences in nations that required 12-14 doses compared to the US and other nations giving out 21-26.

Now I'm not going to go heavily into the toxic ingredients of vaccines and the thousands of studies that prove they can cause disease, injury and death, but instead, give you a brief overview of the exact dangers of vaccines. However, I have to say the work done by Dr Alan Palmer who has written the book 'The Truth Will Prevail' which cites over *1400* different studies showing the exact dangers of vaccines is as in-depth as anyone would probably want to go! Awesomely he is giving the book away completely for free with no strings attached. The book is fully searchable if you don't want to read the full thing. It is in the Resources section of my website, and I would urge everybody to check it out obviously after finishing *this* book. Now onto some of the ingredients which are all listed by the CDC on their page titled, 'Vaccine Excipient Summary Excipients Included in US Vaccines', which makes for scary reading;

- **Mercury** - In 1996, The US Environmental Protection Agency set a new guideline for methyl mercury in the diet: 0.1 ug (micrograms) of mercury per kilogram of body weight per day. The average vaccine is a 0.5 ml dose which is 25 ug of mercury. The average six-month-old baby weighs around 7.5kg. That is more than *three* times the recommended amount of mercury for a 6-month-old in *one* vaccine. But what about a 2-month-old baby? The Director from the Institute of Vaccine Safety at Johns Hopkins University, Dr Neal Halsey had this to say about the subject, "Exposure to a fixed dose (e.g. 62.5 ug) of mercury at two months of age poses a greater potential risk than the same dose administered at 6 months of age because a child weighs more at 6 months and the target organ, the brain, is more vulnerable early in life."

- **Aluminium** - As vaccine manufacturers have reduced the use of mercury, they have increased the use of aluminium, which many scientists believe may be up to *seven* times more neurotoxic than mercury. According to the CDC's schedule as of 2009 and the product inserts from those vaccines, the average child was receiving nearly 5 mg of aluminium by 18 months of age, The FDA says that anything over .85 mg of aluminium can be dangerous. Do the math yourself.

The average child receives approximately 600% more aluminium from vaccines alone than the FDA deems safe.

The first vaccine children receive in the USA is the hepatitis B, which contains 225 mcg of aluminium and is often given within the baby's first 48 hours of life which is five times the total exposure of orally absorbed aluminium through the next six months. Premature babies have to deal with this load with even lower kidney function and lots more aluminium that comes from the medications (such as IV feeding solutions), given in the newborns intensive care unit.

In an eye-opening paper published in Current Medicinal Chemistry in 2011, researchers state that through experimental research, it's clear that aluminium in vaccines has the potential to induce serious immunological disorders in humans. In particular, aluminium carries a risk for autoimmunity, long-term brain inflammation and associated neurological complications. They conclude that 'In our opinion, the possibility that vaccine benefits may have been overrated and the risk of potential adverse effects underestimated, has not been rigorously evaluated in the medical and scientific community.'

They show the amount of aluminium injected into babies is, in my opinion, simply outrageous! 2-month old children in the UK, US, Canada and Australia routinely receive a burden equivalent to 34 standard adult-dose injections of hepatitis B vaccine.

Newborns at birth receive from a single hepatitis B vaccine, a dose equivalent to 10 standard adult-dose injections of hepatitis B vaccine in a single day.

Whether such doses of aluminium are safe even for adults is not known. Infants and children up to 6 months of age in the US and other developed countries receive 14.7 to 49 times more than the FDA safety limits for aluminium. It's *insane*. Consider that in the 1970s, when autism affected 1 in 10'000 children, babies got only four aluminium-containing vaccines in their first 18 months of life, but now they typically receive *seventeen*.

- **Formaldehyde (Formalin)** - Is a proven carcinogen and according to the Agency for Toxic Substances and Disease Registry, 'Formaldehyde is a colorless, highly toxic, and flammable gas at room temperature. Ingestion of as little as 30 mL (1 oz.) of a solution containing 37% formaldehyde has been reported to cause death in an adult. Ingestion may cause corrosive injury to the gastrointestinal mucosa, with nausea, vomiting, pain, bleeding, and perforation.' Sounds like a good idea to inject it then doesn't it!?

- **Monosodium glutamate (MSG)** - More commonly known as a not so healthy food additive that people generally want to avoid. MSG is notorious for causing headaches in some people and can also cause fatigue, disorientation and heart palpitation. MSG has been called an excitotoxin. According to a paper published in the Journal of Neurobiology, excitotoxicity is when there is a death of the central neurons in the brain, causing brain or spinal cord injury associated with several human disease states.

- **Aborted Human Fetal Tissue** -Yes, you read that right. And no, it's *not* a conspiracy *theory*. It's listed in the CDCs list of ingredients, and the use of tissue from aborted babies has been used for decades in the pharmaceutical industry. According to a paper published in the Journal of Public Health and Epidemiology in 2014, there have been distinct spikes in autism rates in the years when vaccines grown in human fetal cells were introduced. This one above all else, for me at least, has colossal *moral* implications.

- **Phenol (Carbolic Acid)** - According to the Material Safety Data Sheet (MSDS) on Phenol, "passes through the placental barrier. May cause adverse reproductive effects and birth defects (teratogenic)." However, it is an ingredient in the recommended vaccines for pregnant women...

- **Sodium Borate (Borax)** - Sodium Borate is a common ingredient found in rat poison, pesticides, and various commercial applications such as flame retardants, enamel glazes, and laundry detergent. The FDA has outlawed Sodium Borate from use as a food preservative in the US...but not for it to be injected directly into people's bloodstreams.

- **VERO Cells** extracted from the kidney of an African Green Monkey, **human and animal DNA** (one study found mouse DNA, and its origin was not known), plus **human, cow** and **pig**

serum proteins. - A study of 7 vaccines done in Italy in 2018 found as many as five do not conform to the guidelines for the quantity of biological material, DNA or foreign RNA of human or animal origin. Scary indeed! What *is* been injected into you or your child?

- ***Plus*** - A load of other chemicals I didn't cover and many other synthetic ingredients that are not listed on the ingredients list. A 2017 article published in the International Journal of Vaccines and Vaccination revealed a shocking cocktail of non-biocompatible substances in 43 different human vaccines and one veterinary vaccine. Ironically, the veterinarian vaccine checked out to be cleaner than all of the human vaccines! The researchers stated, "all samples checked vaccines contain non-biocompatible and bio-persistent foreign bodies which are not declared by the Producers, against which the body reacts in any case."

In addition to aluminium, which is disclosed in some vaccines, they found it in some vaccines that don't even list it in the ingredients list! Also discovered was lead, stainless steel, tungsten, silicon, gold, silver, nickel, iron, chromium, copper, zirconium, Hafnium, Strontium, Antimony, Platinum, Bismuth, and Cerium. Phew, a few heavy metals there then...

As well as the toxic ingredients we also (again) see financial interests ruling over people's safety. Glaring conflicts of interest were found in a congressional investigation done by the Committee on Government Reform within the House of Representatives into the rotavirus vaccine. The vaccine was approved in 1998 but pulled in 1999 for fears of safety. In the report's findings was that three out of five members of the FDA's Vaccines and Related Biological Products Advisory Committee (VRBPAC) "who voted to approve the rotavirus vaccine in December 1997 had financial ties to pharmaceutical companies that were developing different versions of the vaccine", while four out of eight members of the CDC's Advisory Committee on Immunization Practices (ACIP) "who voted to approve guidelines for the rotavirus vaccine in June 1998 had financial ties to pharmaceutical companies that were developing different versions of the vaccine". My word it gets worse doesn't it? Wherever you turn when following the money, you will see the same faces sat on advisory boards for both private companies and government agencies.

With hundreds of new vaccines constantly in development at least you never need to worry about any upcoming diseases, cancers, or viruses;

"150 people die every year from being hit by falling coconuts. Not to worry, drug makers are developing a vaccine." - Jim Carrey

As mentioned, none of this is an attack on doctors as people; I'm simply reporting the facts and looking at an industry as a whole.

Doctors Are Only Human

Now what I'm *not* saying is that all doctors are bad people. I've Personal Trained doctors who are good honest people. However, I always ask them; "How long did you learn nutrition for at university?" They answer anywhere between zero nutritional training and a maximum of two days. They are doctors of *medicine*. They get taught what drug to give for what problem, or what body part to remove in surgery, and unless they've gone out to self educate on subjects such as what I discuss in this book, then they know nothing of what health really is.

Doctors can be sincere people, but they can be sincerely wrong with what they are recommending.

You've got to ask yourself, why do drugs have so many side effects? Because pharmaceutical drugs are the purest form of acid that people regularly put into their body. And acid causes 90-99% of disease. They are acid-forming in the body because they are *always* synthetic. They are always synthetic because you cannot patent nature. No one has a patent for an almond or an orange. It's the patents that bring about the big bucks. And I mean the BIG bucks.

I've not had a pharmaceutical drug for over ten years. People often ask if I ever take a headache pill? I say no. It's masking a problem. You might get rid of the pain, but the problem is still there. You need to get to the root cause of the problem. Don't treat the symptom. Besides, a lot of headaches are actually caused by dehydration, so when someone takes their headache pill with a large glass of water, what is really curing the headache?

Now I'm not saying to quit taking your prescribed medication. Not without a doctors help anyway. If you feel like you want to get off of your medication and you've been implementing the Action Steps so far in this book, then that is a *real* possibility. Approach your doctor and say, "I'm practising a new healthy lifestyle, I'm eating better, I'm exercising more, and I would like to get off of the medication I'm on."

Their response should be, "Absolutely, that's the plan." If it is not, they refuse or say that you can't because you need it, find a new doctor. Get at least a second and if needed a third opinion. In fact, keep going until you find a doctor that will help you.

It is *your* body and it is *your* health. Take charge of it.

An Alternative Health Plan

So, what can we do other than take pharmaceutical drugs and go on prescription pills? Well, the first and foremost thing for lasting change is to make the lifestyle changes in this book. Step by step, chapter by chapter, make the changes.

If you want something to change, you have to first change something.

This will have the most profound effect on your health in the long term. However, there are different herbs, plants, spices and the like that can have a huge impact on your short term wellbeing and long term health, many that can replace the drugs you are currently turning to. Let's take a look at some alternatives to pharmaceutical drugs that you can use. There are thousands of remedies out there from throughout history and from every corner of the world. Because this book is not purely about natural remedies, I won't be filling the book with all of them. I'm only going to talk about some that have a personal story attached to them, to give you an idea of how powerful Mother Nature can be. Keep an open mind and keep reading beyond this chapter as many more will be presented to you throughout this book. Read every chapter, and you'll have some huge 'Aha!' moments. Many more will be revealed to you that you can use for ailments or diseases that you have.

Alternative Medicine

I have to admit it. I, just this month, as I come to the end of writing this book, took my first pharmaceutical drugs for many, many years. It was something I had to think seriously about. It took me a while to come to my conclusion that yes, it had to be. You see, I was in Manila, Philippines and needed to get to Alaminos City in Pangasinan. A 5-hour drive if there's no traffic. However, if you've ever been to Manila, you'll know that this is an *extremely* rare occurrence. The whole no traffic thing. In fact, I have driven in big cities on almost every continent, from London to Sydney, and Miami to parts of Mexico. As far as traffic goes, Manila beats them all *hands down*. In fact, if you asked me to describe Manila's roads and traffic situation, I'd describe it as being absolutely flipping nuts!

And so why I turned to drugs. The evening before our journey, it seemed that something I'd eaten did not agree with me, and I sat on the toilet a little while. Throughout the night and all the way into the next morning, the situation got no better. And so, I faced driving to Alaminos City with a rather upset tummy. Not too bad, I could pull into each and every service station once I was on the highway if needs be, but that wasn't what concerned me. The *ESDA* did. According to a 2015 survey done by Waze, the ESDA road has the "worst traffic in Southeast Asia". The first time I tackled the ESDA, I travelled 20km in 3 hours. Not only is it extremely slow, but it is also hair raising in the madness that you witness. There are four distinctly marked lanes, which seemed not to be used. At times there were seven lanes of traffic magically created from the cars, buses, motorbikes and even bicycles using the busiest road in one of the most densely populated cities in the world. Never in any other country, have I been able to see the dirt under other drivers' fingernails as he traverses the lanes without a care in the world for his or anyone else safety. Not a place to be stuck for 3 hours if diarrhoea has a grip on you.

And so, the only solution I had beyond crapping my pants or getting arrested while pooping at the side of the road was to take something that was available to me in Manila, a pharmaceutical drug that would clog me up until I arrived in Pangasinan. I took the capsules that were presented to me by the chemist, and I have to say they worked. That is until about 2 hours from the end of what ended up being a 7-hour journey thanks to the EDSA that day; the now-familiar whirling in my stomach started up again. Now, at this point of the journey, we were off of the highway and heading through the province. There wasn't a service station or indeed a toilet of any kind insight. I decided to take one more pill to get me to the end of our journey. And again, it worked. However, it did nothing for the severe stomach ache that had developed. It had treated symptom but not got to the root cause. As I pulled into the house, which was my destination, the lady who is known as Mama (May's mother) noticed I was in some discomfort.

Kardis Leaf - aka Pigeon Pea *(Cajanus cajan)* Tea

A few moments later, she presented me with tea. I asked what it was, and she described it as Kardis, which is known as 'pigeon pea' in other countries. Kardis is a legume that is consumed all across the face of the Earth, especially in India and South Asia. Mama had made a tea out of the leaves for me, claiming it is good for stomach aches and diarrhoea. Within 5 minutes, my stomach ache was gone. I drank the tea again in the morning and had no more diarrhoea or stomach pains. Wow! Where was Mama when I needed her in Manila? This experience showed me again, as I have witnessed many times throughout my life; there are natural alternatives to almost every pharmaceutical drug. In fact, many modern Western medicines are based on herbs, plants and botanicals the world over, but are made synthetic in order for it to be patented.

Ice

Just wanted to throw this one in early to help the minds of any doubters. Ever heard of RICE? Of course, you have. Rest, Ice, Compression and Elevation - taught everywhere to budding First Aiders. Ice (frozen water, not the illegal street drug!) is a *natural alternative* to reduce swelling and inflammation. It is also used to relieve pain.

Calendula *(Calendula officinalis)*

While living in Australia, I had developed some sort of skin growth on my back. Anytime anyone has anything on their skin in Australia; everyone thinks the worse and panics. I was sent packing to the doctors. Reluctantly off I went to see a GP for the first time in years. He looked closely and said it's nothing to worry about, just that one of my hair follicles had an infection. Simple solution, take a course of antibiotics. Simple for some, but not for me! I had put *a lot* of hard work in to reversing the negative effects of the antibiotics (as described later in the book) I had taken years earlier, and as such, I was extremely reluctant to take any. I knew he wouldn't understand, so I thanked him and took his prescription, folded it neatly and tucked it in my pocket, knowing it was never going to be seen by a chemist, I politely said, 'goodbye" went on my merry way.

I headed straight to my friend, who was a naturopath and told her about my plight. She took one look at it and said, "Here, try this cream". It was made from Calendula which she said had some of the same properties as antibiotics. Within seven days, the lump on my back was gone. Phew! Another near-miss with the pharmaceutical industry.

Banaba Leaf *(Lagerstroemia speciosa)* Tea

According to some people in the Philippines, another tree with similar properties to antibiotics is the Banaba Tree. As well as my stomach troubles in the Philippines, I also had to deal with an infected injury. What started as a cut on my big toe turned into a considerable wound that got heavily infected. I wish I'd taken a photo to show you because I genuinely thought I was going to lose my toe. After a clean-up operation using no chemicals or pharmaceutical drugs, that ended with an application of 'Magic Juice' which was a locally made ointment consisting of various plants, I was instructed to drink Banaba Leaf Tea day and night until my toe had recovered. Again, everything turned out fine.

The Banaba Tree is native to the Philippines and Southeast Asia. However, there are leaves of trees and plants in your home country that will have similar effects, ones that I write about in a later chapter (so keep reading, wink, wink). In the Philippines, the Bananba Tree is used to treat diabetes and has been proven to do so successfully. Researchers at the Suzuka University of Medical Science in Japan found a growing body of evidence that Banaba leaf extracts exert antidiabetic and antiobesity effects.

Oregano *(Origanum vulgare)* Tonic

Back to something that is accessible to almost everyone reading this and it's the herb oregano. Buy or even better yet, grow fresh oregano in your garden. Once you have the plant an amazing home remedy that helped me tremendously with fighting infection was an Oregano Tonic made for me daily by Mama. Oregano has been shown to have powerful antibacterial and antivirus effects. As my body was fighting the infection in my big toe, I developed a sore throat and flu-like symptoms, to which Mama did the following;

- She took 9 Oregano leaves and held them individually in BBQ tongs over an open flame on the stove for around 2-3 seconds each side.

- Once all nine leaves were warmed up, she pressed them out using her hands into a small bowl, rinsing them until every last drop of juice was squeezed out.

- She then poured the liquid into a shot glass, which I downed in one.

Again, within 5 minutes, I began to feel better. My sore throat and flu-like symptoms were persistent and hung around for a few days, but every time I had Mama's Oregano Tonic, I felt instantly better for many hours, doing such things as driving long distances and writing this very book. Something that I wouldn't normally be able to do with flu-like symptoms.

Vitamin C

Still not convinced? This is for those who call natural cures bullshit and Alternative Practitioners snake-oil salesmen and quacks. Some people are so adamant that only Medical Doctors can be right, and modern-day science is the only way to go about healthcare that they are blind to the truth all around them. Well, something that cannot be argued is that the treatment for scurvy is Vitamin C. Centuries ago, sailors developed scurvy while travelling over long distances and did so because of a lack of Vitamin C in their diet. In those times, they were not given synthetic Vitamin C tablets that I see in every drugstore and supermarket today, something that will be discussed at length in the very next chapter. They were given fruits and vegetables, which had a high Vitamin C content, like oranges. So then, what's the cure for scurvy?

Saltwater

Most people know of using salt water to heal wounds. And it works, far better than soap and water according to a paper published in 2015 in The New England Journal of Medicine. I used this method twice a day to help heal the wound on my big toe. I also used the ocean as part of my eczema healing journey with massive success. When my wounds were open all over my body, it was incredibly painful, but after 10 minutes of feeling like I was on fire, my skin always felt better. The next day it looked far healthier too.

Many people use the power of the ocean to heal different skin conditions, partly because of the minerals that are naturally found in seawater. There's just something about being in and even just around water (oceans, rivers, lakes) that just feels 'right'. That's no accident as we will discuss a later when you are ready to hear how nature can heal.

Taking Natural Cures To The Next Level

For now, I want to introduce you to a man that when I met him only last year I knew immediately upon meeting him that I wanted him to write me something for my book. My little stories of healing scabby toes and stomach pains don't do natural healing any justice whatsoever when there are far bigger stories out there. Even my very personal story of naturally healing eczema and the journey I went on that inspired me to write this book pales in comparison to the story of Tom Dennis. When I was presenting one of my health seminars I was breaking down the pH Scale as I do, and when it came to talking about Otto Warburg showing the world that cancer cannot live in an alkaline state, I heard a voice say quietly, 'I did it.'

I looked around the room, unsure as to where the voice came from and asked out loud, 'Did what sir?'. The voice came back, 'I cured cancer by getting my body back into an alkaline state.' I was like, *wow!* This has happened to me a few times over the years of presenting, someone stating they healed their body by getting back into an alkaline state, but

I had then never gotten a chance to chat to the person who made the claims. With Tom, however, I did. And boy what a joy it was. As we talked, I learned so much from him, and I asked if he would be comfortable to share his story in my book. He agreed and so, without further ado, I introduce Tom Dennis and his story written in his own words.

My Healing Journey By Tom Dennis

The road to a natural cancer healing for myself began in my childhood. I had several members of my family in the medical professions, so I was always made very aware of the ways of Western allopathic medicine to treat serious chronic disease like cancers or other immune-related diseases. Most of my childhood was spent being treated for minor ailments with Western medicine such as antibiotics, sulpha etc. I had a relatively healthy childhood on a physical level with no broken bones and only one major illness, a serious intestinal blockage at 13. Which in retrospect may have been related to my cancer diagnosis 13 yrs later.

However, I also had the luxury of several close relatives in the arts who had an interest in alternative treatments and cures, especially those listed in the readings of the psychic healer Edgar Cayce. While in college, I also made the acquaintance of a coworker who encouraged me to try a few of Cayce's remedies for my slow thyroid and other simpler ailments which I used with great success. Having grown up in the midwest suburbs, alternative holistic medicine was something only beginning to be distantly heard about in the 1970s but was regularly discussed by my artist relatives when visiting them.

As I matured into adulthood and left the midwest after college for the Pacific Northwest and California, I began to be exposed to magazines and articles, and even radio programs in the late 70s related to natural living, organic whole foods, and alternative treatments for illness and disease. Of particular note was my making friends with a local health food store owner in Alaska in 1979. She wisely fed me not only her newest delicious treats but also numerous magazines and books that I devoured in my downtime.

I went from eating a SAD diet (Standard American Diet) of mostly meat, carbs, and sweets to a mostly vegetarian diet rich in fruit, whole grains and vegetables. I was still eating milk, eggs and occasionally poultry, as well as frequent junk food but I, thought it was okay because it was "natural junk food "...chips, crackers, ice cream, and sweets...the best of alternative snacks. I lost 25 lbs without trying and felt more energized than with my previous diet. But still, something felt off-kilter in my life, and my needs for junk snacks, however, rationalized as "health food" occupied a large part of my diet...especially sweets.

Reality was to set in a year later after a move to Hawaii for work. At first, Hawaii seemed a dream come true with warm, tropical weather, beautiful beaches and welcoming people. But after about three months of long workdays and several hours of bus commuting daily, something seemed wrong. I no longer had unlimited energy like before when I was first eating "healthier"...I began feeling sluggish, bloated, and distracted. I was having trouble making it through the day. Often I wanted to sleep in my off-hours, regardless of how much I had had each night.

Then I noticed blood in my stool. A tiny amount at first...maybe just a haemorrhoid...but then it got heavier and didn't improve over the week. I began to feel seriously concerned. After a visit to a gastrointestinal doctor and some testing, my worst fear was confirmed. I had a tiny but malignant polyp in my colon, that was recommended to be surgically removed along with possibly a portion of my intestinal tract...followed by chemotherapy and radiation. The good news was that it was discovered very early, and the chances of a full recovery were high. I was only 26...(a very rare occurrence in 1980) and time was on my side.

To be truthful, I dropped into a serious depression for a bit, not uncommon with a cancer diagnosis. And so, I decided I wanted a second opinion and that I'd leave Hawaii for the Pacific Northwest where I felt more at home. Besides, I could stay with friends while I figured out my best options. My somewhat depressed state continued despite improving a bit from living with supportive friends, who were terrific to have as I looked at treatment options. I knew what chemo and radiation meant from growing up in a partially medical family. Not an inviting future and that knowledge contributed to my depressed state. Yet I didn't have much awareness of alternative treatments either. I was praying and deeply meditating daily...but for what? A miracle? Something...anything that would heal me without destroying my body in the process. I felt completely discouraged and very desperate.

Then, incredibly, my "miracle" arrived sooner than I could have wished. A month after my arrival in the smaller NW town, by total chance, I wandered into the local library one evening. In their vestibule area, they had a "swap table" of magazines and paperback books people left to be traded. Amazingly on the top of the pile, that evening was a bright yellow covered paperback entitled; "How I Conquered Cancer Naturally".

Every hair on my arm stood up as I looked through the book. It almost seemed like it had been waiting for me. I took the book home and sat up all night reading it. It was a revelation in its simplicity in offering another way to heal a serious cancer. It was easy to read, very straight forward and incredibly inspiring, especially since I had been recently so depressed about treatment options. The author told of similar moments in her healing and especially noted the difficulty she had had with initially using standard treatments that had serious side effects and no assurance of addressing the real cause of her illness.

Yet once she fully committed to a somewhat intense but entirely holistic treatment (involving deep detox cleansing and a mostly raw, vegan diet), she immediately began to feel better and better. She ultimately triumphed in completely healing and felt compelled to share in writing a number of years later. And so, by morning, I was now seeing the first glimmer of light again, feeling that perhaps my prayers had indeed been answered.

But it would take much more than reading. I still needed to commit 100% to the plan outlined in the book. Not an easy task as it was so different from anything I'd heard of, with the program being one I wasn't sure I could handle alone given the need for regular medical testing to ensure that the healing was really happening. And what about finding a medical professional who was competent AND open-minded enough to agree to assist with the then highly unorthodox program? This was a small university town in 1980...not LA or Boston.

I must have had great guardian angels that fall because amazingly only three blocks from my home was a new naturopath who was also a fully trained Medical Doctor. Not only that, but they had also recently completed the exact same detox/raw diet training program in San Diego that the author had undergone as the cornerstone of her healing! Not only could his office offer support through initial cleansing assist (a high colonic cleansing series) but also medical testing and follow-up. Even informal support as he and his wife were also beginning their new raw food lifestyle. How lucky could I be??!

Suffice to say that although my cleansing and then changing my diet to 100% raw vegan overnight was occasionally a challenge, the huge return of energy and mental wellbeing within me kept me both motivated and encouraged. I began not only to feel better than before but better than I had EVER felt. Follow up testing at 3 and 6 months confirmed my hopes that the polyp was shrinking rapidly, and finally had completely disappeared, yet I waited a good two years to resume my fully active life. In the interim, I read and learned much more and collected even more living food recipes and techniques to enhance healing.

I began to exercise and deeply meditate daily; I believe both were an integral part of my full healing. I took a position where I could be of service to others, and that helped heal my spirit as well. I let go of a lot of childhood anger and allowed myself to forgive old grievances. I also gave myself permission to be less than perfect and "cheat" on my new raw diet from time to time (not too much though). Over time, the urge to eat forbidden foods naturally diminished as I discovered new raw treats and foods that tasted wonderfully satisfying in new ways, not missing the old foods much at all.

All this happened over 40 yrs ago. I've been blessed since to have many years of enjoyable, health-filled living. At 66, I take zero prescription medications, but I still start most days with a raw green drink and a handful of wholefood-based supplements and continue to follow my raw vegan diet 99% of the time. I do allow myself a tiny bit of organic raw milk goat or sheep cheese at holidays followed by enzyme caps and lots of tropical fruit to assist digestion. At annual checkups, my doctor marvels at how perfect my blood work numbers are, especially as a senior.

Later tests confirmed that my system still does not create the enzymes necessary to digest heavy proteins, especially animal-based...and most likely hadn't since well before my diagnosis. Hence my colon blockage at 13...which, by the way, was heavily x-rayed at the time. Could both perhaps be leading causes of my illness? Enzyme deficiency leading to toxicity, then heavy irradiation that began cell mutations? And a subsequent immune system dysfunction that allowed my cancer to grow? I'll probably never know exactly which or if it were perhaps a combination of all three.

I'm just glad I was able to find a way to heal through an amazing series of events, just when I needed them, and I'm especially happy to have been able to stay around to enjoy such a blessed, fantastic life!!

Tom Dennis

I hope you all enjoyed hearing Tom's enlightening experiences as much as I did. During our conversation together, Tom recommended three herbal remedies he uses as soon as he feels there is any chance of him getting a viral infection. You know, the usual signs of a cough starting up or a runny nose. He told me to take the following three herbal remedies as soon as I feel any symptoms, and that I'll be highly unlikely to get sick. Since that day, I have, because I definitely needed something! I can tell you that because of the amount of time I spend dealing with the public, on cruise ships, sharing the same air-conditioned air and in between contracts spending *a lot* of time on planes, I am very susceptible to different viral infections. The following three ingredients have been a strong addition to my health regime and have seen that I have not gotten sick in spots that I might have in times gone by.

Antiviral Herbal Remedies

- **Oregano Oil** - One herb that has already made an appearance in this chapter and one that I know will make another appearance later on in another chapter for its antibacterial and antifungal properties is Oregano. Here we see that it has high antiviral properties just as Tom Dennis suggested. Many studies have been done on the effectiveness of oregano fighting disease as it has been used in traditional Chinese medicine for centuries for the treatment of heatstroke, fever, vomiting, acute gastroenteritis, and respiratory disorders. My first experience of Oregano Oil (and way before Mama's Oregano Tonic for flu) was during a Candida Cleanse which I write about in much more detail later in this book. As Tom Dennis mentioned it in our conversation, I was immediately taken back in my mind to my experience of trying to swallow the tiniest amount in a large glass of water. This stuff is so strong that one single drop can easily be tasted in half a litre of water. Absolutely mind-blowing stuff! So, Tom, in all his wisdom, recommends having Oregano Oil *capsules* rather than a tincture as I was attempting! Then you barely taste the stuff. If you can't find the capsules; however, you might need to harden up a little, pinch your nose and simply get it down as fast as you can. This will also help you increase your water intake!

- **Goldenseal (*Hydrastis canadensis*)** - Another popular herbal remedy Goldenseal that is traditionally used to treat skin infections. Researchers at The University of North Carolina Greensboro and the University of Iowa, found that the alkaloid berberine within Goldenseal leaf extracts possesses direct antimicrobial activity which can successfully treat skin infections. Goldenseal has proven to be antibacterial, antifungal and antiviral. Another potent medicine from the plant world, Tom again recommends taking it in capsule form because of its strong taste. But then again, if it's good for you, you'll just have to get it down regardless!

- **Wormwood (*Artemisia*)** - Already seen to save the lives of those at risk of malaria, wormwood is now being studied for a whole host of amazing anti-disease properties. In a paper published in Clinical Infectious Diseases, researchers show Wormwood has activity against malaria, cancer cells, and schistosomiasis. They also see it as having the potential to considerably contribute not only the desperate challenge the world faces in malaria, but to other viruses such as herpes and hepatitis.

And so here again we have three more herbal remedies that have been proven to be effective by science. However, it took science decades to prove what people like Tom and Mama have known for years. Worse than that it is literally *thousands* of years after they were first used regularly in Traditional Eastern Medicine for the exact reasons that science is now proving for which they work! My point here is that science is often built up to be a religion of sorts that cannot be argued against. If you do put forward ideas of plants healing diseases, you are often met with ridicule and shunned by people both in the professional realm and in everyday life. Many a time I am met with comments such as, "Snake oil salesmen used to recommend things like that!" or "Yeah but is it proven by science?".

To which I say; You can wait around for decades for so-called 'modern' science to prove ancient natural remedies really work, and without all the side effects of synthetic drugs. You can do this while watching your health deteriorate. Or instead, right now, trust thousands of years of records and human knowledge and do something good for your health without a doctor, a scientist or a so-called 'knowledgeable, well-read friend' telling you that it's a good idea. Which is a conclusion they *might* come to if they decide to go against everything they think they already know. Meaning going against everything they got taught in medical school, anything they read in (most) science and medical journals, or on scientific and medical websites (which go out to 'debunk' anything natural and not patented for profit). Plus, anything they have discussed with small-minded individuals in the same professions who only believe what they got taught at university or medical school, or what they hear at medical conferences and the like.

What I'm saying is, it's tough for someone to turn round after years of medical school or university and say, "You know what, a lot of what I got taught is bullshit." I've been lucky enough to meet a fair few doctors who had the guts to tell me that. And when someone who is a doctor comes out and tells me that, I know I'm on the right path with my own research. And kudos to those doctors and scientists who go against the mainstream. Those who actually study and say things that aren't going to make them a ton of money. Because plants won't make anywhere near the money synthetic drugs do, as mentioned already in this chapter. And that's the reason it takes decades for 'ancient remedies' to be proven correct in today's day and age. Anyway, rant over.

In the next chapter, I'm going to explore a billion-dollar industry and save some of you loads of money in the process. I will go out to prove how you can dramatically improve your health while lowering your bottom line. Along with that expect big increases in energy and feelings of wellbeing. For now, let's look at the Action Steps needed to turn this chapter from words on a page to a full-force tornado of health and wellbeing...

Resources

Go to **www.TomBroadwell.com/resources** to see;

- A link to Dr Alan Palmers free book 'Truth Will Prevail'.

- A video on how to make Mama's Oregano Tonic with Mama!

Action Steps

- If you are on prescription medicine, approach your doctor and tell them you would like to get off of it. If the answer is no, find a new doctor.

- Stock up on Oregano Oil, Goldenseal and Wormwood - (at the time of writing you could well do with these things with all the 'viruses' going round...)

- Do some research and see if any herbs, leaves or other Eastern medicine ingredients will help you with your health problem.

- Stock up on herbal medicine available in your country that will alleviate simple ailments like belly aches, diarrhoea, headaches etc. If you have a medicine cupboard, start switching out toxic Western medicines for healthier Eastern alternatives. Ask at your local health food store for advice if you are confused.

- However, keep some antibiotics, antibiotic ointment, antihistamines, anti-inflammatories, anti-diarrhoea medication and laxatives aside for a first aid kit in case of emergencies.

Chapter Nine

Supplement*Nation*

*"If you think you don't have time to live a healthy lifestyle and that it costs too much, try living in sickness for a while and then get back to me."— **Tom Broadwell***

Mr Jones walked into the drugstore.

He used a stick as he walked, huddled over from the pain in his joints.

He was at 'that age' when arthritis was common.

His memory had started to desert him too.

He pulled a list out of his jacket pocket and turned to the sales clerk;

"Can you point me in the direction of the calcium, magnesium, one a day multivitamin, glucosamine, vitamin D3, fish oil, zinc and vitamin C please. Doctors' orders."

"Yes sir, start by heading down the seventh aisle, on the right."

Mr Jones joyfully shuffled down the aisle, thinking of all the wonderful benefits he would feel from taking this concoction of vitamins and minerals.

His aches and pains would disappear.

He would now wake up with a spring in his step.

He would rediscover the energy of his 25-year-old self.

The doctor said his immune system would be boosted with his vitamin C, putting a stop to his annual cough and cold.

His brain function might even return to somewhere near its original state.

Exciting times...

Before we get onto the subject of which vitamins and supplements you should be taking, why are they needed at all? Surely if we are sticking to fresh produce, eating all of our vegetables, nuts, seeds and some wild-caught fish, then surely we are getting everything we need from food, right? Wrong.

Everything from the quality of the soil, to farming methods, to how far food travels and stays in storage before we consume it, to the vast amount of pesticides used all play a role in the massive depletion of nutrients in our food today. A study published in the British Food Journal looking at data from 1930 to 1980 found that in 20 vegetables, the average calcium content had declined 19 per cent; iron 22 per cent; and potassium 14 per cent. That was 1980. Things have gotten far worse since then. One study found that we have to eat 8 oranges today to get the same amount of vitamin A as our grandparents did. Yikes! One of the solutions to this is improving the soil quality by using far less (preferably zero) pesticides and switching to more organic farming. This will be discussed at length in the next chapter. Instead of waiting around for the powers that be to wake up to the fact we are screwing up the world that we live on and the quality of the food that comes from it with current farming methods, start to get the nutrients you need in supplement form.

However, most people think all supplements are created equal, and as long as you are putting them into your body, the health benefits will follow. Sorry. Simply not true.

Synthetic Vitamins

Please consider the following fact.

The vitamin industry is dominated by the pharmaceutical industry who supply around 97% of the ingredients used in synthetic vitamins.

I ask many a client. Do pharmaceutical companies profit from healthy people or sick people? After a little pondering, sick people are the answer that always follows. Hmm. So, would they ever supply a supplement that benefits your health? The answer is...No. So why would you take a pill on a daily basis that is created for the most part by the pharmaceutical industry? I explain to them; it is not only not good for you, but it's bad for you. Shocking, again, I know because people are spending their hard-earned money on something because they think it is good for them...

Consider yet more amazing facts. Synthetic vitamin C is simply ascorbic acid, which has little value to the human body, of which more than 80% is produced in China in the most polluted areas of the country. From which only 2% of imported vitamins ever get checked for safety. Another shocking fact is that most of the vitamin E in the US was first found as a byproduct of when Kodak makes camera film. After purification, it gets sold to the supplement industry. Gob smacking.

Under a microscope, a lot of chemists can't see the difference between synthetic vitamins and naturally occurring vitamins in food sources and whole food supplements. It has been proven time and again that the body does not absorb synthetic vitamins in the same way as natural vitamins, which puts a massive strain on the liver causing more problems than not having the vitamin in the first place.

Synthetic vitamins are missing vast amounts of additional ingredients such as minerals and bioflavonoids, that make the naturally occurring vitamin what it is and recognisable to the human body. The process changes the atom structure, which turns synthetic vitamins into yet another toxin that the body has to deal with. And it's not just supplements where you will find these damn awful additions to the ingredients list.

Synthetic Vitamins In Food And Beverages

Look at cereals and beverages such as vitamin waters, and you'll find ingredients such as niacin, thiamine, riboflavin, B6 and folate added. This process is called fortification and the replacement of those lost during making it a heavily processed food is called enrichment. Makes it look like the company has your best interest at heart, doesn't it?

It's not just me who has a problem with it. Lawsuits aplenty over the years have shown that consumers need to read between the lines of clever marketing and which companies that actually have your best interests at heart. In 2015 Coca-Cola Co agreed to change labels on its Vitaminwater beverages admitting it was not as healthy as they'd been advertising. Amongst the changes were that they now had to tell you that you got a nice dose of artificial sweeteners along with your synthetic vitamins and that Vitaminwater did not improve metabolic or immune functions because well, it doesn't! To which I will point out, *natural* vitamins absolutely would improve your immunity. Meaning right here we have a lawsuit admitting synthetic vitamins do not work in the same way natural vitamins do.

And if you're still wolfing down cereal on a morning thinking it's the healthiest option for breakfast you have been falling hook, line, and sinker for some seriously brainwashing marketing ploys that have been going on for decades! The UK and Ireland consume more puffed, flaked and sugared breakfast cereals than anyone else in the world at 6.7kg (14.8 lbs) and 8.4kg (18.5 lbs) per person per year! The UK market alone was worth over £1.27 billion in 2005 and is maintained through very clever advertising. Understand that alongside the synthetic vitamins added for 'your benefit' the large manufacturers have to add synthetic flavourings. This is to make the cereal taste how it's actually meant to taste! All this is added along with a good dose of sugar because the flavour and nutrients are lost during the processing. So, in your 'healthy, fitness, slimming' cereal we have starchy, high glycemic carbohydrates, refined sugar, synthetic vitamins and flavourings, stripped-down table salt and I've not even got started on the pesticides and GMO's yet! We will discuss that at length in the next chapter.

Back to vitamins in supplement form now, and I have a quick question for you. Do you take a multivitamin purchased at a drugstore or supermarket? Now ask yourself; have you ever felt *any* different after taking it? Do you feel more energy, clarity, focus and vitality? The answer in my experience after asking thousands of people in health seminars around the world the same question is a resounding *no*! The following is a table showing all the synthetic counterparts for nutrients. If you see any of these on the label understand it is not doing, you the good you thought it might be.

Table Of Synthetic Vitamins

Nutrient	Synthetic Name
Vitamin A	Acetate Palmitate - if source not given
B1 Thiamine	Thiamine Thiamine Mononitrate Thiamine Hydrochloride
B3 Niacin	Niacin Nicotinic Acid
B5 Pantothenic Acid	Calcium Pantothenate d-Pantothenate Panthenol
B6 Pyridoxine	Pyridoxine Hydrochloride
B9 Folic Acid	Folic Acid Pteroylglutamic Acid
B12	Cyanocobalamin
Vitamin C	Ascorbic Acid - if source not given
Vitamin D	D2 Ergosteral (Bad Yeast) Calciferol
Vitamin E	dl-Alpha Tocoperoldl-Beta Tocoperoldl-Delta Tocoperoldl-Gamma Tocopherol
Vitamin K	Menadione
Choline	Choline Chloride Choline Bitartrate
Biotin	d-Biotin

Other Ingredients

We then have to look at *what else* is in most supplements on the market today. When you're reading a label on a supplement, understand the company will always list the good stuff at the top. Usually in a panel titled 'Supplement Facts' or 'Nutrition Facts' depending on where you come from in the world. Here you can see the Daily Values of vitamins and how much the amazing product you are buying supersedes all the values by far! Usually, the Vitamin C will amount to 4000% of your Daily Value, making most people think they're going have a superhero immunity. However, it's the synthetic vitamins pumping up the numbers which are really just toxic mess made in a factory somewhere. This labelling system, by the way, is a directive of the very caring FDA... ahem.

Something else you need to understand is that seemingly 'natural' brands will have what looks like great ingredients listed there. You'll find all sorts of exotic fruits and superfoods that are making the headlines that year, but now take a glance down to somewhere below that grid, and you'll find the Other Ingredients. This is where you'll find all the nonactive ingredients. It is something people rarely look at unless someone tells you to do so. I've had many clients who are buying organic food, who don't eat sugar, wheat or dairy. People who seem truthfully clued in with what is going in their body, and then they bring me their 'healthy, high quality, natural' supplements to take a look at. I point out the Other Ingredients to them, and it's full of fillers, binders, colourings, preservatives and the like. Shocked is a word I'd use to describe their reaction when they see what is in their 'expensive', 'premium' supplements from doctors they trust or companies with the word 'natural' or 'organic' in their brand name. Some of the following ingredients can appear in food too, so take this as a 101 in reading labels for all edible products. Below are some added major ingredients I would avoid like the plague, but please note there are many, many more which again I can't fill the book up with. So as always, do some of your own research beyond this brief overview:

- **Artificial Food Colourings**: Used to make the supplements look pretty. As if the colour of a pill that goes down in one, is of any concern to most people who are spending their hard-earned money to become...healthier? They can be used if active ingredients in the vitamin have been degraded by exposure to light, air, moisture, heat, or poor storage conditions, which makes it even worse when you think about it! Artificial dyes are derived from *petroleum* and are found in thousands of foods such as breakfast cereals, candies, beverages, snack foods, baked goods, frozen desserts, condiments, and even pickles, salad dressings and loads of other products mainly aimed at children.

You might be shocked to find some *fresh* oranges have colour added to both brighten them up and uniform their colour!

The Center for Science in the Public Interest wants them banned by the FDA. Their report, *Food Dyes: A Rainbow of Risks*, further concludes that the nine artificial dyes approved in the United States likely are carcinogenic. They also cause hypersensitivity reactions, ADHD and behavioural problems, or are *inadequately tested*. There are more natural ways to make food have brighter colours. In 2008, a ruling was passed banning the use of the specific food colours in the UK, and so manufacturers turned back to using *plant-based* colourings. As reported in a 2010 paper published in the journal Environmental Health Perspectives for example, in the United Kingdom, Fanta orange soda is coloured with pumpkin and carrot extracts while the US version uses Red 40 and Yellow 6. McDonald's strawberry sundaes are coloured only with strawberries in the UK, but Red 40 is used in the United States. If you are wondering why your little ones are going hyperactive crazy after eating candy, take a look at the ingredients list. If containing any of the following artificial dyes, now you know why: Food dye consumption per person has increased fivefold in the United States since 1955, with three dyes—Red 40, Yellow 5, and Yellow 6—accounting for 90% of the dyes used in foods. Also keep your eyes peeled for Blue 1, Blue 2, Citrus Red 2, Green 3, Orange B, and Red 3.

- **Hydrogenated Oils**: Here you are thinking you're avoiding trans fats since Chapter 5: You Are What You Eat...and then they turn up in your supplements! Usually in the form of partially hydrogenated soybean and corn oil which are both pretty much always a Genetically Modified Organism, the scary-ass dangers of which we will cover in the very next chapter!

- **Artificial Sweeteners**: Already covered in Chapter 5: You Are What You Eat...but just know they are in many, many supplements. Why? Because most people only look for information like the sugar content, and they don't think about why it still tastes sweet...or they simply don't care. But it still tastes sweet because of the use of these heavily toxic, fatally sweet, zero calorie abominations.

- **Magnesium Silicate or Talc**: Again, used to make supplements and food a pretty white colour for reasons that will never be clear to me. Yes, I know people shop with their eyes, but is it worth the health risks for the consumer, if they are buying products to be...more healthy? You may recognise talc as it has been used as a hygiene product by ladies and for their babies for more than 125 years! You might also recognise it because of the many lawsuits around it potentially causing women ovarian cancer and major health issues to their babies. As per a study done by the World Health Organization International Agency for Research on Cancer; 'Perineal use of talc-based body powder is possibly carcinogenic to humans.' So, something that could possibly cause cancer to humans when we apply it externally is in our food and supplements to be taken orally, wow, just wow! Even more gobsmacking is that to this day, talc products can be tainted with asbestos. That sounds tasty! And it is one of the possible reasons why it may cause cancer.

- **Silicon Dioxide**: Do you know the excitement when you open a new wallet, purse or pair of shoes and you get a whiff of fresh leather, and then you have to remove that little white packet in there. The packet that says, 'Do Not Eat'. Yeah, that one. That's silicon dioxide. So, if we can't eat it when it's in our new wallet, why should we be ingesting it when it's in our supplements? Or our foods like flour, baking powder, sugar and salt. Apparently, it stops all the powder sticking together, which is great, but I've had many an organic supplement in powder form and also alternative grain flours that don't have it in. So, there must be another, healthier way, and so now you as a newly educated consumer can avoid which may be sold to you as unavoidable...

- **Titanium Dioxide**: Another little wonder that allows our supplements to be a fantastic white. Not so fantastic when you consider it's shown to cause lung damage and researchers at the Southeast University, in Nanjing, China showed it could cause marginal damage to your DNA. Ohh not a problem, I'd take some

DNA damage to potentially (probably not) feel better with my supplements...

So, what are you saying Tom? You've already told me food quality is crap, so I need to supplement. Now you're saying I can't take my one-a-day? What the hell do you want me to do? Okay, calm down, calm down. It's all good, I've got you covered. When don't I? Don't answer that. It might cause me stress...

Whole Food Supplements

Listen, it's just as easy as that one-a-day and all the other pills you are popping. There are vitamins from natural, whole food sources readily available which are actually good for you. I suggest taking at the very least the following supplements and then using the information in this chapter to decide if anything else you need or desire to take is good for you or not. Basically, learn to read the labels of everything you buy and not just trust it will be good for you!

Whole Food Vitamins And Alkalising Greens

These can come in in different forms, I prefer either a liquid form you shoot down each morning or a powder that you can add to your morning juice or smoothie. You can get one or the other, or if your budget allows both. The basic rule is, it has to say; 'from whole food sources' on it, for you to know it's actually from the good stuff like vegetables, herbs, spices, grasses and the like. I also prefer it to be raw and organic. This is where your budget will come into play (and to be honest it is where you *choose* to spend your money because most people could afford the monthly outlay of 50-100 dollars it costs to get the good stuff by giving up one or two things that are not so good for the body...just sayin').

They are proven to make your body more alkaline too. In a study done at Florida University, 'To examine the effects of a green alkalizing dietary supplement on urinary pH levels in individuals with lower than average pH levels'. The dietary supplement contained certified organic ingredients such as whole food vegetables, fibre, algae, and fermented cereal grasses. To give you an idea of what to look for it included, kale powder, broccoli powder, spinach powder, carrot powder, parsley powder, dulse, chia seed powder, inulin powder, sea algae, organic spirulina, barley grass, wheatgrass, oat grass, and alfalfa grass. Phew!

The results were as per the researchers, 'Compared to baseline, mean urine pH levels in all volunteers were significantly higher following the supplementation' (after only three days), 'Participants pH levels were also significantly higher than baseline on days 5, 6, and 7 of the treatment period. Noteworthy, on day 7, participants' mean pH levels were significantly higher than at the beginning of the treatment period.' This was done using urine tests which as mentioned are not as accurate as testing blood, but it is still well worth taking into consideration, especially since all the ingredients come up as alkaline when tested in blood.

Fish Oil And Flaxseed Oil

What are other supplements worth taking I hear you ask? Well, I'm glad you asked. Going back thousands of years, the ratio of omega 6 to omega 3 was 1:1. Fast forward to now, and it's 20:1. Omega 6 comes from sources such as red meat while omega 3 comes from fish. The number of meat products we eat has gone up dramatically. The massive difference in the ratio has been linked to obesity and many health issues. Autoimmune illnesses like asthma and eczema are heavily contributed to by these dietary changes.

As such, supplementing with a good quality fish oil (or flaxseed if you are vegetarian or vegan) is essential for your health to bring that ratio back into balance. If you were in need of further convincing omega 3 has shown to be good for your heart, brain, eyes, nervous system, joints, skin, hair, and nails, to name just a few...However, yet again we must be careful because where you source your supplements from is crucial. For example, when choosing fish oil, you have to take into account the cleanliness of the water, because in some parts of the world, you risk poisoning from mercury and other nasties. Great stuff! So, look for pure fish oil from the Arctic Circle where there's not so much pollution. Don't buy the cheap stuff; it'll do more damage than good.

Prebiotics, Probiotics And Digestive Enzymes

For gut health, these are all essential, as we've already seen and as we'll soon learn in even more depth, good gut health is critical for overall health. I personally think any supplements are best used after a good cleanse, especially anything for the gut. However, as we have yet to cover cleansing then give them a shot now and see how you feel. They might just work for you right now.

The great news is there top quality products available in health food stores now that have all three of these in one convenient supplement. The reason these are so important is that if you've ever done a course of antibiotics, then it might well have killed the bad stuff, but also all the good bacteria in your gut. Once this essential bacteria is lowered, a yeast known as candida slowly starts to take over. Candida yeast overgrowth has been linked to almost every disease in Eastern medicine, but Western medicine pretty much ignores it...go figure.

These digestive aids will help with the breaking down of food, which of course feeds your body with more nutrients and more energy and helps to get your gut balance back into a healthy ratio. However, as mentioned, a candida cleanse will be essential to getting your digestive health truly back on track. That's going to be discussed later as it's probably the most hardcore thing you'll attempt in this book and so needs some mental preparation before we go there. Exciting times indeed. No?

Raw Organic Vegan Protein Powder

Now this one is not particularly essential unless you have smoothies or juices for breakfast or you are smashing out the workouts over at TomBroadwell.com, and you needed a little extra muscle recovery and repair. ;) The reason I say this about smoothies and juices is that they are mainly carbohydrates, especially if you have any fruit in there. Which means they will spike your insulin levels and end up making you fat, which is not what we want if we want to look better naked. The protein will slow down that insulin response we mentioned in Chapter 5: You Are What You Eat...

Why do I want you to fork out for Raw Organic Vegan Protein Powder? It all comes back to the pH Scale and gut health. You can buy huge tubs of Whey Protein for next to nothing, but that doesn't mean it's either good for you or giving you the amount of protein, it says on the container. The process of making cheap protein powders kills almost all of the nutrients before it even goes in your mouth. And so because your body doesn't recognise it as natural or whole, absorption is much lower.

Besides that, most of the supplements in the Fitness Industry use artificial sweeteners to lower sugar content, which of course if you've made it this far into the book you know they should be avoided at all costs. Even if you find a more natural product, Whey Protein is dairy which is acid-forming in the body. Then if you want to know how good (or not so good) it is for your gut health, simply go take a deep breath in through your nose in the weights area of any large gym. After a while, you'll think some of the members have had a small creature crawl in their ass and die. You'll hear whispers of 'protein fart' because digestive issues are such well-known side effects of whey protein it has developed its own nickname!

Raw Calcium

A lot of older people take calcium on doctors' orders because they are concerned about health issues such as osteoporosis. And while this has merit, there is little point in a.) taking calcium if your body is constantly flooded with acid-forming foods and drinks. It will not go to patch up damage already caused in your bones and increase bone density; it will instead be used in the fight against the acid. Therefore, make sure your food intake is mainly alkaline, remembering this is only a supplement (to good nutrition) And b.) taking calcium recommended by most doctors which is nothing more than chalk which you would write on a blackboard with and often contains heavy metals such as lead.

There are fantastic alternatives out there that are pure, raw calcium made from things in the sea, which will hold far more health benefits than chalk. The better companies will also include the other natural ingredients that are needed for maximal absorption, such as naturally sourced Vitamin D and magnesium.

Individual Vitamins And Supplements

As you go along your health journey, you might be recommended individual vitamins by your doctor or other healthcare practitioners which I would never go against if they have a good reason for it. However, at the risk of repeating myself, do not take the *synthetic* version of any vitamin. There is always a natural alternative available. And whereas the synthetic version will be seen as a toxin by your body, along with its many fillers and binders, the natural one will work far better and do what it is supposed to do. Of course, there are better natural vitamins available compared to other brands, and you can find the brand I currently recommend in the Resources section.

At this point, even if we have given up the processed foods and turned to a mainly fresh produce diet, full of vegetables, herbs, nuts, seeds and some meat and fish, there is still more to consider if you truly want optimal health. In the next chapter, we are going to explore the world of organic, as we ask ourselves the question; is it really worth it? Before that, let's take some potentially painful Action Steps and make our supplements worth the money we are currently spending on them.

Resources

Go to **www.TomBroadwell.com/resources** to see;

- The current brands of supplements and vitamins I recommend and use.

Action Steps

- This might be an expensive and painful thing to do but throw your synthetic supplements in the trash (or you could always give them to someone you don't like).

- Master reading labels and knowing which brands are being honest with you and then change over to using the best brands straight away.

Chapter Ten

Grown By Nature

"Essentially, all life depends upon the soil... There can be no life without soil and no soil without life; they have evolved together."– Dr Charles E Kellogg

The journalist for the local school newspaper walked through the farm and thought it represented some sort of colossal factory more than a farm.

He was writing a piece that had simply started as reporting on the life of a dairy cow in America.

He initially thought he might be walking through green fields, something like out of Little House on the Prairie.

Oh, how wrong he could be...

He was back after three months to check up on the dairy cow he had named Daisy.

The smell was sickening as he looked around at the rotting carcasses being fed to the cows.

He heard the cries from the mothers as their newly born calves were taken away.

The mothers seemed more stressed than he could possibly imagine a cow could be.

He thought back to nature programs he had seen, where mothers of all the animal kingdom fiercely defended their young, sometimes carrying a dead baby around with them for days in some sort of grieving process.

Of course, a mother cared...

The steak he ate last night suddenly had a whole different back story to it.

The hugely obese cows seemed to have grown at an obscene rate since his last visit, something that only the bovine growth hormones would be capable of.

The carcasses that were currently being fed to the cows were cats and dogs killed by euthanasia in pet homes, best not go to waste, let's feed them to the herbivore cattle.

He looked at the mountains of grain that the cattle were also feeding on, asking himself if a digestive system designed only for grass could handle it?

He then noticed Daisy had not moved; she was in the same pen as three months ago.

"Wow", he wondered aloud, no exercise, no sunlight, and force-fed massive amounts of food it was never meant to eat.

Steroids, growth hormones, unworldly amounts of stress, and not to mention the enormous amount of antibiotics it was consuming because of its poor health...

...All going into the meat and the dairy that we consume...

No wonder his classmates were looking more like men and women than the teenagers they were meant to be.

He wondered why he didn't choose the local organic farm now, at least there the cows walked around in a field eating grass without the steroids and growth hormones...

What I have just described is not a story; it is the reality to differing degrees depending on the country you live in, in the Western world.

Animal Products

A fact that see's chickens grown at up to 65x faster than they would naturally. A world that has seen the demand for fast (literally) food implement a whole new methodology on the way that animals are farmed. A whole new world that now more resembles that of a Frankenstein horror movie than it does real life.

And it really is horrifying if you take the time to look at how the nonorganic meat you eat ends up on your plate. Chickens, for example, regularly die from heart failure due to their still baby hearts not being able to deal with their adult bodies. At least 12.5 billion chickens per year suffer from serious leg problems, bucking under the gross weight from genetically manipulated growth. Ammonia burn and respiratory fatalities are commonplace from the build-up of faeces in the large shed housing thousands of birds that are usually cleaned only every 2-4 *years*. Laws state that chickens must have enough space, which ends up each chicken having the same space as a piece of A4 paper when they are fully grown.

Their journey to the slaughterhouse is brutal, to say the least, with them roughly being shoved into cages by human hand or vacuumed up by a 6-ton machine that can capture and then automatically blow up to 7000 birds an hour into crates. This process will see millions of birds a year die before even reaching the slaughterhouse. If they live, many will suffer from broken wings and legs, haemorrhages, lacerations and dehydration. They will stay in cages for hours at a time without food or water. Chickens deemed too sick or injured to be sold as food will get thrown away like trash, sometimes into mass graves while still alive. For the animals that make the grade, it has been shown that animals do have feelings and have a complete sense of knowing what will happen to them.

"They try everything in their power to get away from the killing machine and to get away from you. They have been stunned, so their muscles don't work, but their eyes do, and you can tell by them looking at you, they're scared to death."
– Virgil Butler *(former slaughterhouse worker)*

Now I'm not saying the organic industry is all butterflies, rainbows and unicorns. It's not perfect, and the animals still die a painful death. I'm not saying go vegan either, but if you truly want *perfect* health, then the evidence points that way. However, this book is not about being perfect all the time and taking away all of life's pleasures, because at the end of the day what would be the point in having perfect health but not being happy? And if you're not happy, are you healthy anyway?

If being vegan makes you happy, then go for it. If you still want to eat meat, then go organic as much as possible. Why? It is healthier, it tastes better (most of the time) and the animals have a far better standard of living while they are alive. To become certified as organic as per the California Certified Organic Farmers website; 'organic meat, poultry, eggs, and dairy products come from animals fed 100% organic feed and forage, given no antibiotics or growth hormones, and raised in conditions that follow their natural behaviors.'

As well as chicken, beef and the other farm animals too, you have to consider only ever eating wild-caught fish. You may have noticed in the Acid vs Alkaline Food table in Chapter 7: The perfectHealth Scale that wild-caught fish was way out on its own as the best form of animal protein. Fish, in general, is easier to digest than other meats and contains more beneficial nutrients such as the inflammation lowering omega-3 fatty acids. One of the main reasons that wild-caught is better is because farmed fish has a far higher content of inflammation producing omega-6 fatty acid. Beyond that, we've got to talk about the contaminants found in farmed fish. In 2004 researchers at Indiana University determined that PCB concentrations in farmed salmon were *eight times* higher than that found in wild salmon. PCBs and the effects on human health will be discussed at great length in an upcoming chapter, but just know that they have been strongly linked to cancer and many other health issues, and that eight times the amount is massive. So much so that if the EPA guidelines were applied to farmed salmon, people would be encouraged to restrict salmon consumption to no more than once per *month*.

For evidence of what the hormones in farmed meats, in general, are doing to us as human beings, you simply have to look at the average age of children hitting puberty versus when even I was growing up. Looking at statistics provided by German researchers, who found that in 1860 (before the synthetic chemical age we are now in), the average age of the onset of puberty in girls was 16.6 years. In 1920 the use of synthetic chemicals was in its infancy, but it had already dropped to 14.6 years. By 1950, it was down to 13.1 years. By 1980, it had fallen to 12.5 years; and in 2010, shockingly it was down 10.5 years. Similar sets of figures have been reported for boys, with a small delay of around a year. The real trouble is the decline was expected to stop, but it has continued at the same constant rate of a decline of 4-5 months in age for each passing decade.

Who knows where we will be in 50 years? Well, to be honest, there's mountains of evidence already presenting itself. In the medical journal Pediatrics it was reported that in a study of 17'000 girls, by eight-years-old, one in seven white girls and one out of every two African-American girls had already started puberty. However, that is not the most shocking finding, as 1 in 100 white girls and 3 out of every 100 African-American girls had already started puberty at the age of 3 years old! The main reason was thought to be their *diet*. I will present evidence later in the book that it's not just down to hormones in the meat we are eating, but other synthetic chemicals that are used in everyday modern life (but don't have to be).

As well as the health benefits for you and your family, when eating organic, you are not funding huge corporations that demand meat and dairy at a far quicker rate than what is possible to do naturally. Corporations such as massive supermarket chains and fast-food restaurants. For me to fund and empower small farms and local businesses (such as health food stores and local grocers), means I am doing some good in the world, and I am voting for what I want and believe in with my money.

Fruits And Vegetables

What about fruits, vegetables, nuts and seeds I hear you ask. Is there a difference? Well put it this way;

If I was to pick an organic apple from a tree, then spray it with insecticide in front of your face, would you eat the apple?

When I put this question forth in my health seminars presented to thousands of people across the world, I've only had someone answer, "Yes" three times. In my opinion, that person when questioned by me sounds a little bit uninformed, but of course, that is only my opinion. One lady said it's designed only to kill small bugs and not humans. Okay, but taken on in a huge dose all at one time it would kill you too or at the very least make you incredibly sick. So, if in a higher dose it causes an acute reaction right now, then a little bit at a time over the course of years will surely increase the chance of you developing a chronic disease at some point in the future.

I often hear; "How do you know it's organic? It's got chemicals on it too." I agree that in today's modern world, it's difficult for anything to be truly organic. Most crops will have some form of contamination from either pesticide being blown in the wind from neighbouring nonorganic fields or having pesticides being present in the soil from previous crops being planted there.

However, looking again at what it means to be certified organic on the California Certified Organic Farmers website; 'The use of sewage sludge, bioengineering (GMOs), ionizing radiation, and most synthetic pesticides and fertilizers is prohibited from organic production. Certified organic produce is grown on soil that has been free of prohibited substances for three years prior to harvest to ensure that the crops will not be contaminated. Focused on the use of renewable resources and conservation of soil and water, organic farmers enhance and sustain the environment for future generations.'

That's one reason I'd never buy nonorganic carrots. They have shown a tremendous ability to soak up pesticide residue from the soil, and so are used to do so by nonorganic farmers. In one study done by The University of Wisconsin, one variety of carrot soaked up to 80% of the pesticide residue that was found in the soil! And so even with possible contamination in organic fruits, vegetables and crops, when grown in organic conditions, the amount of pesticide is always going to be *far* less. The fact also remains that time and again organic food has far higher nutritional content too.

A summary of a large number of studies done at The University of Otago in New Zealand found this to be true when comparing the nutritional value of organically and conventionally grown food as purchased from retailers. One study found that organic green beans, beetroots, peppers and tomatoes had a considerably higher mineral content. Another study of apples, pears, potatoes, wheat and sweetcorn showed significantly higher levels of some minerals in all the organic varieties. A third study showed higher levels of all minerals in biodynamic (a form of alternative agriculture very similar to organic farming) cauliflower, red radish, celery, carrots and lettuce versus the conventionally grown vegetables. I could go on, but you hopefully get my point!

GMOs

This is another area of great concern for many, regarding the health of humanity and the environment. Someone somewhere decided they wanted to play God and started changing plants and animals from their natural state by introducing genes from other species into their genomes. Firstly, you have to be somewhat worried as an American because somewhere between 60 to 70 per cent of processed foods in grocery stores contain at least some genetically modified ingredients. The majority of GMO crops are grown in just five countries around the world, the United States, Argentina, Brazil, Canada, and India, with most countries around the world outlawing it. Which has to tell you something about its safety.

Everywhere you look, science papers say many more years of testing needs to be done to really see how significant the effects on human health could be. That means once again. You are the chemistry test. Scary stuff indeed. In 2009 researchers at the University of Athens, Medical School, Greece found that the results of most studies with GM foods indicate that they may cause some common toxic effects on the liver, kidneys, pancreas and reproductive organs. They go on to state, 'However, many years of research with animals and clinical trials are required for this assessment.' Yikes. In something that doesn't need any further testing is the fact that in March 2015, the World Health Organization (WHO) classified Glycerophosphate as carcinogenic. Glycerophosphate is a toxin that is greatly used in GMO foods and has been linked to many illnesses such as Parkinson's disease and Alzheimer's.

The major problem with GMO is that there is a massive amount of money behind it. Virtually every major food corporation is behind the movement, and with that amount of money, they can be very persuasive to an unsuspecting public using every marketing trick in the book. One of the angles is that GMO is meant to 'feed the world'. However, we have two *major* problems with that. Studies show that organic farming without the need for both GMOs or pesticides can accomplish far greater results. For example, in one of the *largest-ever* studies of commercial rice growing, researchers found that thousands of Chinese farmers using organic farming techniques saw yield increases of 89% while completely eliminating some of their most common pesticides.

In one of the most perversely sick discoveries, it was found that biotech companies unleashing GMO crops on the world, sometimes in the poorest nations such as India, have dozens of patents for 'terminator genes' which make the crops sterile after the first harvest. It was created to ensure farmers can not reuse the seeds, and so we now have over 1.5 billion people lives who rely on this as their food source who could go hungry all for the sake of profit—farmers who if they stick to their roots, and natural methods of farming would do absolutely fine. Talk about 'feed the world', more like 'line my pockets'.

Packaged Foods

Not only fresh food, but when it comes to packaged foods such as cereals, bread, pasta, chocolate, and cookies buy *organic*. You are then avoiding many of the harsher chemicals that are in their mass-manufactured counterparts. Which means you are avoiding many of the additives that make you *addicted* to the foods we need to be cutting down on.

I'll often hear people saying; "If I live for 10-15 years longer but can't have chocolate or eat cookies, then I'd rather die young and enjoy life." Of which I say; "You *can* have those things, and you know what, they even taste better!" To which I add that eating sugar in any form is not good for you and will add on the pounds if you eat enough of it, but 'Raw Organic Cane Sugar' is far better than 'White Refined Sugar' you'd find in all foods produced by large food manufacturers.

Cost

So, the choice is yours. Invest now in your health and your future, or spend time and money being sick and on medication. A story I often tell in seminars is when I arrived to live in Australia; I had zero clients. I had to slowly build my business from the ground up, one client at a time. I did this rather quickly and had a decent income by the end of my first year, doing around 50-70 sessions per week. Building that up to around 100 sessions per week.

Why I am I telling you this? I didn't own a car while I lived there and for the most part, the reason was simple, I couldn't afford to even when earning a lot of money. Why? Because I invested so much money into my health. I had regular chiropractic sessions to make sure my nervous system was running smoothly, acupuncture to control my skin condition and a monthly sports massage to keep my body mobile and injury-free. There's much more on these therapies and what they can do for you, written by the experts themselves in the next chapter. So, you'll get a break from me for a while, which will be nice!

Another example of this is in my apartment; I lived a purely organic lifestyle. Everything from the food I ate, to the sheets I slept on, to the cleaning products in my bathroom. I was even a member of an organic winery in The Hunter Valley wine region. I drank far too much wine, but that's beside the point! And don't worry, there's a lot more to come on why I was laying on organic sheets, cleaning with natural products and drinking too much wine later in the book!

The point is this. Where are you choosing to invest your money?

Most people can afford to eat organic; they just *choose* not to. They *choose* to drive a nice car rather than eat organic food.

They choose to wear expensive jewellery rather than to spend money on organic sheets. They choose to eat in fancy but nonorganic restaurants when they could actually save money and cook organic food at home.

So, the choice *really* is yours. For now, take the following Action Steps and start feeling the benefits to your health, the increase in your energy levels and the taste sensation that organic food brings!

Action Steps

- Go online and search for local farms or companies that deliver organic food to your door in your area. This is a surefire way to guarantee what you buy is both organic and local, and an awesome way to support small businesses. Search for organic farmers markets in your area, which is another way to support local businesses.

- Search for organic health food stores or independently owned organic supermarkets in your area.

- Search for organic butchers, bakers, and greengrocers in your local area - meaning; shop local to support these small business owners. Yes, it might be more expensive than the supermarket, but wouldn't you rather give your hard-earned cash to a small business owner than a multibillionaire who pays their staff a pittance?... Do something good in the world and start voting with your money.

- Search for organic cafes and restaurants in your local area, and anytime you travel, search them out and eat there too.

- If struggling for money, start by replacing long-lasting food items first. Buy organic herbs, spices and condiments. It's often not much more expensive and will last a while, meaning the extra cost is spread over a longer time.

- Only buy organic canned food from here on out. Kidney beans and chickpeas, for example, are usually less than a dollar more expensive than the nonorganic variety but come without the harsh preservatives, colourings and additives.

- Buy organic packaged foods such as cereal, health food bars and chocolate. Try different brands and find one you like. If anything, at least you'll be lowering the amount of refined sugar you're consuming, as organic varieties will only use raw sugar which is better for you.

- As soon as you realise that you'll either pay now or pay later (with your health and medical bills) start buying organic meat, fruits and vegetables.

Chapter Eleven
Alternative Therapies
"Medicine's a funny business. After all, dispensing chemicals is considered mainstream and diet and nutrition is considered alternative."– **Charles F. Glassman**

The disgruntled young man would not be deterred,

He had ripped up the piece of paper that the dermatologist had given him,

It was the prescription of which was as promised by his GP,

Just stronger steroid tablets and steroid cream.

Surely there must be something else he thought to himself,

His eczema had gotten to such a bad state and was so painful at times he wished he was dead rather than alive,

And now this,

Another stumbling block,

No doctor with any information other than to hand out a stronger form of the medicine which had done very little for him over the last year when his skin had become terribly painful.

Fast forward almost another year and there in Cozumel, Mexico he was trying an Alternative Therapy he had read all about,

He had originally booked in for a Chiropractic session understanding the relationship between his nervous system being aligned and the condition of his skin,

But then after the treatment, the chiropractor surprised him by asking him to sit at the end of the bench with his eyes closed,

The young man did as asked and sat quietly for what seemed like an age, which turned out to be only ten minutes,

Then the chiropractor asked;

"Did you feel that?"

The young man's entire body went ice cold,

In the heat of the Mexican summer,

In an office that had him sweating profusely with no air conditioning and no windows, this seemed impossible,

"Yes, I'm freezing!"

"That's what happens when we harness the power of the Universe I guess", was the response.

"Well, what happened, what did you do?"

"I used Reiki, a form of energy healing. I imagined showering you with a waterfall of aloe vera. It seems to have worked. I'm just studying it at the moment, but it really is an incredibly powerful form of healing. I suggest carrying on with someone at home."

Wow, this had just opened up a whole new world...

There are so many opinions around Alternative Therapies that it has all pretty much become like assholes. Everyone has one. I urge you, and I mean it, try it for yourself. Don't let other people's opinions sway you from something that might be good for your health, heal your body or help you lose weight because of their bad personal experience. You *have* to choose a therapist that is great at what they do, and I'll teach you how to spot them, and then it could change your life. The good ones will literally blow your mind. You will be left wondering; "How the hell did they know that!?!" or "Oh my, I feel fantastic, I feel so freaking amazing right now!" or "They literally just described everything that was wrong with me, and I didn't even tell them a single thing!'

The example in the story above is a true story and the young gentleman (I was one once upon a time!) was me. I even use exact words that were said in the chiropractor's office, because although it was more than 12 years ago my first experience of Reiki was so mind-blowing, I still remember it like it was yesterday. However, I'm not going to start with Reiki because for most people it will be the hardest to get your head around and therefore the hardest to believe, and if you don't believe, *nothing* will work. So, to start let's look at the most well-known in my opinion and then work our way down:

Massage Therapy As Described By **May Estrada**

I first met May Estrada in 2017 while working on a cruise ship. For me, it was love at first sight! Not only that, but she is an excellent Massage Therapist. You can book in and see her in our upcoming beach and forest spa retreat (or already up and running retreat, depending on when you are reading this!). You will learn more about this in the very next chapter. Here in her own words, she is going to describe the benefits of massage, and what a regular massage can do for you;

Massage therapy can help the body in *many* ways. It can help to relax your muscles and decrease any nerve compression that happens when muscles are overused, tight, or full of lactic acid. A good massage will increase the range of motion of your joints and reduce pain.

Massage is a fantastic stress reliever which in itself is terrific for your health. It will also help to improve your blood circulation and lymphatic flow, which will enhance the delivery of oxygen and nutrients to the muscle cells and help to remove waste products. In fact, *every* cell in the body will benefit from better circulation and improved lymphatic drainage.

From my personal experience of working in massage over the last seven years, I have seen some amazing things. One story I would like to share with you to show you the power of massage is this; I once had a guest while working on cruise ships which had a frozen shoulder. His was shoulder was so immobile he couldn't even put his shirt on alone; his wife needed to help him get dressed. His shoulder had been bothering him for a couple of months already. He had booked a massage simply to relax as he believed there was nothing that could be done for his shoulder. He told me that he would do surgery when he got home.

Massage can come in many different forms. I knew I had a limited amount of time to work with my guest as he was on his vacation and would soon leave, so I chose to combine the massage with heat therapy using hot stones. The heat helps me work far deeper into the muscle belly, helping me to release the tension without causing too much pain.

He came back to see me again for two more massages that week as he felt much better and had a far greater range of motion after the first treatment. On his second visit, we did another heat treatment this time with a poultice, which is a combination of different herbs and ingredients wrapped in a muslin cloth. Herbs can include turmeric, which is excellent for the treatment of inflammation and improving circulation, lemongrass, which helps regenerate connective tissue and ligaments, and it can also contain ingredients like coconut, which is hydrating.

As he came in for his third treatment, he referred to me as 'The Witch Doctor' and was very excited to tell me that his wife didn't help him dressed or undressed anymore. I was thrilled to hear that. After three sessions, his range of motion was vastly improved to the point he felt he didn't need surgery anymore.

A regular massage will help keep you relaxed, pain-free, injury-free and mobile. It could also quite possibly work miracles on your body. I look forward to seeing you in the Philippines for your health retreat or vacation.

May Estrada

Chiropractic As Described By Dr Darren Little

In September 2012, Dr Darren Little was awarded International Chiropractor of the Year by SORSI (Sacro Occipital Research Society International). He has speaking engagements all around the world and was my chiropractor over the four years I spent living in Australia. Along with his wife he owns Central to Health, which has three practices in Sydney, Australia. To look them up if you are ever in the area and to learn more about Chiropractic, visit their website www.centraltohealth.com.au - their whole philosophy around holistic healthcare is phenomenal. Here is what he has to say about chiropractic care;

Chiropractic has been helping people of all ages with a variety of health issues for over a century without the use of drugs or surgery. They use the best available evidence from research, the preferences of the patient and their own expertise and personal experience to help the spine and nervous system function optimally.

Chiropractors thoroughly assess the spine and the person as a whole, to determine the effect of spinal misalignment on the function of the nervous system.

The chiropractic philosophy is based on the following simple, common-sense principles.

Being healthy is your normal state - When everything works correctly, proper adaptation to the environment and health is the result.

Your nervous system controls everything - Your brain, spinal cord and nerves control and regulate every cell in your body.

Stress can overload your nervous system - Physical, chemical and mental stressors all impact our nervous system.

Spinal joint dysfunction results as a coping strategy - These can be acute or chronic, depending on the level of stress or when they were established. Postural imbalances and patterns of compensation are formed in the body, and the body's ability to adapt correctly is reduced. Pain, functional loss, and other symptoms and disease processes can result. Over the years, spinal degeneration may be sped up, and a person's health slowly declines.

Adjustments help reduce spinal dysfunction - There are many chiropractic techniques designed to address these areas of dysfunction or "subluxations". There are manual techniques such as Diversified or Gonstead technique. The adjustments are done by hand and often result in a "cracking" noise, which indicates joint cavitation. Another common technique is Sacro Occipital Technique (SOT) where pelvic wedges and musculoskeletal indicators and cranial function are all addressed for proper function and balance.

With the reduction of the spinal dysfunction or postural imbalances that have arisen from compensation for stressors on the body, the brain can start communicating better with the rest of the body. Muscles and joints work better and more efficiently. Many symptoms that have manifested as an expression of a health crisis can repair through the body's innate ability to self-heal and self-regulate. Chiropractors believe that this natural expression of the nervous system just needs no interference to work properly. The ultimate goal of the chiropractor is to work with the patient by administering gentle adjustments to achieve the optimal expression of their body. Through regular care, the adjustments provide ongoing assistance to the journey towards better health and vitality.

Dr Darren Little B.S. (Syd Uni) MChiro (Macquarie Uni)

Traditional Chinese Medicine and Acupuncture
As Described By **Dr Hanh Tran**

I first met Hanh while living in Australia. She was teaching an outstanding yoga class at the same gym I was a Personal Trainer at. After speaking to her, I was surprised to learn she was a pharmacist, as many Yoga Teachers are more into holistic remedies. All became clear as she was going on to study Traditional Chinese Medicine and Acupuncture and so with her experience in both worlds of medicine is the perfect person to introduce us to Eastern Medicine.

Traditional Chinese Medicine is an Eastern Medicine modality that includes acupuncture, herbal medicine, and body healing practices such as qi gong, tai chi, and massage which are all aimed to improve the quality of life of all living beings.

There are two central ideas behind Traditional Chinese Medicine: qi and yin & yang. Qi is the life force or vital energy that sustains life in the body and is constantly moving and changing. Yin and yang describe the quality of qi, which can also be seen in nature; day and night, masculine and feminine, hot and cold, light and dark. When the yin and yang of qi are balanced people would feel healthy and well, but when the flow of qi is disrupted, then disease can enter the body.

As a practising pharmacist with over ten years of experience, I have seen many ill patients that I have attended to. I noticed chronic and acute illnesses had emerging patterns and thought that was quite interesting, as that is what Chinese Medicine is - patterns of diagnosis and syndromes.

By doing my masters in Chinese Medicine, I was able to be more useful to patients coming in with symptoms and provide more tools and answers for people. It is an exciting time for the world of holistic practices where patients are able to explore what works for them personally, rather than being given a 'magic bullet' drug of which only treats the symptoms and not the root cause.

Dr Hanh Tran

Holistic Dentistry As Described By Dr Charlotte de Courcey-Bayley

I first went to Charlotte while living in Sydney to get my amalgam fillings taken out after learning about the ill effects mercury and other heavy metals have on the body. She is the owner of St. Leonards Holistic Dentists and is also the wonderful lady I mentioned in Chapter 2: Stress Less who got me to tape my mouth shut at night to invoke nasal breathing. She is an absolute wealth of knowledge and if you are ever in need of dental work or thinking of amalgam filling removal and anywhere near Sydney, Australia, go and see her. She's comfortably the best dentist I've ever met. Her website is www.holisticdentist.com.au if you need anymore information. Here's what she has to say about Holistic Dentistry and safe amalgam removal;

Holistic Dentistry is a philosophy of practice that stems from the observation that the health of the body impacts on the health of the mouth, gums and teeth and vice versa. Most people acknowledge that the food we eat can directly impact our teeth; sugar is known to cause decay. However, what does sugar do to our immune system? How does it increase inflammation in the body? What does it do to the microbiome of the mouth and the microbiome of the gut? Does dental disease predispose a person to gut problems or do gut problems initiate dental disease?

As researchers start to unravel the complex and critical mysteries of gut health, dentists hold a unique advantage to be able to observe the impact of gut health in action. Dental decay and acid erosion of teeth are barometers for gut health. The presence and severity of gum disease tell us about the functioning of the immune system and its interplay with tissue inflammation in the body. These diseases, therefore, need to be thought about holistically for treatment to be effective in the long-term and for well-being to be optimal.

Over the last 20 years, the field of sleep medicine has developed rapidly, and dentists have come on board to assist with providing certain types of treatment for snoring and sleep apnoea. Every dentist is trained in examination not only of the teeth but also of the area at the opening to the throat as well as the soft tissues of the mouth. A dentist trained in the area of sleep medicine understands that there are often indicators in the shape and size of these tissues that can show a patient may be experiencing impaired breathing when asleep. Working together with a sleep physician, the dentist provides valuable insight and can assist in the early detection of snoring and sleep apnoea.

Most commonly holistic dentistry is thought of in relation to the removal of mercury amalgam fillings. If this is something you are considering undertaking it would be worth reviewing the website of the IAOMT (International Association of Oral Medicine and Toxicology) www.IAOMT.org, to understand the correct protocols for the safe removal of amalgam. Ask the dental practice or the individual dentist exactly what their protocol is for managing this treatment. If they don't have a protocol, then you may need to rethink your plan, especially if you have health concerns to start with.

A holistic dentist, therefore, is someone who thinks beyond the obvious disease they see in the mouth. They can help their patient connect the dots on the journey to better health. In most countries, traditional university training and Dental Board registration requirements limit specifically what treatment dentists can deliver. However, a holistic dentist should have within their circle of practitioners, many other health care providers to help address other aspects of well-being that become apparent through a dental examination and discussion. You might, in fact, be surprised to discover how widely an experienced holistic dentist might think in the areas of healthcare and your well-being.

Dr Charlotte de Courcey-Bayley BDS Hons (Syd Uni) MSc Med (Sleep Medicine)

Reiki As Described By Reiki Master Mariesa Matire

I first met Mariesa when I was Personal Training in the gym she owned. I noticed she was 'different' you might say and as we became good friends, we had many a conversation about energy, the universe, positive mindset, meditation, natural healing and many more subjects besides that! Since then, she has gone on to become a Reiki Master and is the perfect person to introduce us to the wonderful world of Spiritual Energy Healing. You can find her over at www.happihealings.co.uk

Allow me to introduce myself. My names Mariesa and I am a Spiritual Energy Healer. "What's that?" I hear you say. Well, using my intuition, I am able to tap into the bodies energy system to help give messages to clients about how they can improve their physical and etheric health. I absolutely love working with the main Chakra system in the body, which are the energy centres, where intelligent energy from outside of your body enters the physical body. This energy is here only to serve your highest good.

There are seven main Chakras in the body, and I will briefly tell you about each one. I say 'briefly' as you can write a whole book and more on these amazing magical centres.

I will start right at the bottom of the spine in between your genitals the perineum area. We call this the Root Chakra. As everything is vibration, this includes colours too. Each chakra holds a resonance of a vibrational colour when it is spinning in harmony, therefore balanced and healthy. The Root Chakra is Red. This area is said to represent survival, career, your finances, home and a sense of belonging.

Next, we have the Sacral Chakra, which is situated just below the navel. The colour of this chakra is Orange. Its function is sexuality, desire, pleasure, physical energy and power. If you have a lack of energy, you may find your Sacral Chakra is out of balance.

Moving up above the navel, we have the Solar Plexus Chakra. The colour of the Solar Plexus is Yellow. Here you will find your humble personal power, confidence, self-esteem and happiness.

Then we reach the beautiful Heart Chakra. The colour of the Heart Chakra is Green. This chakra brings love, compassion and forgiveness.

Next, we move up to the Throat Chakra, which is the colour Blue. Here we find being able to speak our truth and to be heard by others. It is also linked to communication and listening to others too.

Next, we have the Third Eye. It is situated between the eyebrows. The colour of the Third Eye is Purple. It represents our psychic abilities, telepathy, our visions and intuition.

As we move right to the crown of the head, we have just that The Crown Chakra. The colour here is Lilac although I personally feel a lot of white light here. This is where we allow universal knowledge to enter our bodies, as a gateway to the 8th chakra, which is situated 3 feet above the head and is the gateway to other dimensions. When this chakra is balanced, we have a sense of all-knowing.

The Chakra System helps to explain the movement of life force or 'energy' and can help us understand ourselves in many ways.

The Energy Healing I serve can rebalance these beautiful energy centres helping you lead a healthy life but more than that helping you to have more control of the life you are living.

Where focus goes energy flows. So, if you practice a simple meditation such as sitting in silence, back straight, closing the eyes, you can become aware of the breath for a few moments. Now starting with the Root Chakra simply think about this area. We don't have to try or do anything but as we think about the Root Chakra area energy begins to flow here. How amazing that?

You then take your awareness up to the Sacral Chakra for a few minutes and repeat this process for all 8 Chakras that we have spoken about. You could even take this a step further once you have practised this a few times. We can add in the feeling of Joy or Gratitude while thinking of the Chakra area, repeating the process of working your way up all 8 Chakras.

Mariesa Matire

And there we have it. I want to thank all of my contributors for sharing their wisdom on these very pages. In the next chapter, we will cover what is maybe the most eyeopening information in this whole book. It's a subject I have presented hundreds of seminars to thousands of people around the world about and is something I am incredibly passionate about. Not only because of the mind-blowing information that I love sharing, but because it was one of the most effective things I did when healing my body from the condition eczema. Before we head on to that potentially life-changing information, first follow the Action Steps in this chapter.

Resources

Go to **www.TomBroadwell.com/resources** to find;

- A link to the website of all of this books contributors.

Action Steps

- Search online for a local, recommended performer of all the Alternative Therapies mentioned. Just remember when reading reviews online, that most people who leave reviews online are negative. Even if you look at reviews of the finest restaurants in the world, many are negative because of this reason, and if you base your actions purely on what is written online you will miss out on some amazing experiences in life...

- Because of the above, speak to people. Maybe try asking people in your local yoga or meditation class that have tried such things as Reiki or Acupuncture for their recommendations.

- Or simply go out and try for yourself. I tried seven different chiropractors in Sydney before finally finding Darren. When I met him, I simply knew he was the one! On the flip side, Charlotte is the only holistic dentist I've ever met, but when I first spoke to her she impressed me far more than any other dentist before her, so I knew I'd found a great one right off of the bat!

Chapter Twelve
You Are Also What You *Don't* Excrete

"Because we cannot scrub our inner body we need to learn a few skills to help cleanse our tissues, organs, and mind."– **Sebastian Pole**

He inhaled a big breath of fresh, clean air,

Today was the first day of spring,

The migration from the warmer climates of Africa to the harsh winters of Europe had brought about the first real day to day stress mankind had felt,

But the fire he had built and maintained had kept his family warm throughout the entire winter and food was plentiful,

His strong, lean and flexible body had made hunting easy even in the harsher climates,

He decided to go for a drink of spring water to start his day and to then see what fruits were beginning to come through in the natural woodland that surrounded them,

His mind was clear, and his body was healthy; he was excited to see what the spring would bring...

That was then, the time of the caveman. Today's world is very different, however, the inner workings of our body, and what it is designed to deal with when it comes to stress, synthetic chemicals and 'toxins' of any kind are the same. The liver is the same exact organ, doing the same role as a filter inside of a human body that we now overload with toxicity from all angles.

Toxins appear in everything from the air we breathe, to the food we eat, to the water we drink and bathe in. The day to day stress which we *don't* offload with physical activity gets worse year on year. The pharmaceutical drugs and the cosmetics we use load our body with synthetic chemicals which are toxins that it was simply never meant to deal with.

What Is A Toxin?

Let's first look at what 'toxins' are. The Cambridge Dictionary describes a 'toxin' as; 'a poisonous substance, esp. one that is produced by bacteria and causes disease'. This stems from times before the advances we see in chemistry today when a toxin encountered by humans would predominantly come from poisonous plants and venom. Now we can also look at synthetic chemicals used in pharmaceutical drugs, cosmetics, our food and water supply as toxins.

We can do this because if we then look up 'toxic' in the dictionary, we see the words 'biology' *and* 'chemistry' and then poisonous. 'Poisonous' is described as; 'a substance that can make people or animals ill or kill them if they eat or drink it'. Which, for example, you could describe pharmaceutical drugs as because if you took thirty high blood pressure pills all at once, what would happen? You would become extremely ill or die.

If you were wondering why I've gone into so much detail about what a toxin is, it's because if you type the word detoxification (detox for short) into a search engine, there are a lot of medical doctors, so called scientists and keyboard warriors who are calling bullshit on the entire idea. They also do it sometimes in an unnecessarily aggressive way, basically trying to publicly shame anyone for even trying it, never mind someone writing books about it. One was so over the top aggressive about the entire premise of detox; he told his large audience of muppets to challenge anyone who mentions the word detox to ask what a toxin is. If they couldn't repeat perfectly word for word what the dictionary says, then they should shove a camera in their face and take a picture and put their face on your wall...not sure why? But there you go.

Or maybe, just maybe, *some* doctors are so egotistical that they believe everything they got taught at university and nothing else. Anything that doesn't fit into their extremely rigid belief system (what the pharmaceutical companies taught them) cannot *possibly* be true. Or maybe, even worse than that is the fact that doctors do earn a living from people being sick. Many patients are sick from the toxins that are at detectable levels in their body and so helping someone get better through an alternative method (i.e. detox), from which they don't profit would negatively affect their income.

Now, I'm not saying all doctors are either one of the above, far from it. A lot of doctors are good honest people. But a small percentage of them are either stuck in a mindset that allows them only to believe in Western medicine or are simply in it for the money. Just as is the case with *any* profession, there are good people, and there are bad people.

I'm also not claiming that *all* detoxes are good for you or that every single detox out there works. There are lots of terrible products on the market, and some of the ingredient lists I've seen beggar belief. I've seen proven carcinogens making up the majority of the ingredients in some detox products. I've seen corn starch used as a bulking agent, talc, Red 40 and Yellow 5 used as colourings and artificial sweeteners used to make it taste better. These are just a few of the many toxic ingredients that are regularly used in detox supplements today. These I remind you are in products that are supposed to 'detox' you. Putting more toxins in, to detoxify, obviously makes no sense. Once again, we see the Western world fucking up what something is supposed to do, all because of greed. I urge you to read the labels and look at the 'Other Ingredients' and if you see any artificial colourings, synthetic additives, preservatives, artificial sweeteners etc. in there, run a mile!

Now, all I ask is for you to open your mind and do what feels right to you. Don't let *anyone*; even a doctor put you off doing something that could be good for your health and something that could change your life. Because detox certainly changed mine, in fact, one of the things that I attribute to helping my skin the most was detoxification.

So, what effect do these toxins have on the body? As mentioned, taken in large quantities, they will make you either seriously ill or kill you. But what about in smaller quantities? Because that is the stance that most people who call detoxification 'pseudoscience' take. In smaller amounts, all the chemicals we take on board in our everyday lives are safe. Hmm really...Let's take a look at the evidence, shall we? Of course, we shall.

A Brief History Of Toxins

In 1907 the first-ever plastic, based on a synthetic polymer, was invented by Leo Hendrik Baekeland. In 1939 the first significant synthetic organic pesticide, DDT was discovered by a Swiss chemist Paul Muller. If you are wondering how something can be both synthetic and organic at the same time, let me briefly explain. Synthetic organic chemicals are manmade substances that contain carbon atoms. All organic compounds are organic because they have a carbon atom in their structure. Carbon is a primary component of all known life on Earth, representing approximately 45–50% of all dry biomass. A natural organic chemical is ones that are already present here on Earth such as oxygen, diamonds and gold. A synthetic organic chemical is made by man, but usually is actually an imitation of a natural organic chemical. Such as synthetic vitamins which as discussed are missing all the stuff that makes them healthy, versus the naturally occurring vitamins in sunlight and food. Today the Environmental Protection Agency (EPA) holds a list of over 86'000 different chemicals used by manufacturers, many of which have never been tested for safety as they get new chemicals submitted every day.

At the turn of the 20th Century production of synthetic chemicals in the US was less than 1 million pounds per year. Fast forward to today, check out what the website worldometer.com has to say on the subject. (Their counters, by the way, have been licensed for the United Nations Conference Rio+20, BBC News, and World Expo so are seen as being rather accurate); 'every second 310 Kg (682 pounds) of toxic chemicals are released into our air, land, and water by industrial facilities around the world. This amounts to approximately 10 million tons (over 21 billion pounds) of toxic chemicals each year of which over 2 million tons (over 4.5 billion pounds) are recognized carcinogens. This amounts to about 65 Kg (143 pounds) each second.'

Looking at those figures in a different light, we've gone from 1 million pounds to more than *21 billion* pounds per year in a little over a century.

The difference between a million and a billion is far more substantial than most people think. Put it this way, 1 million seconds in time is 11 days. One billion seconds is 32 years...

Richard Denison, Senior Scientist at the Environmental Defense Fund, estimates that chemicals are used in 96 per cent of manufactured materials and products today. In 2009 the Fourth National Report on Human Exposure to Environmental Chemicals was compiled by the Centers for Disease Control and Prevention (CDC). Polybrominated diphenyl ethers (PBDEs) were found in nearly all of the participants that were tested; with the test being done on people aged six years and up. PBDEs are fire retardants used in the manufacture of numerous polymer-based commercial and household products, such as clothes, furniture, and electronics.

Sounds like fun having that in my system, especially when current thinking points to chemicals like this being the leading cause for the massive increase in childhood cancer we see today. Why do children have flame retardant in their body? One reason is that it's in their *pyjamas*. Ahh makes sense, protect the children against fire with highly toxic material. Yeah, but hang on, isn't it usually the smoke that kills and not the fire? Besides that, I've never seen a child randomly combust...sorry just thinking out loud, but really, why is it in there? In a 2016 study performed in Oregon by the Environmental Health Sciences Center at Oregon State University, 92 children aged 3–5 years old were involved in a test to see how many flame retardants they were exposed to. Researchers found a total of 20 different types of flame retardants, with over 60% of the children exposed to 11 or more. Keep that in mind for what's to come.

Another chemical the general population has exposure to in vast quantities is Bisphenol A (BPA) which can occur through ingestion of foods that are in contact with BPA-containing materials such as aluminium cans and absorption through the skin by handling receipt paper.

CDC scientists found BPA in more than 90% of the urine samples representative of the US population.

The problem with BPA is that it is an endocrine-disrupting chemical (EDC). Just like the fire retardants mentioned above, as was DDT, the pesticide that got banned in the US in 1972. It's not only the current use of these chemicals that are a cause for concern, as reported in 2005 by the CDC, 'nearly all US residents have measurable serum p,p' - DDE levels'. DDE is what DDT breaks down into in the body. Amazingly it was still in almost every living person 33 years later. Hmmm, maybe I'd like to detox... since obviously the human body and our environment are having a hard time breaking down these things naturally.

Okay so, check this out; in 2002 a report entitled; 'Global Assessment of the State-of-the-Science of Endocrine Disruptors' was compiled for the World Health Organization (WHO) and the United Nations Environment Programme (UNEP). In the upcoming paragraphs, the underlining of words has been added by me for emphasis. They stated that; 'although it is clear that certain environmental chemicals can interfere with normal hormonal processes, there is weak evidence that human health has been adversely affected by exposure to endocrine-active chemicals.'

Now keep up with me here, because I know there's a lot of long scientific words and acronyms which can be an absolute ball ache to read. Trust me, I know; as I've gotten many a headache and had to walk away many times to rest my brain from reading the hundreds of medical papers and government reports that I had to endure during the research for this book. But it's all well worth it in the end. Why? Because this section will not only show you how vital it is to your health to avoid as many toxins as you can but also the importance of helping your body get rid of them.

Without a healthy endocrine system, reproduction and normal development are not possible. Worldwide, endocrine diseases are on the rise at alarming levels. Now for the fun part, because in 2002 there was weak evidence it had sweet f. a. to do with human health, but just ten short years later in 2012, the same group revisited the initial 2002 report and stated amongst other things that;

'Human and wildlife populations all over the world are exposed to EDCs. Unlike 10 years ago, we now know that humans and wildlife are exposed to far more EDCs than just those that are persistent organic pollutants (POPs). New sources of human exposure to EDCs and potential EDCs, in addition to food and drinking water, have been identified. Close to 800 chemicals are known or suspected to be capable of interfering with hormone receptors, hormone synthesis or hormone conversion. However, only a small fraction of these chemicals have been investigated in tests capable of identifying overt endocrine effects in intact organisms. The vast majority of chemicals in current commercial use have not been tested at all. This lack of data introduces significant uncertainties about the true extent of risks from chemicals that potentially could disrupt the endocrine system.'

Oh, and they also stated;

'Internationally agreed and validated test methods for the identification of endocrine disruptors capture only a limited range of the known spectrum of endocrine-disrupting effects. This increases the likelihood that harmful effects in humans and wildlife are being overlooked. Disease risk due to EDCs may be significantly underestimated.'

Toxin Synergies

Another thought within the same report that needs to be taken seriously is;

'A focus on linking one EDC to one disease severely underestimates the disease risk from mixtures of EDCs. We know that humans and wildlife are simultaneously exposed to many EDCs; thus, the measurement of the linkage between exposure to mixtures of EDCs and disease or dysfunction is more physiologically relevant. In addition, it is likely that exposure to a single EDC may cause disease syndromes or multiple diseases, an area that has not been adequately studied.'

Some of the above revelations are absolutely stunning, such as no one really knows the risk when it comes to these types of toxins. The fact that the synergy of multiple chemicals reacting in the human body is something that isn't even considered when testing for safety is quite scary. In a world of thousands of different chemicals, most of which have never even been tested individually, can you imagine the work involved to test them in combinations?

However, let's look at why they will likely never check for combinations of chemicals by taking the above example where most children were exposed to 11 flame retardants over just seven days. If we were to check every possible synergistic interaction of every flame retardant found in most children in the study, there are more than 700'000 combinations. That's for 11 flame retardants...found in children...age 3-5 years old...over just seven days...

Now let's look at the 9282 people who were tested for pesticides by the CDC, who found at least 13 different pesticides in 100% of the participants. You now have over 10 million possible combinations to test, just for the 13 different pesticides...Add them together, just the flame retardants and pesticides mentioned above. Forgetting about the additives, preservatives, sweeteners and colourings used in our food. Forgetting about the combinations of chemicals used in pharmaceutical drugs, the pollution in the air, the fluoride and chlorine and other chemicals found in our water supply etc. etc. etc. Just adding simply, the 11 flame retardants and the 13 pesticides found in most people, and you now have a possible 620,448,401,733,239,000,000,000 combinations. I do not even know how to say that number in words, but it's bloody big! And that is why they will likely never check the combinations of how chemicals react synergistically inside of you. Which means one thing.

You are the chemistry test.

Now I don't know about you, but I am not taking the risk of exposing myself to said chemicals, neither singularly or in synergy. I am also not willing to risk, not even trying to get rid of them through safe, effective detoxification methods. Fuck what some angry doctors say, there is plenty of scientific evidence to suggest that we need to take our health into our own hands because research seems to come too little, too late for my liking!

Endocrine Disrupting Chemicals

Okay, so going back to those pesky Endocrine Disrupting Chemicals (EDCs), and yes I am putting a lot focus on this type of toxin. The reason is that frankly there are so many different types of chemicals that affect the body in so many ways, I feel it essential to drive home the importance of only one in great detail. I'll let you make up your own mind about if it applies to the rest of the synthetic chemicals out there! My mind is made up, that it surely it does, and I will not be the chemistry test that these huge companies and the government want me to be.

I mentioned earlier that endocrine diseases are on the increase and below are a few of the health issues that are happening the world over, from the same 2012 report done for the WHO and UNEP; 'Global Assessment of the State-of-the-Science of Endocrine Disruptors'.

- Large proportions (up to 40%) of young men in some countries have low semen quality, which reduces their ability to father children.

- The incidence of genital malformations, such as non-descending testes (cryptorchidisms) and penile malformations (hypospadias), in baby boys, has increased over time or levelled off at *unfavourably* high rates.

- The incidence of adverse pregnancy outcomes, such as preterm birth and low birth weight, has increased in many countries.

- Neurobehavioural disorders associated with thyroid disruption affect a high proportion of children in some countries and have increased over the past decades.

- Global rates of endocrine-related cancers (breast, endometrial, ovarian, prostate, testicular and thyroid) have been increasing over the past 40–50 years.

- There is a trend towards the earlier onset of breast development in young girls in all countries where this has been studied, which is a risk factor for breast cancer.

- The prevalence of obesity and type 2 diabetes has dramatically increased worldwide over the last 40 years. WHO estimates that 1.5 billion adults worldwide are overweight or obese and that the number with type 2 diabetes increased from 153 million to 347 million between 1980 and 2008.

We can also look towards a paper published by The Journal of Clinical Endocrinology & Metabolism and the Endocrine Society, which presented yet more evidence that endocrine-disrupting chemicals (EDCs) contribute substantially to disease and disability. In the paper, they show how EDCs contribute to everything from autism to ADHD to obesity to infertility and more. They estimate EDC exposure costs hundreds of billions of Euros per year. Researchers produced a median cost of €157 billion annually across the EU from this exposure! Holy smokes! So, not only is being exposed to these chemicals costing us our health, but also our wealth. However, I always say health really is wealth. It doesn't matter how much money you have if you are not healthy enough to spend it. Experts also think EDCs are making us more stupid too. IQ's are lowering because of the chemicals. I'm not going to lie and say I didn't notice...

Looking again at fire retardants and the statement I made about refusing to become the chemistry test that huge companies and the government want me to be...See, it's been shown time and again that the government and large corporations are actually one and the same. Most people think the government have their best interests at heart when really, it's been shown many times that they simply don't. As a perfect example of this, as if fate would have it while researching I came across a very recent story in the British newspaper 'The Guardian', showing that the government would much rather protect the interests of massive corporations than the very people it is meant to serve.

Boston firefighter Jay Fleming is trying to get flame retardants banned in the state of Massachusetts. It seems counterintuitive for a firefighter to be campaigning for such things. However, after seeing many of his colleagues die from different cancers that firefighters simply did not regularly die from - at least until the introduction of fire retardants in household goods in the 1970s.

First, let's look at the huge corporations who proposed the use of fire retardants in the first place; The Tobacco Industry. Yes, you read that right. To stop house fires caused by cigarettes, rather than taking the cigarettes away, changing their products or even promoting smoking outside, the Tobacco companies wanted to add more chemicals so you can use their...well...chemicals, in your own home. They chose to blame the furniture rather than cigarettes. Ha! You couldn't make this shit up.

Now you have people like Jay Fleming who are faced with the obvious dangers of these chemicals, wanting to have people around him stop becoming sick and dying. But he has faced massive opposition when doing so, from the American Chemistry Council (ACC) for one. The ACC represents huge corporations from oil companies to pharmaceutical companies and have lobbyists employed all over America to fight against bills that would not benefit the corporations that they represent. Now for the interesting bit, the bill was 'pocket-vetoed' by the governor, which means he let it pass without signing it but without saying why. It was found that he had had a face-to-face meeting with the ACC but never with the firefighters. Interesting.

The same was said of the ACC when they sent lobbyists from Washington to Hawaii, "They will send a lobbyist from DC to Hawaii at the most local level of city and county to try to stop plastic bans here," said Rafael Bergstrom, executive director of Sustainable Coastline Hawaii. Trying to stop a ban designed to help with the major problem of plastics washing up on Hawaiian beaches, sounds like a lovely bunch of people.

So, all in all, we now have evidence of chemicals that are barely ever tested for safety. We also have chemicals that are going from being seen as safe to highly toxic in the span of ten years and politicians allegedly not banning chemicals because it would affect the profits of large corporations. So now I put it to you; Are you ready to detox?

Awesome. Now, not only are we looking at purging our bodies from harmful chemicals such as DDT, DDE, PDBEs, EDCs and BPAs....did you get all that? I just want to brush over some other things that are toxic to our body both to cement my case and to be able to show you different types and methods of detox that you may (or may not), want to embark on.

Detoxification

To start this process, I am going to bring in another expert, this time of the digestive system and the practice of Colonic Hydrotherapy. My longtime friend Jane Barber, who I first met when she inserted a long (and thankfully thin and well-lubed) object into my anus...during my first colonic! With nothing more to do than chat as the system worked it's magic, we quickly became friends as we realised we were on the same wavelength and we have been good friends ever since. How about that for the start of a friendship! I have to say that my fondness for Jane only grew as I walked down the road from her clinic in Leeds, England, as I felt like I was floating home on a cloud!

Here I'm going to have Jane explain all about the gut, and why it is so important to cleanse it. Some of this information you will notice is repeated from what I've already taught you, which is always nice to have an expert in a certain field agree with what I've said, and is good for you as it is a friendly reminder to make the changes if you haven't already. Nudge, nudge, wink, wink. Some of it I am learning for the first time too! Which is amazing and fits in with my whole philosophy, never stop learning and growing. You can find Jane over at www.detoxonline.co.uk for more information or if you want to book in and go see her.

Cleansing The Gut As Described By Jane Barber - Colon Hydrotherapist

Something Hippocrates, who is considered the father of modern medicine, knew 2400 years ago and now mainstream medicine and science have begun to realise is that "All disease begins in the gut", or the version I prefer, which is "Health begins in the gut".

Each day heralds fresh reports of studies that have found connections between poor gut health and serious health conditions. If you are not working on your gut, then everything else you do in pursuit of glowing good health will be compromised. Good guts can't be taken for granted.

What Does The Gut Do?

Digestion starts in our head, literally. During the cephalic phase of digestion (imagine you are preparing food and the delicious aromas are making your mouth water and your tummy rumble), your stomach floods with gastric juices which start the digestive process. In order to maximise digestion, food should be a feast for all the senses.

Chewing is of paramount importance. There are no teeth in your stomach. Any chunks of food which arrive in your stomach are likely to stay that way. When we chew properly, the food is ground to a paste and mixed with saliva so that it moves easily through the oesophagus.

The bolus of food is then sent to the stomach, which is highly acidic. The acid forms a barrier preventing harmful bacteria from entering the digestive tract and softening proteins ready for digestion. The stomach churns the food and gastric juices together, ready for digestion.

The resulting chyme (a mix of the juices and the mashed up food) is then squeezed from the stomach into the duodenum which plays a vital role in chemical digestion. Secretions from the pancreas, liver and gallbladder mix with the chyme in preparation for absorption in the small intestine.

The small intestine is where most of the digestion and absorption of food occurs. It starts off highly acidic but becomes less so the closer it gets to the colon. Bacteria in the small intestine regulate both the digestion and absorption of lipids (fats).

What's left after digestion and absorption of nutrients then heads to the colon which is way more than just a poop shoot. The first section of the colon also absorbs and synthesises nutrients. B vitamins from the diet are absorbed in the small intestine; however, bacterial B vitamins are produced and absorbed mainly through the colon. The colon is teeming with bacteria which forms a significant portion of your immune system when the balance is healthy. The colon also reabsorbs water from the waste matter. So, the slower your waste moves through your gut, the drier and harder it will be.

Modern Life Is Bad For Your Gut

Life in the 21st century is seriously bad for your gut. We live in a toxic soup, but to top it off, there is a range of lifestyle and health choices that are damaging. How many on the following list are potential issues for you?

- **Stress**: Keeps you in a permanent state of flight or fight and shuts down digestion/elimination functions as part of your survival mechanisms. Very disruptive to gut bacteria.

- **Artificial sweeteners**: Have been found to decimate good bacteria and encourage bad bacteria to flourish along with a whole range of other health issues, including potentially bringing on a pre-diabetic state quicker than actual sugar.

- **Sugar**: Slows the movement of the gut leading to sluggish elimination of waste which provides an unhealthy environment for gut bacteria. It also encourages the overgrowth of yeasts and bad bacteria, leading to lots of issues.

- **Antibiotics**: Despite warnings (even Fleming warned against the overuse of antibiotics more than 100 years ago), antibiotics continue to be overprescribed. In some circumstances, they are essential, but issues would often resolve if just given some time. Ask your doctor that antibiotics are absolutely essential before popping those pills. Antibiotics, as the name suggests, kill probiotics.

- **Pesticides**: Kills pests and gut bacteria.

- **EMF pollution**: In the form of mobile phones, computers and smart devices. We are electrical beings, and messages are sent around our bodies by electrical pulses. Being constantly surrounded by alien electrical fields has negative impacts which have barely been researched as yet.

- **Air pollution**: Who knows what we are breathing in and what it is doing to our overall health!?

- **Processed foods**: Do not provide the required nutrients for our bodies to work as they should. Refined carbohydrates don't provide enough fibre for the bowel to work correctly and flood the body with sugar. When we consume insufficient fibre, the gut is left littered with food remnants.

- **Pharmaceuticals**: Especially focusing on antibiotics, NSAIDs and PPIs. Antibiotics kill off good bacteria. NSAIDs (such as Ibuprofen) have been found to make the gut permeable allowing food particles and bacteria to pass into the body. PPIs (such as Lanzaprazole and Omeprazole) inhibit the production of acid which impairs digestion.

- **Lack of exercise**: Being active keeps the gut mobile. Good core muscles provide support for your gut and keep it where it should be. In addition, the peristaltic action of the gut is supported. It's the difference between keeping your many yards of entrails in a supermarket carrier bag versus a good, strong suitcase.

- **Antibacterial cleaners**: Kill the bacteria in your home and your gut.

- **Dehydration**: Impairs all digestive functions, thickens the blood, ages skin, can lead to joint problems, cognitive impairment, depression and anxiety.

- **Excessive alcohol consumption**: Studies have found that some alcohol, gin, for example, kill off useful bacteria whilst red wine, in moderate amounts, was found to be beneficial to gut bacteria. Drinking too much, however, floods your system with empty calories and sugars. It also removes your willpower, leading to eating the wrong things.

- **Food sensitivities**: Becoming increasingly common and more complex. We are not designed to eat the same things all the time. Supermarkets becoming the primary source of food, importing foods from far and wide, has removed seasonal eating (eating what's grown in your home country when it's in season). This has led to us eating the same things year-round which would have only been available for a short time previously. Strawberries are a great example. In the UK they were only available for about two weeks of the year and so were a massive treat to eat.

- **Bad dental hygiene**: This is a rarely considered factor (covered in Chapter 3: Sweet Dreams in this book though! -

Tom). Gum disease and decaying teeth will pour a constant supply of bad bacteria into your gut.

Indications That Your Gut Is Not Happy

If you eat three meals per day, packed with fruit and vegetables providing abundant fibre, and your gut is working optimally, you should be evacuating your bowels two to three times a day. Certainly, judging by the people who visit my practice, very few people in the Western world are achieving this.

While sluggish elimination is a sound indicator of less than happy guts, there are also other symptoms including:

- Reflux, indigestion, and heartburn

- Bloating

- Diarrhoea

- Stinky breath

- Abdominal pain or discomfort

- Fatigue

- Anxiety and depression

- Skin breakouts

- Candida

- Urinary tract infections

How To Restore Your Gut

If you read the myriad of adverts on Facebook and Google, you'd think restoring your gut is just a case of chucking down a few probiotics. There are a few issues with this approach. If you really want to work on your gut, then you need to correct every aspect of the process and in the right order.

How's Your Digestion?

There is a really easy way to test the acidity of your stomach. First thing in the morning before you eat or drink anything put a heaped teaspoon of bicarbonate of soda in a small glass of water, stir briskly and drink. If sufficiently acidic, as soon as the bicarb hits your stomach, you will start to belch: a lot and loud. If you do a couple of polite little burps or nothing at all, then you would benefit from supplementing with digestive enzymes.

Gut Integrity

Many people have leaky gut. Your gut is a barrier between you and the outside world. In a healthy gut, the nutrients, in a molecular state, are carried across the gut wall by good bacteria. If the gut is leaky (has holes), and especially if both digestion and chewing are poor, the partially digested food and bacteria, both good and bad, can pass across the gut wall and into your body. Even good bacteria, when it's in the wrong place, is not good at all.

Heal your gut by changing your diet and supplementing with L-glutamine, which rebuilds your digestive tract. Taking Slippery Elm powder before eating a meal helps to prevent bacteria and undigested food crossing the gut wall.

Hydration

It is impossible to be healthy and dehydrated. Drink 35mls of good quality water per kg of body weight. If you have been drinking less, then you will need to add an extra litre to repay your hydration debt. It can take up to a year to fully hydrate on a cellular basis (which means that all cells are fully operational, taking in clean water and nutrients and flushing out waste).

Food Sensitivities

Food sensitivities will generally cause some disruption to the gut so you will probably experience:

- Constipation and/or diarrhoea

- Bloating

- Abdominal discomfort after eating

- Weight gain or loss

- Skin issues

- Itching

- Emotional issues

- Inflammation

If you suspect you may have food sensitivities, then get tested and remove the foods. Even very healthy foods can be disruptive to your gut health if they don't agree with you.

Diet

Every choice you make is going to either heal or harm your gut. There is no one size fits all diet; however, there are foods that don't work for any of us. Eliminate these foods from your diet:

What *Not* To Eat

- Sugar

- Fizzy drinks

- Artificial sweeteners

- Refined carbohydrates (white rice, pasta, bread)

- Grains (with the exception of millet)

- White potatoes

- Dairy

- Sweets, cakes, and biscuits

- Damaged fats (vegetable oils, hydrogenated fats, and margarine)

- Excessive alcohol

What *To* Eat

- A wide variety of green vegetables: Greens support your body to create its own good bacteria.

- A wide variety of red, green and yellow vegetables: To make sure you are getting plenty of antioxidants.

- Purple/blue veg: Great for your heart and brain.

- Resistant starches: Such as sweet potato, parsnip, turnip and persimmon (sharon fruit) and legumes (be sure to pressure cook beans). Resistant starches provide nutrition for good bacteria.

- Protein: Eat small amounts of good quality protein. If you eat meat and fish, eat less and buy the very best quality. Eat only wild-caught fish and meat that has been raised on grass. Go vegetarian or at least flexitarian.

- Fruit: Vegetables are four times as nutritious as fruit so eat less fruit than vegetables. You can eat fruit every day but don't go crazy on it.

- In addition: Small amounts of nuts and seeds as snacks. If you are a chocoholic, then you can allow yourself a small serving of at least 72% dark chocolate.

Detoxification

So you've eliminated unhelpful foods from your diet, boosted your digestion, getting plenty of fresh, pure water and started working on healing your gut. Now it's time to start cleansing (although you could have kick-started the whole shebang with a good cleanse) and the best way to do that is colonics all the way. There is no better way of removing old, stagnant waste, dead and dying bacteria, yeasts, and if you are very lucky, the odd parasite. In addition, colonic irrigation will give your gut a workout a bit like sending it to the gym and with regular sessions, the muscle will be strengthened.

How many colonics will you need? More than you think. If you imagine your bathroom is old and in a state of disrepair. The walls are stone, so there is no clear line to meet with the floor, which is made of wood and has plenty of nooks and crannies for dirt and germs to get stuck in. The whole room is a haven for bacteria. If you throw in a bucket of water, will you remove all the bacteria? Most definitely not. Well, your colon is a bit like that dirty bathroom. It twists and turns through your abdomen, creating lots of places for things to hide. Old waste can be harbouring bad bacteria, excess mucous (in the form of mucoid plaque which mainstream medicine does not believe in, but I have to believe my own eyes) and parasites. Have your first three sessions close together (3 – 5 days) in order to clear out your colon and then progressively remove whatever was chugging its way through your system. Then have sessions a week apart, progressing to monthly as your gut starts to work properly. Commit to having regular colonics as part of your health and beauty routine.

Probiotics

Your gut will start to heal in as little as three days (on the downside, it only takes three days of eating rubbish to undo all your good work and create lots of bad bacteria). I recommend leaving it until two weeks into the healing process before you start to take probiotic supplements.

- Choose probiotic supplements with a wide variety of strains.

- Make sure the amount of live bacteria they contain is stated one year from the date of manufacture. Many probiotic supplements advertise the number of live bacteria they have on the day of manufacture. By the time you get them, they may have little or no bacteria alive.

- Rotate brands of probiotics and look for different strains. Diversity is more important than the dose.

Remember...

- Everything you put in your mouth will either harm or heal you.

- It only takes three days to undo all your good work.

- Looking after your gut is ongoing not something you can do once and forget about.

- Love your gut, and it will love you back.

Jane Barber - Colon Hydrotherapist

Thanks to Jane for some invaluable insight into gut health. It was shown in a paper published in the International Journal of Molecular Sciences just how important gut bacteria are to human health. Researchers showed it has a hand in *everything* from nutrient absorption to nerve function and when out of balance due to antibiotics, stress and a lousy diet, it could cause many chronic diseases, such as inflammatory bowel disease, obesity, cancer, and even autism.

Intermittent Fasting

As part of our gut detoxifying section, we need to talk about something that has gotten a lot of press in recent times, but once again we see the West screwing things up. Intermittent fasting is an eating pattern that involves not eating for a period of time, *without* starving the body of essential nutrients. The most popular ways of eating are alternate day fasting, 5:2 intermittent fasting (fasting two days each week with a restricted calorie diet on those two days), eat stop eat which is a full 24 hours fast for two days of the week and daily time-restricted feeding (such as eating only during a six to eight hour window). Going on the evidence I am about to present I feel the best two options are doing a full 24-hour fast twice per week or if that is too daunting to you, eating in a small window, with the best option being an 18/6 hour ratio. During your time of fasting you can drink water and some black coffee, black and herbal teas. Do not add anything such as milk or sugar to your hot drinks. You can add a little lemon to your water if you prefer.

There are hundreds of studies that have shown that intermittent fasting can lead to improvements in health conditions. In a paper published in The New England Journal of Medicine in 2019 researchers found it would help with ageing, brain function, losing weight and diseases such as diabetes, cardiovascular disease, cancers and neurological disorders. The obvious fantastic health benefits, however, are if it is done *properly*. By that, I mean what we see promoted in the West is the fact you can eat *anything* in your window, and still lose weight. Firstly, this way of eating is not and never was *just* about losing weight, but of course, that's where the money is, so people will keep pushing that agenda. When it comes to this, yet again, the mainstream talks about caloric restriction, which of course we now know, you'll lose weight on *any* calorie-restricted diet (only to put it back on again). But as already discussed, you are losing *muscle* and screwing up your health. And then eating fast food, sugary snacks and soda in your eating window is not going to lead to abundant energy and optimal health even if you do lose weight (temporarily).

What you should be eating in-between is what we have already discussed in this book. Fresh, organic produce - without getting too obsessed about it and enjoying the odd treat now and then, something we will discuss in the next chapter. As far as health benefits go, intermittent fasting will give the digestive system a rest, allowing it to detoxify your body regularly. There is a reduction in the production of damaging oxygen free radicals, which lowers inflammation levels. During fasting, cells activate pathways that enhance the body's natural defence against oxidative stress, and the body is also better able to remove or repair damaged molecules. These cellular responses happen during fasting, which will lead to improved mental and physical performance, as well as resistance against disease.

Any way of eating that you implement should be part of a healthy lifestyle, rather than a set period of time with the goal being to simply lose weight in that time.

Rather than focusing on losing weight to be healthy, focus instead on being healthy to lose weight...permanently.

While fasting, triglycerides that are stored in fat cells are broken down into fatty acids, which are used for energy. The liver converts fatty acids into ketone bodies, which provide a major source of energy for many tissues, especially the brain. This is why people report boosts of energy and more intense focus and clarity of thought while fasting. In a paper published in The Journal of Lipid Research in 2012, researchers found that ketone levels in the blood are highest after 24 hours of fasting, showing not only intermittent fasting but 2-3 day fasts are a good way to start a weight loss plan and detoxify the body. So intermittent fasting will use what fat cells are made up of (triglycerides) for energy, leading to fat loss. Not only that, but in a paper published in The British Journal of Nutrition in 2013, researchers compared a group of people who did a period of intermittent fasting with a second group who simply lowered their calorie intake by 25%. They lost the same amount of weight, but the intermittent fasters lost more *belly fat*. As you will soon see, to lose stubborn belly fat you need to lower inflammation levels and one way to do that is to detoxify. This will explain why intermittent fasting is more successful at lowering belly fat than just dieting. A paper published in The International Journal of Obesity also showed that intermittent fasting was better than simply reducing calorie intake for glucose regulation, blood pressure, and heart rate; plus, the performance of endurance training.

In one of the earliest studies of intermittent fasting, published in the journal Mechanisms of Ageing and Development in 1990, reported that the average life span of rats is increased by up to 80% when they are maintained on a regimen of alternate-day feeding! This has been shown in subsequent studies, maybe not quite 80% but vast improvements to ageing and health overall. So, if you want to lose weight from the right areas, improve health, physical and mental performance and detoxify your body, intermittent fasting is a proven method that you can incorporate into a new healthy lifestyle.

Detoxifying The Liver

This is a subject that has intrigued me for more than a decade - the detoxification of the liver. The liver is the largest digestive gland in the body, playing a major role in metabolism and has more than 500 vital functions. These include detoxification, synthesis of proteins and hormones, storing glycogen, as well as holding a reservoir of blood. On a very basic level, the liver is your fat-burning organ with its other primary function being a filter for toxins. Now, if you are struggling to lose weight just think for one moment, if the liver is focused on breaking down synthetic chemicals, do you think it is busy breaking down fat? Your body is built for survival, and so breaking down toxins that could kill you is going to take precedence over breaking down fat.

A lot of people tell me they have a slow metabolism; however, no animal in the wild that has never been exposed to synthetic chemicals has ever had a slow metabolism. I've seen overweight domestic animals which *we* just happen to feed, which to me at least points to the fact that it is a man-made problem. Overweight people has only become a common thing since the dawn of the chemical age we are living in.

Common sense points to the fact that we have *created* 'slow metabolisms' and now we have to turn back to nature to right the wrongs.

The liver is an incredible organ and is the only one that can completely regenerate, even after a massive injury. It has been shown that you can lose up to 75% of your liver, and it will completely regenerate back to its full size and function. Because of its role in detoxifying and dealing with acid, it goes through a process of cell renewal, with every cell in your liver getting replaced every 150-500 days. This brings me to a major point in that a true cleansing of the liver will take a *minimum* of 6 months as it takes just short of this time to replace cells. Your skin has to deal with the environment and so goes through the same process of cell renewal. You have brand new skin cells on the surface of your skin every 14-28 days. My point here is that if you had your hand in a trash can for 28 days, would you expect the new generation of cells to be healthy? The answer you've come to is hopefully; "No".

Your liver is basically the trash sorting area of your body. Every single toxin that enters your body has to confront the liver at some stage. Whether it's in the air you breathe, in the food you ate or from a product that you put on your skin (more about that in a later chapter). Now, if you embark on a liver detox that lasts in the region of 7-21 days (most of the detox products I've seen in stores and online are within that timeframe), this is as if you've cleansed the skin on your hand for around 1-3 days. From there you shoved your hand into a trash can for the remainder of your cell renewal process, still expecting your the new skin cells to be healthy.

And so, cleansing the liver is going to take a little while, especially knowing some of the bad habits my clients have had! Haha! Me too, don't worry, I ain't judging. And so, we need to establish some habits that remain for the next six months while taking supplements that are renowned for cleansing over, at least, that period of time. Both the habits we create and the supplements we take are also going to help us cleanse on a cellular level, which is all the better for us. More about that in a moment but let's continue talking about the liver.

Green Juices

Again, when looking at the liver, we see a lot of health issues that arise related to a lack of oxygen being present. Which I suggest as others do, happens anywhere and everywhere in the body. In a 2015 paper published in the journal Evidence-Based Complementary and Alternative Medicine researchers at Sichuan University found that reduction-oxidation (redox) represents a crucial background of various liver disorders. The answer to this is our good friend's *anti*oxidants. The research reveals, as suggested elsewhere in this book, that green leafy vegetables are the best for liver health. The flavonoid saponarin, which gives leaves their green colour, was shown to demonstrate powerful antioxidant potencies with therapeutic effects on various cancers and inflammations. Besides that, there is the saying in traditional Chinese medicine: "the dark-green coloured falls into liver meridian." And who am I to argue with ancient people who seem to know a little more than us 'modern' humans about how to tackle healthcare!

And so, at least while detoxifying the liver make a green vegetable juice part of your daily routine. It would be awesome if this simply becomes part of you and your family's life forever. Best if made at home, but if not possible, then buy from an independent organic cafe that you trust. Oh, and make sure the vegetables they use are actually organic. I have seen dodgy business practices aplenty even at the local level of business. While I was living in Sydney, there was a rapidly growing chain of health food stores and cafes that used organic coffee, but cleverly made their sign and menus to look as if the entire menu was organic when in reality it was only the coffee! They have since been served their rather large dose of karma and went from 9 stores to zero overnight because of lawsuits aplenty...

Detoxification Of Fat Cells

Back to detoxifying on a cellular level and what you can do. The scariest toxins are those that are soaked up by the fat cells in your body, which are known as persistent organic pollutants (POPs). These are the harshest of man-made chemicals such as DDT, that accumulate over time in the adipose tissue and cause a multitude of issues including weight gain and reproductive, developmental, behavioural, neurologic, endocrine, and immunologic adverse health effects.

You'll find most POPs in the non-organic food that you eat...mmm tasty!

One thing we need to understand is that the toxins that head to your liver are broken down into water-soluble toxins. This means you can eliminate the toxins through perspiration, urination, respiration and excretion. That is how your body becomes *pure*. The toxins that are soaked up by your fat cells are fat-soluble. The difference is like having a dirt stain on your white shirt versus an oil stain. You can run a dirt stain under a tap, and the water will help clean the stain. You can run an oil stain under a tap for a week, and it won't make a blind bit of difference!

The same can be said of water-soluble toxins versus fat-soluble toxins. Water-soluble are relatively easy to remove. To help your body in the elimination of said toxins, you can sweat them out in an infra-red sauna or exercise session. And drink more water to urinate them out. Fat-soluble toxins that are bound to your fat cell membrane can be a little more difficult.

In a 2013 paper published in the journal Environmental Health Perspectives, it was proven that Adipose Tissue plays a central role in POP toxicology. As your liver struggles to deal with synthetic chemicals that it was never designed to break down in the first place, it becomes overloaded and backs up into the lymphatic system, which is the sewage system of the body. Fat cells are then used as a buffering system to limit the number of toxins in the blood and to prevent them from accumulating in vital organs such as the brain. It is shown that your metabolic programming is then affected, which leads to obesity and metabolic diseases.

As the fat cells soak up the toxins, this causes inflammation (water surrounding the cell), which then inhibits your body's ability to burn the fat cell. Chronic inflammation is another buffering system that your body uses in your fight against toxins and acidity. It does this to neutralise the acidity of the toxins (body water is at seven on the pH scale, which is neutral).

"Inflammation leads to every one of the major chronic diseases of ageing — heart disease, cancer, diabetes, dementia, and more. It's also by far the major contributor to obesity. Being fat is being inflamed — period!" - Mark Hyman

Burning fat is so-called because you need the same three conditions as starting a fire. You need fuel (*most people have plenty of extra fuel they could do with burning!*), you also need heat and oxygen to reach a fat cell to burn it. When you workout, the body is attempting to burn fat for energy, and so your breathing rate increases to get more oxygen into the body. Your core temperature also increases, and you start to sweat as your body generates more heat. However, when trying to burn the fat cells that are inflamed, it may seem an impossible task to do so.

Just like you struggle to breathe underwater, your cells struggle to receive the optimum amount of oxygen when they are inflamed. And so chronic inflammation links back to every major disease, including obesity because oxygen is, of course, key to life. That's why throughout this book, we keep seeing studies showing lack of oxygen equals ill health and disease.

Now try this, place the back of your hand on your forehead, it's warm. (Hopefully, otherwise, this is one of the times Western Medicine has its place, and you need to go and see a Medical Doctor immediately!) Your forehead is warm because it has great circulation and therefore a good supply of oxygen and heat. Now place the back of your hand on your upper arm near the armpit. It's cool, because of the water surrounding the fat cells. What you see here is inflammation near the major lymph node area of your armpit, where around 100 lymph nodes are located close to the surface of the skin. As your lymphatic system slowly becomes sluggish and overloaded with toxins, it has to start storing the toxins elsewhere, and since fat cells are not a vital organ, they become the perfect place. The lymph nodes become an exit point of the lymphatic system at which point the fat cells in the lymph node areas start to soak up the toxins. Have you ever seen anyone with a fat forehead? Nope. Ever seen anyone (especially the ladies, sorry ladies) with large upper arms that no amount of tricep exercises seem to fix? Of course, you have.

Other problem areas for the ladies are the inner thighs. Another major lymph node area, having another 100 located close to the surface of the skin. As inflammation rises from the fatty adipose tissue holding onto POPs in these areas, it makes it damn difficult to burn the fat. It also makes it impossible to tone because water has no frequency. No amount of sitting on the silly leg squeeze machine at the gym trying desperately to work the adductor muscle will ever tone a wobbly inner thigh! Because the muscle is not the problem, it's the *water*. No amount of cardio exercise will burn the fat, because it's not fat, its inflamed fat cells surrounded by water, and because water has no calories, you can't burn it. The fuel within the fat cell needs heat to burn, to which I ask a simple question, have you ever managed to start a log fire underwater? I'm guessing not.

Half of your 500-700 lymph nodes are located in the abdomen area. Where's most people's biggest problem area, men and women alike? That's right, the abdomen area. Think about it for a moment. Where is the first area of the body that people lose weight from when they go on a diet?...That's right, the *face*. People go on a diet on the weekend and already on Monday morning people are saying, "My word, you look incredible! Have you lost weight?" You're looking down at your belly saying, "Noooooo"...but they are looking at your face. An area again with excellent circulation. Another area ladies always complain about losing weight from is their *boobs*. Ladies let me tell you *one* thing; No one wants you to lose weight from there...No one!

Your mind is incredible. You can have goals, dreams, wants and wishes. But your body is built for two things: reproduction and survival. You get frostbite, and your fingers fall off. That's how good your body is at surviving and keeping the vital organs going. Yet when it comes to losing weight, you lose weight from your chubby cheeks and not the abdomen? An area that is putting huge amounts of pressure on your heart and other vital organs. It makes no sense. Your body wants to lose the fat that is the biggest danger to your survival first, but it can't, because of the *inflammation* caused by *toxins*.

We get rid of the toxins; we get rid of the water; we lose our belly fat.

It really is that simple. You see women (used to be) of a certain age with cellulite (that lumpy, dimpled flesh that begins to look like either orange peel or in some cases cottage cheese...). Where do we see it? The buttocks, thighs, upper arms and abdomen area, exactly where your major lymph nodes are located closest to the surface of the skin. Why only (usually) women, one reason is that men's skin is 25% thicker. And so as inflammation rises from toxicity; nonetheless, women with their thinner skin start to see dimples in their skin. That is not to say men don't have 'cellulite'. Maybe not where it is visible on the surface of the skin, but inflammation around the fat cells in the abdomen is undoubtedly there, and so they will struggle with all their might to burn that fat just like women find it a struggle to get rid of cellulite. It ends up being far more dangerous to men than women, as the inflammation and thicker skin create a large hard belly, almost like a balloon. This then puts immense amounts of pressure on the heart, and so in general men suffer hearts attacks at a younger age than women.

You may have noticed I said, 'used to be' women of a certain age because as we see obesity rise in children, I am also regularly asked by teenage girls about the cellulite problem that they have. More often it's slimmer girls, as I think larger set girls think it's normal to have cellulite at any age when they are overweight and so don't even question it. This in itself shows cellulite is not a fat problem; it's an *acid* and a *toxicity* problem. It used to be ladies who had reached the menopause who struggled with cellulite, because of lower collagen levels, the accumulation of toxins and an increased rate of skin thinning. But each year that has passed cellulite has affected younger and younger people.

People used to talk about a middle-age spread and used the excuse that they had become 40 years old. Then thirty became the new forty. Now, sadly, we see weight problems and toxicity problems in teenagers and even children. It's so sad, and now as you'll see since you've had your eyes opened, the media try to pass it off as being 'normal'. Fuck that it's not normal, no matter what, for teenagers to have cellulite and children to be overweight. For yet more proof that this is an inflammation problem, grab the fat around your thigh near the knee. This is a place where lymph nodes are *not* situated near the surface of the skin. You can also pinch the fat on your forearm. Both will feel firm because it's fat. Now feel the fat around your belly. It feels like a waterbed because that's exactly what it is!

Again, there are many a medical website who say toxins do not cause cellulite. However, they go on to give either no or half-arsed explanations for what causes it, usually stating that no one knows! I feel like the explanation I gave makes the most sense. Researchers from the University of Pavia, Italy found that areas of cellulite have a significantly reduced amount of adiponectin, a hormone that has anti-inflammatory effects and one which increases blood flow to fat cells. However, no one says why that might be. If I may theorise for a moment; that may be because the fat cells are now dealing with manmade chemicals such as endocrine disruptors in such vast quantities, it struggles with its usual function.

Can we really load the body with more and more synthetic chemicals, that don't break down in the body or the environment and expect it to be all *fine* and *flipping dandy*, and continue on as normal?

Now, if like me, you want to cleanse your fat cells, you have to limit your exposure to POPs. Don't worry, I've done the hard work and found out where the majority of POPs occur. There was a list of the dirty dozen POPs released in 2001 at the Stockholm Convention. 10 of the 12 were pesticides, insecticides and fungicides.

Plain and simple, if you want to lose weight and dramatically improve your health. *Go Organic!*

To make up the rest of the list, one was our old friend PCBs, and the other is from pollution in the air. There's no point cleansing if toxins are coming in as quickly as you get rid of them. It has been shown that weight loss reduces the appearance of cellulite and has been shown in a separate study that burning fat gets rid of toxins, namely PCBs. So losing weight will help the body get rid of POPs, lowering inflammation levels and therefore the appearance of cellulite.

A paper published in The International Journal of Cosmetic Medicine showed weight loss improved the cellulite severity, although in obese subject's skin dimpling does not seem to change appreciably. They also showed cellulite had been treated successfully through massages. Yet more evidence that we need regular massage while detoxing and on an ongoing basis. *At least* once per month (if finances allow once per week is preferable) and more often than that if you are detoxing. The other thing to take note of here is the fact that the appearance of cellulite doesn't seem to change purely through weight loss in the obese. Meaning, do not let it get to that stage if you are not already. And if you are obese don't worry, we are not simply losing weight here, we are also going to purge your fat of toxins giving you the greatest chance of at least decreasing the appearance of cellulite and more importantly improving your health.

Researchers at Skidmore College, New York found that intermittent fasting not only achieves long-term weight loss but also helps release toxins from the body fat stores in the form of PCBs. It also enhances heart health and reduces oxidative stress. Intermittent fasting we know has a detoxifying effect by giving the digestive system a rest allowing it to eliminate backed up waste and now we can see it lowers inflammation by releasing at the very least PCBs from fat stores. We know this because it was shown to reduce oxidative stress and where you find oxidative stress, you find inflammation.

And finally, a brilliant bit of research that ties it all together. You see, all over the internet, you are told that cellulite is purely cosmetic, which of course is completely unacceptable in today's world of vanity! However, you are also told that it is nothing to worry about from a health perspective if you can't afford the expensive and unproven methods. Which of course I believe to be completely untrue as the changes that we are seeing in people of a younger and younger age, in a world that is more and more toxic leads me to believe that it is a *health* problem and not just a cosmetic problem.

Researchers the Medical University of Lodz, Poland completely agree, and I have to say this is the most in-depth researched I've found on the subject. They found where there was cellulite there was also circulatory problems and disorders in the endocrine system. They state, 'The involvement of many complex mechanisms of the body implies that cellulite is not only a cosmetic issue but also develops as a result of interdisciplinary homeostatic disorders.' At last, some common sense! Great work.

So, cleansing the fat cells will help both men and women to lose weight from the 'stubborn' areas such as the hips, thighs, arms and abdomen. It will also help women reduce the appearance of cellulite. Detoxifying both the liver and the fat cells will, of course, dramatically improve your health, metabolism, energy levels and lower your risk of many lifestyle diseases. We've already seen to do this that we need to lose weight. Implementing intermittent fasting as part of your healthy lifestyle (and not a diet) is a great way to do this. We also need to add green juices into our daily routine. A regular massage will help too. Daily exercise would be amazing as well, even if it's just a walk to get your heart rate up, body sweating and lymphatic system moving. Park your car further away from work. Get off the bus a stop early. Take the stairs. Whatever it is, *move* your body daily.

Detox Supplements

Back to the subject of supplements of which I have seen with my own two eyes and felt in the very depths of my body are absolutely essential when it comes to detoxification. Food and exercise just are not going to cut it. I point out to people who claim, 'I'm going to detox through food and exercise' - There are more gyms and more diets and information about nutrition in the world than ever before. Yet, more people are overweight than at any other point in history. That is why in this book, on my website and in seminars, I go into so much more detail than the usual subjects of diet and exercise.

If you've tried some of the plants and herbal extracts already mentioned in this book, you'll know the power of plants. You can taste just a couple of drops of Oil of Oregano extract in half a litre of water, yet to get the same power from oregano the herb will take you eating a small mountain of the stuff. Eating tons of alkaline spinach is okay, but at the end of the day, you are simply piling more food onto a problem caused by food. That's why we need something far more potent to detox properly. Then the alkaline food you eat and the exercise you do is your maintenance program.

As previously mentioned the use of medicinal plants based on ancient teachings is an excellent, drug-free (therefore mostly side effect free) and scientifically proven method to healing disease and ailments. Similarly, other organisms coming from all over Earth show properties we need for detoxification, and we will use both in our quest to detoxify the body.

Find the following in supplement form, either individually or in specialised detox blends using the same rules when reading the labels as described in Chapter 9: SupplementNation. There are many hundreds of plants and organisms I could write about, but I don't want to fill the book with pages and pages of proven remedies. The following plants and organisms have been used successfully for thousands of years by people, based on both ancient and modern 'scientific' reports and so are a fantastic place to start. I'll also throw in some botanical detoxifiers that you can go straight out into your garden and find right there amongst the grass. You can make your own detox teas to help things along, with some of these cost-free little beauties.

Algae

As part of a detoxification program, the first organism you may want to consider supplementing with is algae. One of algae's major roles in nature is to clean the lakes, rivers and oceans from pollutants. Algae help to purify water by absorbing pollutants such as heavy metals, which is something we most definitely want to rid the body of. Algae has even been shown to soak up oils spills in the ocean. A word of warning though, if allergic to seafood and especially iodine, algae might *not* be the best choice for you.

Microalgae have been used as a supplement for nutrition for thousands of years. Chinese populations used it two thousand years ago to survive during famine. Spirulina is a highly popular source of algae today but was first harvested from lakes by the Aztecs in the sixteenth century. Spirulina (*Arthrospira*) is the algae that are most well known for its benefits and helping human survival or wellness in today's day and age. This is due to it having every vitamin, mineral and trace element needed on a day to day basis and its exceptionally high protein content and beautifully balanced essential amino acid composition.

Now back to those persistent fat-soluble toxins that can hang around for years if we don't help the body get rid of them and the fact that algae clean up oil spills. Researchers at the Indian Insitute of Technology showed the sorption rate of algae on diesel was *instant*. The toxins around your fat cells are fat-soluble as is oil. To help the body get rid of fat-soluble toxins we need to introduce something that has the ability to break them down. Nothing in nature cleans quite as well as algae does.

As already shown, there's increasing concerns over oxidative stress-mediated diseases and so in Eastern medicine at least there is a natural gravitation to herbal and botanical medications rich in antioxidants. There's now lots of evidence in some cases that algae are even more potent than medicinal plants, and that's one of the reasons it tops our list of natural detoxifiers. An in-depth joint study from the Universiti Putra Malaysia and the University of Texas found marine resources such as microalgae have compounds with higher bioactivity than terrestrial plants. This is generally attributed to their ability to survive under extremely oxidizing conditions which increase cellular antioxidant contents, which is exactly what we need to detoxify. We need something that can survive the harsh environment of firstly the acid in the stomach, followed by toxin soaked fat cells and finally, the chemical filtration centre of the body - the liver.

There's plenty of evidence that algae are amazing for human health, with more than 4000 studies now having being performed. Algae has been found to have many bioactive compounds that are needed for optimal health, including various carotenoids and previously, mentioned omega-3 fatty acids. Algae has been proven to be a natural source of potent antioxidant, anti-inflammatory, anticancer, and antiviral properties which can prevent disease rather than turning to synthetic supplements and drugs to cover up symptoms. You can buy algae supplements in either capsule or powder form, again, following the usual rules of adequately reading the labels and avoiding toxic ingredients. Once again, just like fish oil, you need to be clear where your algae are sourced from, as the cheaper stuff will usually be from dirty waters. The more expensive stuff, but far more effective and safe will be either from organic sources or places like Klamath Lake, Oregon that sits high up in the mountains with minimal pollution. Many scientists have proven once again that supplements are absolutely necessary not only for detoxification but overall health, and algae supplements are potentially the most powerful of them all...

Milk Thistle *(Silybum marianum)*

Milk Thistle is the most well-researched plant in the treatment of liver disease and is used all over the world to treat liver problems. Interesting fact; traditional stories say it is so-called because a drop of Virgin Mary's breast milk fell upon the leaves. How does it help your liver detox along, I hear you say? Researchers at University Magna Graecia, Catanzaro, Italy found the three main active compounds in Milk Thistle, known as silymarin act as an antioxidant by reducing free radical production. It also has antifibrotic properties and inhibits the binding of toxins to the liver cell membranes. Antifibrotic means Milk Thistle stops the scarring and damage of tissue, this along with it inhibiting the binding of toxins means the liver can run smoothly and get its many roles in the body done without having damage inflicted on it.

You can take Milk Thistle in a variety of ways. I like the tincture approach, which is how I like to take Tom Dennis' three recommended herbal medications from Chapter 8: Trust Me, I'm *Not* A Doctor. However, if the taste completely repels you, try taking capsules with 150 milligrams twice a day while detoxifying the liver. Of course, read the label and make sure it is pure Milk Thistle; otherwise, that would completely go against the entire idea of detoxification!

The next three supplements will make most people think I've finally lost it! Mainly because if you had a childhood like me, these were seen as weeds. Unsightly things to have in the garden! And if I were seen blowing the little white poofy looking seeds from one of these 'weeds' as we used to when we wanted to 'make a wish', my father would be very upset as I was spreading the 'weed' everywhere. However! All three of the following have huge amounts of health benefits and will most certainly help your body detoxify.

Make sure you are not picking any of the following medicinal plants from an area that has been sprayed with weed killer. If searching anywhere near roads, pick plants as far back as possible from the road as they will readily soak up pollution. Basically, go organic when picking your 'weeds'.

Dandelion *(Taraxacum)*

Dandelion has been used as a medicinal herb from as early as 900 AD in many different cultures. Researchers at Sichuan University, China list dandelions as a plant with protective effects for the liver. In a paper published in the Journal of Pharmacy and Pharmacology looking at the effectiveness of herbal teas and their ability to detoxify, researchers found a dramatic increase in the activity of a detoxifying enzyme in a group of people drinking dandelion tea. In another paper published in the Journal of Alternative and Complementary Medicine looking at the diuretic properties of dandelion found a significant increase in participants urination and so it decreased water weight and bloating. And because of dandelion having high amounts of potassium, the electrolytes are replaced immediately making it far more effective and beneficial than synthetic medication. So go on out into the garden and get yourself some dandelions!

To make **Dandelion Detox Tea**, you can try the following simple recipe;

1. Thoroughly clean your dandelions.

2. Use it all. The flowers, leaves, stems, and roots are all beneficial.

3. Place about 2 cups into a saucepan.

4. Cover it with 4 cups of water.

5. Bring to the boil, then take off the heat and cover using a lid.

6. Allow to steep for 3 hours or even better, overnight.

7. Strain out the dandelions and use water for your Dandelion Detox Tea.

8. Dilute with more water if it's too strong.

If you want to dry the flowers to use later on in herbal teas, it's best to use **The Solar Method**. See below on how to best dry the roots in the Burdock section.

1. Inspect the flowers for any insects and wash thoroughly.

2. Spread the flowers out on a flat surface inside that gets direct sunlight.

3. The flowers will dry in as little as 1-3 hours.

4. Don't over-dry as the flower will seed and turn into a white poofy looking thing, the one we used to love blowing all over my father's garden.

5. You will know they are ready when the flowers close slightly, and the petals look dry.

Burdock *(Arctium)*

Another ghastly 'weed' with detoxification properties is burdock. Burdock has been used therapeutically in Europe, North America and Asia for hundreds of years. Researchers at The Hong Kong Polytechnic University found that the root has active ingredients that detoxify the blood and promote blood circulation to the skin surface. This, in turn, improves the quality of the skin and can help heal the skin from diseases like eczema. Again we also find potent antioxidants and even anti-diabetic compounds. In the seeds, there can be found active ingredients that possess anti-inflammatory effects and can even have potent inhibitory effects on the growth of tumours.

To make **Burdock Detox Tea**, you can try the following simple recipe;

1. Wash the roots thoroughly.

2. Cut them up into small pieces.

3. In a saucepan, combine 3-4 tbsp of fresh burdock roots and 3 cups of water.

4. Let simmer for 10 minutes, covered.

5. Add fennel seed and let simmer for an additional 5 minutes.

6. Strain herbs and drink your Burdock Detox Tea.

There you have it. As simple as that and you can have cleaner blood flowing to every cell in your body. I even learned something new during my research about eczema there! I'll let you know how I go if my eczema ever flares up again and I use some Burdock Tea to clear it up.

If wanting to dry the roots and use later, not only in tea but soups and stews etc. roots are best dried using **The Oven Method**.

1. Wash the roots thoroughly.

2. Cut up the roots or grate them.

3. Place on an oven tray.

4. Heat up the oven to 200°F and then turn the oven off.

5. Leave the door open for air to circulate.

6. Store the roots in an airtight container. If well dried they won't rot.

Stinging Nettle *(Urtica dioica)*

This one has some painful memories for me. Many a time being stung as a child while out playing, building dens etc. Not knowing that this sometimes irritating 'weed' had so many health benefits. So when going out to harvest some Stinging Nettles make sure you are wearing long clothing and gloves! And a little tip from my proofreader (my father), the sting of nettles can be eased by using another common 'weed' and rubbing dock leaves (*Rumex obtusifolius*) onto the area. I remember doing this, and it worked a treat!

Again for centuries, different cultures around the world have used the Stinging Nettle for detoxification. In a paper published in the Journal of Ethnopharmacology, researchers at the Université Mohammed Premier, Morocco showed it's diuretic properties during testing. For ladies who suffer from painful premenstrual symptoms, it's been shown to give relief from cramping and bloating. It has also been used to help asthma sufferers for generations in Australia, as shown by researchers for the HerbalScience Group in Florida who found it to be effective in reducing allergic and other inflammatory responses.

To make **Nettle Tea**, you can try the following simple recipe;

1. Thoroughly wash the nettles wearing gloves!

2. Place about 2 cups into a saucepan.

3. Cover it with 4 cups of water.

4. Bring to the boil, then take off the heat and cover using a lid.

5. Allow to steep for 3 hours or even better, overnight.

6. Pour through a strainer and use the liquid as your tea.

7. The sting should be gone from the plant which can be used for soups or stews but check with your fingers first.

8. Dilute your tea with more water if it's too strong.

If wanting to dry the nettles for use later, it's best to use a dehydrator if you are fortunate enough to own one or using **The Hanging Method** which is as follows;

1. Place into bunches of 5 stems that are tied together using kitchen string.

2. Hang in a clean, dry and dark place.

3. It can take anywhere from 1-3 weeks to fully dry, depending on moisture levels in your chosen room.

4. Make sure they are completely dry before storing in airtight containers.

And there you have it, three detoxifying plants with lots of other health benefits that most people can find in their very own garden. The next method of detoxification that we would benefit hugely from incorporating into any detox you do, should be easy enough to find for most people. Now onto what tools you can use to detoxify your body.

Detox Tools

Infrared Sauna

Before the invention of infrared saunas, hot air baths and sweat lodges were used by various cultures, including Native Americans, Eastern Europeans and the Chinese to relieve stress and detoxification. Infrared Saunas are now seen as the best type of sauna as they have the ability to penetrate through the skin and have positive changes in the body on a *cellular level*. They have been shown to remove harsh toxins stored in your fat cells.

Researchers at RMIT University, Melbourne, Australia found considerable evidence to suggest that sauna bathing can induce profound physiological effects. On a cellular level, they found a reduction in oxidative stress and inflammation and a significant improvement in circulation. An Infrared Sauna delivers far-infrared light wave radiation (FIR) deep down into the body, without any need for bands (which have commonly been used and are widely recognised as having healing effects especially on inflammation). FIR is a natural and beneficial type of radiation. Researchers at Harvard Medical School found FIR stimulates cells and tissue and considers it a promising treatment modality for certain medical conditions.

Infrared saunas are capable of causing dramatic changes in body chemistry. They have helped people with many chronic problems related to pain, inflammation, low energy and poor circulation. It is a fast and easy way to help your body detoxify on a cellular level, with 15-20 minutes being a sufficient amount of time to see positive changes. Unlike other types of saunas, infrared lamp saunas penetrate the skin and heat the body from the inside-out, which means they don't cause too much heat in the room and so are far easier to bear for some people who can't deal with too much heat seen in traditional saunas. When doing a detoxification program, having a sauna on a daily basis is best, however, if this is a struggle time wise, aim for at least three times per week. In a world of constant exposure to synthetic chemicals, having regular saunas is something necessary to keep the body healthy.

Dry Skin Brushing

As far as dry skin brushing (sometimes known as body brushing) goes, it is a simple two-five minutes that you should add to your daily morning routine as part of a detox protocol. It is also something that I would carry on as a daily habit. When people are getting swollen ankles, most of the time it is down to poor circulation and poor lymphatic drainage. To combat this and to help exfoliate your skin, aid digestion and help almost every bodily system - dry skin brush. The simple act of brushing lightly over your skin upwards on each section of the body *at least* ten times towards your heart each morning will help boost your circulation, improve lymphatic drainage and aid the body with detoxification.

Dry Skin Brushing Method

1. Start by brushing the bottom of your feet, where there is a map located of the entire body as per reflexology; this will help stimulate every organ and system to get you going for the day.

2. Move onto the top of the feet and ankles.

3. Then the calves.

4. Followed by the thighs and buttocks (paying special attention and a little more time on any areas where you suffer from cellulite).

5. Then do the upper arms.

6. Followed by the back.

7. For your abdominal area brushing 20 times in a clockwise direction will help digestion and your body to eliminate first thing in a morning.

Having a bowel movement first thing is something that a lot of people struggle with and so to give your body a natural, helping hand to make you go first thing on a morning is an amazing thing. When you are asleep, this is when a lot of detoxification happens as your body is at rest, and it can focus on the breaking down of toxins. And so, eliminating said toxins on a morning is key to better health.

Dry skin brushing will help this process along with another little trick. Every single 'hippy' type I've spoken to has done this, and it works fantastically well! That thing is to sit on the toilet for 5 minutes every morning until your brain connects with your body (your intestines are a muscle, and so that mind to muscle connection is a very real thing) and you poo. If you don't go the first time, don't worry, keep repeating the 5 minutes per morning until it becomes a natural thing for you to have a bowel movement first thing.

Finding a good body brush is not as simple as buying the first one you see. It needs to be made of 100% natural ingredients, have tough bristles and be built to last. That means there are not many out there that are any good. One rule to keep it performing at its best is to not get it wet. If it gets wet, it goes soft. Much like a particular male body part, the benefits will be not as apparent if it has gone soft. I use **Tea Tree Spray** to keep my brush clean. Simply add filtered water and some pure tea tree (*Melaleuca alternifolia*) essential oil in a spray bottle to make your own spray. A couple of pumps each time you use it *without* soaking the brush will kill any unwanted germs.

Detox Protocols

Let's talk about detoxification programs you can go on starting with the shortest and easiest to complete, ending with the longest one in which you have to be the most dedicated.

Juice Cleanse

Probably the most well-known type of detox is a Juice Cleanse, which will give the digestive system a rest so it can eliminate the buildup of toxins and will flood your body with nutrients and antioxidants. Juices can contain both fruit and vegetables. However, vegetables should be the main component of any juice, with only lemons, limes, grapefruits, rhubarb, pomegranate and melon being the only fruit that can be used regularly.

A lot of people embark on a Juice Cleanse in order to lose weight. This and all the benefits mentioned have been proven in scientific studies. Researchers at the University of California Los Angeles found that a 3-day juice detox aided in significant weight loss because of the improvements in *intestinal health* and a decrease in *lipid oxidation*.

Oxidation leads to one of three things, the first of which is inflammation, causing the fat cell to hold on to water. It can lead to the cells dying, which is ageing or cell mutation, which leads to disease. This process happens through free radicals (toxins within the body that either naturally occur through processes or are introduced from an outside source) stealing electrons from the fat cells leading to cell damage and mutation. To stop this as mentioned, you can detox to lower the number of free radicals and improve nutrition by increasing the number of antioxidants in the body to protect you against oxidisation. The results continued for at least the following two weeks and probably beyond, but the study did not go further.

Remember where you have inflammation around fat cells you also have a lack of oxygen and therefore a lack of fat burning. Where you have an unhealthy gut, you also have a lack of nutrient absorption. The 3-day juice cleanse also improved circulation leading to every cell in the body, getting more oxygen and nutrients.

At the beginning of your health and detox journey I would recommend doing a 3-day Juice Cleanse twice per year, once in the Spring and once in the Autumn. I would look to slowly build up to doing a 3-day Juice Cleanse once per month to give the digestive system a rest and the body a much needed antioxidant and nutrient boost.

As mentioned, you can also do a 1-day Juice Cleanse as often as once per week especially after a big drinking or binge eating session to help the body recover. If the thought of just having juice seems a bit daunting, have a juice for breakfast and lunch, then a raw, vegan salad with plenty of greens for dinner. Because of the short nature of its length in time, Juice Cleansing is a nice way to dip a toe into the world of detox. It can also be used as part of a lengthier protocol which I regularly will do with clients. As part of your daily routine, I would incorporate a Vegetable Juice as part of your first meal of the day. It is alkaline and will help detoxify the body, especially the liver. Here's my Super Alkaline Liver Detox Juice (a mouthful I know!) recipe with easily found ingredients; here you go...

Super Alkaline Liver Detox Juice

Ingredients

- 1 Large Cucumber (or two small)

- 1 Lime

- 200g French Beans

- 200g Spinach

- Thumb of Ginger

- Thumb of Turmeric

- Fresh Oregano

Method

1. Wash all vegetables and spices thoroughly.

2. Chop cucumber, oregano and spinach into small manageable pieces.

3. Peel lime and chop into small pieces.

4. Leave the skin on ginger and turmeric, just chop into small pieces.

5. Top and tail french beans, then chop in half.

6. Juice ginger and turmeric first.

7. Follow with rest of ingredients.

As always you can check the Resources section to find a fun video of me making this juice. If you haven't already, get started straight away and make juicing a part of your life!

Liver And Fat Cell Detox

Talking of Liver Detoxes, here is what I recommend someone who is looking to properly detoxify their liver and the toxins from your fat cells.

- Go out and get some natural liver detox supplements that are from whole food sources and contain no fillers, binders, sweeteners, preservatives, additives etc. In fact, it should contain no synthetic ingredients whatsoever. The supplements can be a blend of algae and other herbal extracts. Add to this a Milk Thistle extract supplement preferably in the form of a tincture. Do the recommended amount of drops on the label 3x a day. A proper liver detox should, as mentioned last for six months or more. However, if doing this, you need to make sure the supplements you are taking are purely natural. Most importantly make sure they are designed to be taken for that long, and of course, you should consult your doctor first if you have any underlying ailments. If the doctor is completely against the idea because of a lack of knowledge or having a closed mind, then find another doctor.

- Drink at least a gallon of filtered, bottled (at the source) or your very own spring water per day.

- Kick start your detox with a 3-day Juice Cleanse using only vegetable juices. Repeat at the 3-month stage once your body has gone through one of its natural 90-day cycles.

- You have to strictly eat at least 80% alkaline and only drink alcohol for a *maximum* of 2 days per week. Preferably go 21 straight days with no alcohol to develop new habits. No cheating (beyond your 20% treats)! If you are committed, six months is a long time I know, but do it to the very end. The difference you will feel in just energy levels and focus will almost blow your mind if you do this properly.

- Implement the Intermittent Fasting routine that suits you best, choosing between a full 24 hours fast for two days of the week or daily time-restricted feeding. If choosing to do a full 24-hour fast, still take your detox supplements if they contain no calories but look at spreading them out throughout the day so they are not too overpowering to the body. If doing a fasting window, look to eat during a six hour window but have your vegetable juice 2 hours before the window starts on an empty stomach.

- Have a Super Alkaline Liver Detox Juice every morning before any food. You can swap out any of the ingredients for other green vegetables, grasses, herbs etc. you can get your hands on to mix it up.

- Do at least three Infrared Sauna sessions per week.

- Try doing at least three Colonics in your first 7-14 days. This is a must for your next detox, and I know it's strange to ask when doing a Liver Detox but remember everything in your body is connected.

- A weekly massage is best, but if not doable for whatever reason aim for at least once per month.

- Exercise daily. Walking for 20 minutes is enough if you are not able to commit to anything else. The 20-minute workouts available on TomBroadwell.com are the best for overall benefits.

There you have it - a simple, clean way of living for six months that will make you feel incredible. If you think about it, six months is not a large amount of time in the whole scheme of things. But if it adds years, even decades onto your healthspan and years onto your life, allowing you to see your grandchildren grow up, walk your daughter down the aisle and move around freely in a strong, lean body, then it is well worth it, no?

Candida Cleanse

Here we have the daddy of them all which doubles as your Colon Cleanse protocol. It is a must-do if you want to have optimal health. Candida is a yeast overgrowth that happens in the gut in today's world of highly processed, sugar-laden food and pharmaceutical drugs. Namely antibiotics and the massive overprescription and misprespcribing of said antibiotics. The CDC states, 'Antibiotic resistance is one of the biggest public health challenges of our time.' A 2013 report done by the CDC, 'sounded the alarm to the danger of antibiotic resistance, stating that each year in the US, at least 2 million people get an antibiotic-resistant infection, and at least 23,000 people die.'

Studies have shown that antibiotics are misprescribed 30-60% of the time, for viruses when they only have any effect on bacteria. In my research on placebos, I found that it is common for doctors do this on purpose as they know the mind will cure the problem regardless of the medicine prescribed. Next time you are getting prescribed antibiotics, remember to ask if you have a viral or bacterial infection because you don't want to be taking antibiotics for the sake of it. Plus at this point, I've shown you plenty of herbal based remedies that will get the job done when it comes to viral infections without the side effects.

Researchers at the University of Nigeria state, 'Antibiotic use is by far the commonest cause of Candida overgrowth. Overgrowth of candida results from factors that disrupt the intestinal microbial balance, such as the use of antibiotics. Of 208 participants who had taken antibiotics within three weeks of the study, 42.3% had candidiasis compared to 20.8% of those with no recent history of antibiotic use.' Once there is an imbalance of bad gut bacteria versus good gut bacteria inside your digestive system, the bad starts to take over. This overgrowth of bad bacteria is candida yeast overgrowth. Candida lives on sugar, so once antibiotics have done the original damage and basically killed off most of your good gut flora, candida only gets stronger with the massive amount of sugar our modern diet contains.

Eastern medicine recognises that candida albicans and candidiasis are responsible for a vast amount of disease, yet most people reading this from the West will never have even heard of candida let alone have been told by their doctor it might well be the reason for their health issues. Researchers from a paper published in Nature Reviews Immunology found that 98% of patients with cancer had fungi in their blood. *Ninety-Eight Percent.* That's not a small number and should motivate you to remove candida if you want to avoid cancer. It won't be easy, and so I urge you to remember numbers like that one as motivation. Another paper published in Science Translational

Medicine showed that candida is responsible for about 400,000 life-threatening infections per annum worldwide with a mortality as high as 40%. The West admits it's responsible for the obvious health problems such as oral thrush and vaginitis yet rarely mentions it as life-threatening or remotely linked to cancer. Yet it is more than likely the cause of everything from bad breath to diabetes through to every single digestive issue and of course cancer.

You might be ready right now to tackle the Candida Cleanse, or it might be a full year or two until you are ready. If you are new to detoxing, I recommend doing the Liver Cleanse first as you have leeway and don't need to be perfect. The Candida Cleanse, however, is a case of if you fuck up once, you have to start again. I can't express that enough, if you cheat, once, even with a tiny bit of sugar, you have truly screwed everything up, and it's time to start the whole process again. Eat sugar in any form, and you have fed the candida which will quickly multiply. You have to *starve* it to death.

This process literally has you dreaming of accidentally eating a chocolate bar and you waking up so disappointed in yourself because you have to start again. I once had a dream so vivid, which involved me actually queueing up and patiently waiting for my turn, with each person in front of me ordering at the restaurant bar I worked at until it came to me and for the first time in years I ordered and then ate a Crunchie which is an English candy bar. I woke up absolutely gutted thinking it had happened the day before and went to work in a very bad mood, asking myself why did the server even give me the bar when everyone knew I was detoxing. Of course, it was just a dream, but this detox truly messes with your mind. You better be ready for war when you embark on this for the next 3-6 months. I'll get to the protocol in a minute, but I have to say first;

When you do this detox, you will know 100% that detox works.

You will feel your body detoxing in such a way that when you have Candida 'die-offs', you will need to sleep, *right now*. If you are already sat down in a place that you feel relaxed, you might even fall asleep and wake up hours later, not knowing where you are or remembering falling asleep at all. Just a warning, but the sleep is so deep at random points of the day you will struggle to wake up. But as scary as this is, once through the first few weeks, you will sleep better than you ever have. You will have focus and train of thought you'd think was only reserved for geniuses. You will not crave a single food. You will have insane energy levels even on minimal sleep and basically feel better than you ever have. Ever.

The Candida Cleanse Protocol is tough, and you have to be perfect, but my gosh is it worth it.

- Find Candida supplements that contain no fillers, binders, sweeteners, sugar, artificial additives etc.

- Along with these take Oregano Oil in water. (Absolutely horrendous flavour and amazing how powerful so little is in a large glass of water but get it down!)

- Take Garlic Capsules, following the above recommendations for which ones you purchase.

- Drink at least a gallon of filtered, bottled water (at the source) or your very own spring water per day.

- Know that this will take a minimum of 3 months to complete. Most people will need more. You can get tested for Candida Albicans, search for someone near you who does this. If not available, go with how you feel.

- Get a course of a minimum of at least 3 Colonics in your first 3-5 days. After that have one per week for the first six weeks and then one per month as part of your maintenance program.

- Your nutrition must contain NO sugar in any form, meaning zero processed foods, no starches such as rice, wheat, potatoes, cereals etc. Starchy vegetables to avoid are yams, squash, sweet potatoes, peas, parsnips, carrots, pumpkin etc.

- No sugar also means zero fruit!

- It also means no gluten-containing grains such as wheat, barley, spelt, and even rice and oats that get contaminated from neighbouring fields.

- You should not have any unfiltered tap water meaning you need to and hopefully, already own a filter jug and a shower filter.

- You should have zero of the following; caffeine, dairy, alcohol, sugar, sweeteners either synthetic or natural including fructose, xylitol etc. (other than 100% organic stevia)

- Do not consume any non-organic meat. Do not consume pork or shellfish, even if labelled organic.

- You *can* eat organic meat and wild-caught fish.

- You can eat all organic vegetables other than starchy vegetables.

- You can eat the following gluten-free grains - quinoa, buckwheat, millet and amaranth.

- You can eat lemon, lime, grapefruit and rhubarb.

- You can drink filtered water, bottled water (at the source) and organic herbal teas.

- Implement the Intermittent Fasting routine that suits you best, choosing between a full 24 hours fast for two days of the week or daily time-restricted feeding. If choosing to do a full 24-hour fast, still take your detox supplements if they contain no calories but look at spreading them out throughout they day so they are not too overpowering to the body. If doing a fasting window, look to eat during a six hour window but have your vegetable juice 2 hours before the window starts on an empty stomach.

- After six weeks you can introduce one tart granny smith apple per day as a treat. (And my gosh what a treat! At this point, your taste buds will be set alight by even the faintest bit of sugar.)

- After week ten you may introduce tart berries as a weekly treat (not daily and not going wild with portion sizes) - meaning small amounts of blueberries, blackberries and raspberries are allowed. - The first time I did this detox, I remember eating my first blueberry for ten weeks, and I felt like I was having an orgasm. If you want to feel how food is really meant to taste, do this cleanse!

- When you feel ready, or your tests say your Candida levels are down to normal ranges start to slowly introduce foods. One food, one day at a time at the most, but it is best to leave it three days or so if you have the will power (you've come this far so why not?) and see how you truly feel when introducing that food, but do not introduce 3 in one meal!

- Start with things like sweet potato and then oats. Alkaline fruits like melon that you had to cut out are best to introduce near the beginning too.

- Slowly introduce foods and see how your health is. Keep a food diary, taking note of how you feel after each meal and throughout the day. Do symptoms like poor digestion, skin conditions or low energy return after introducing certain foods? If so, common sense tells me you shouldn't be consuming these foods at all. That is why three days in-between each introduction is best, so you can fully digest and then pinpoint what is causing your health problems.

There you go - the toughest but most rewarding thing regarding health that you're ever likely to do. Give it a go, to lose weight, dramatically reduce your risk of lifestyle diseases such as cancer and give yourself demigod levels of energy and focus. If you don't consume antibiotics again or go back to a sugar-laden diet and you follow almost all the Action Steps in this book on a consistent basis, then you should only have to do something this extreme *once*. Good luck and let me know how you go.

Detox Retreat

From the research I've been doing, there is a large amount of evidence showing some amazing things happen over the course of a 3-week (or longer) *detox retreat,* such people reversing the effects of 'incurable' life-threatening, debilitating, chronic diseases. At the most successful resorts, no chemicals whatsoever are allowed on site. At the gate, you will have your deodorants, anti-ageing creams, perfumes, processed food, cigarettes, or whatever you may have with chemicals in, taken away from you. There is daily exercise, meditation, nutrient-rich meals and herbal medicine in abundance. This form of shorter but intense detox that has a sense of absolute purity will be far more manageable and appealing for many of you who are time-poor. It can also serve as the perfect platform to launch a new lifestyle, or a longer six-month liver cleanse, as new habits are developed over 21 days.

May (my partner) and I are planning (as of 2019) on building a retreat on our newly purchased beach and forest in the Philippines. If you are reading this a few years on from 2020, then it might well be already built so check out the links listed below! At least two 3-week detox retreats will be put on per year, with a couple of 7-day retreats thrown in there for good measure for people who don't have 3-weeks to spare or financially it is too much of a commitment. Beyond that, the rest of the year, it will be the perfect getaway from the busy and toxic world we live in. You can come to see us anytime for a relaxing holiday outside of the set retreats. We are away from all the hustle and bustle, somewhere you can wake up in the forest and walk through the organic gardens down to the beach, for morning meditation or yoga classes. You can head to the herb garden to choose which plants you would like for your spa treatment taking place in front of the ocean. Choose breakfast, lunch and dinner from the organic menu, grown either on the land or freshly caught fish from the sea just in front of the retreat. Order organic herbal tea, wine or beer with your meal. Book a sea excursion to go fishing or sightseeing around The Hundred Islands. Join me on social media or on my website to hear more about updates.

Now as we head into the next section and the Roof of your Health House, it's time to realise that we shouldn't be taking life too seriously. If you're wondering, hang on a minute! A detox retreat selling beer and wine? Yes. Not on the detox retreats obviously, but the rest of the time, yes. Because life is about balance, if you try to be perfect all of the time, you are going to cause yourself stress, and it will always blow back up in your face. Life is about enjoyment and if that means having a beer, a piece of chocolate or a coffee, then do it. Enjoy it in the moment and then move on with your life. The next chapter is all about allowing yourself to enjoy the finer things in life while having an abundance of health and wellbeing.

Resources

Go to **www.TomBroadwell.com/resources** to see;

- A video of how to prepare my Super Alkaline Liver Detox Juice.

- Links to all the supplements I recommend to complete any of the detoxes in this chapter.

- A link to the Body Brush I recommend.

- A link to May and my retreats website to book your holiday or detox retreat.

Action Steps

- Choose (if you haven't already) to take at least 20 minutes to eat each meal, taking time to smell, chew and taste your food.

- Start right now by making a vegetable juice with whatever is in the house. Then make it a daily ritual.

- Buy a body brush and start dry brushing every day as soon as possible!

- Add L-glutamine and Slippery Elm into your supplement regime.

- Get checked for food sensitivities and put into practice eliminating the foods that come up for a while and then reintroducing them slowly. Follow the guidelines of the practitioner doing the test for timeframes etc. This doubles as great practice for your future Candida Cleanse.

- Search online for someone who performs Massage Therapy in your local area and get booked in to see them regularly.

- Search online for someone who performs Colonic Hydrotherapy in your area and book straight in to see them for at least three sessions

- Search online for an Infrared Sauna in your area and book straight in to use it on a regular basis

- Now it's time to detox. Start with a 3-Day Juice Cleanse. Be well prepared, go out and get all the ingredients ready before you start.

- If detoxing months on end sounds a little daunting right now, then book in to do a detox retreat. If you fancy a real break with yours truly, then come and stay with me in the Philippines! (When the retreat is ready mind you).

- Once you've prepared yourself physically and mentally (if you've been following the Action Steps in this book, you will more than likely already be ready!) tackle the Liver and Fat Cell Cleanse.

- Because this Action Step may be in the future, mark it in a calendar for some time in the future, to do the Candida Cleanse. Set yourself a reminder that it is coming up one month before, so you can get prepared!

Section Three

The Roof of Your
Health House

*"The shelter of excuses has a leaky roof." — **Ron Kaufman***

Chapter Thirteen
Your Liver Is A Muscle

*"An intelligent man is sometimes forced to be drunk to spend time with his fools."– **Ernest Hemingway***

It was 11:11 pm,

She sat there in the corner,

Looking out at the guests dancing,

Letting their inhibitions go,

Her uncle twirled the bride across the dance floor,

Everyone danced laughing and smiling,

Much like the children around and in between them,

She slowly sipped on her sparkling water,

She scanned the dance floor for her boyfriend,

He was dancing tipsily in a group doing the cancan,

He had sat with her chatting until his third beer and got up to dance when invited by her mother,

Not having the confidence to go out there,

Longing for the evening to be over so she could go home to bed,

She could feel the stress in her chest,

Wondering whether her practice of teetotalism was all worth it in the end...

Don't get me wrong. There are people who can party without the need for alcohol...or so they say. Haha. Joking, of course, there is! And there are certainly people who don't need alcohol to be more interesting. (In my head I think I'm one of them! But that might come up against some opposition...)

Why?

As part of my 80% being healthy and 20% living life to the max principal, you need room to enjoy yourself. If it comes in the form of alcohol, coffee, chocolate (or indeed any food treats), or smoking plants, then, in my opinion, it's your human right to enjoy those things. As well as teaching the 80/20 principle, I practice a certain openness when I both talk and write and want to tell you that my vice is alcohol. I have a drink to relax, and I love socialising with friends. I can go without eating chocolate for months even though I love it and drink one coffee per day and sometimes will go a few days without any caffeine and won't even notice that I hadn't had one. For me to not have a drink takes real will power, but every year I will do anywhere from 1-6 months with no drinking, usually as part of a detox.

I would never pretend to be perfect, as I love to have a good time. Me pretending to be perfect would cause me a great amount of stress and paint the wrong picture for you. You can have everything you desire when it comes to health and looking good naked by being good *most* of the time. The rest of the time *relax*, it's okay not to be perfect. If you have been painted a picture of some celebrities or online health guru being perfect, I can guarantee you no one is perfect all the time. If that's the persona they want to show to the world, then it's okay, but understand you don't need to be that way.

"The worst thing about being an inspiration is that you have to be perfect." - Anne McDonald

If you were wondering about the title of this chapter, it came from when I was living with two of my best friends in Sydney, Australia. They were over there from England for one year, and as with a lot of English people, they like to drink alcohol as much as me. After talking about the shenanigans I'd been up to at the weekend, one of my Personal Training clients said, "Why do you socialise so much?", using as much wit as I could muster in the moment I answered, "Because your liver is a muscle, and just like every muscle in the body it should be trained hard. 2-3 times a week should be enough to make it good and strong."

Obviously, your liver is not a muscle; I know that! However, the amount of times I speak to people and they claim they're on a detox just because they're not drinking for a month is crazy - as if alcohol is the only toxin that goes into the body! We've definitely cleared the fact up that this is far from the case, but alcohol remains the top of the list as far as what a toxin is in most people's minds. Along with smoking, people will claim, "I don't drink or smoke, so I'm healthy." Pardon?

If you ever saw the documentary Supersize Me, directed by and starring Morgan Spurlock, you would know this not to be true. For the documentary, he ate only McDonald's food for 30-days. His doctor practically begged him to stop while telling him, "Your liver is turning into pate." All his health tests beforehand showed he was healthy and within just 21 days, and having consumed no alcohol, he was already showing signs of a fatty liver. He also had depression, lethargy, no sex drive and headaches, which only stopped when he ate McDonald's. So, there you go, another bunch of reasons not to eat fast food!

How Often?

Back on topic now, and I have to say that obviously drinking every day is not recommended and neither is binge drinking. If you do currently drink every day, what I recommend clients is to start by taking one day off per week. Then the following week take two days off. Then the week after that a third day and if you can add a fourth day in by the end of the month that would be amazing. After a big session, have a day or two off afterwards as it is well worth it to allow your body to recover. If you are going to do either a fast or a juice cleanse each week, try and do it after your big night out - this allows the liver to detoxify and recover properly, and it won't hit your health too hard.

As far as why I chose to use a teetotaller as my opening to this chapter, it is shown that low to moderate drinkers do live longer than teetotallers. Researchers in a study published in The American Journal of Epidemiology found a 10% lower mortality risk for a light drinker consuming 1–29 g/day compared with being teetotal. I think it might have something to do with the stress of not joining in in social events, as discussed in Chapter 1: Mindset Mastery Matters Most, stress is a silent killer. However, if not drinking makes you happy, then stay with it, because I would never recommend anyone to start even light drinking if they currently don't drink.

However, I have to be realistic here. After training and consulting thousands of people over the years, it's clear to me most people are not going to give up their favourite vice. Whether that is alcohol, coffee, or whatever it might be, no matter how many studies are published on how bad it is for them. So, taking that into account let's look at what to drink, as I get asked this question all the time! "So, Tom, if I *do* have a drink, what's the best drink?" Haha! As if I don't know you're going to go out from my Nutrition Consultation and head straight to the bar!

Which Drink Is Best?

My rules go for alcohol (as it does actually for coffee, or chocolate, or smoking plants) as it does with the rest of the food industry. I try and never drink alcohol from large corporations which have all sorts of preservatives, colourings and additives in there, and so if I'm in a bar, I'll ask what the local beer is. If there is an organic option available, I go straight for that. If wine more your thing, look for organic wine or again from smaller independent wineries, with red wine being better than white. If you like to drink hard alcohol with a mixer, anything with sparkling mineral water and some form of citrus is best. But look, if you are on a night out that happens once in a blue moon, and you fancy a whiskey and coke, have it, enjoy it and move on with your life.

As for drinking at home, as mentioned, I was a member of an organic winery, who would send me crates of wine upon request. I have taken many a tour and a tasting with the winery, and they showed me the entire winemaking process and explained how they used organic fertiliser and natural ways of keeping bugs at bay. The most mindblowing thing on any tour I've personally ever done was when the winemaker produced a shiraz from 2003, which was a year when a massive bushfire decimated most winemakers crop. Of the vines that were saved that year came an organic shiraz in which you could still smell the smoke from the fire, which is something I never smelled at any of the other nonorganic vineyards. It makes you think if pesticides and preservatives can kill that, then what else are they killing?

Nutrients, antioxidants and vitamins come to mind straight away. Amazingly organic wine is no more expensive than it's nonorganic counterparts. Also, in the same wine valley, there is an organic vodka distillery. Which is genuinely the finest vodka I've ever tasted!

As for making cocktails at home, get out the juicer, and you can make some truly amazing, fresh and (almost) healthy cocktails. When you come to see May and I at our resort, there will be plenty of super fresh cocktails and mocktails (contain no alcohol) available for you to taste, plus Cocktail Making Classes so you can learn what to do at home. If you want to get started straight away, here is a recipe for my very fresh Almost Alkaline Bloody Mary which is rather tasty I must say!

Almost Alkaline Bloody Mary

Ingredients

- 1 Large Cucumber (or two small)

- 21 Medium Tomatoes

- 7 Sticks of Celery

- 6 Carrots

- 3 Red Bell Peppers

- 1-3 Fresh Chillis (optional and to taste)

- 2 Limes

- 2 tbsps Worcestershire Sauce

- 2 Pinches of Salt

- Black Pepper to taste

- Premium Vodka

Method

1. Wash all vegetables and spices thoroughly.

2. Chop cucumber, tomatoes, celery, carrots, and red bell peppers into small manageable pieces.

3. Peel lime and chop into small pieces.

4. Chop and deseed chillis (or don't if you are a bit of an idiot like me).

5. Juice all the ingredients.

6. Add salt, pepper and Worcestershire sauce to the juice, then stir thoroughly.

7. Pour a 50ml shot of Premium Vodka into a glass then add the juice on top.

8. Stir thoroughly again.

9. Garnish with lime and a celery stick.

10. Enjoy!

If you check out the Resources section there's a fun video of me making this recipe for Papas (May's father) birthday!

So, it really is all out there. If you want pure, organic alcohol, it's available. You simply have to search for it. And as mentioned, beggars can't be choosers so if there's no organic wine or beer available in the bar that you're in, go with a small, local company, and it will likely have less of the bad stuff in there. Same for coffee, chocolate and ice cream, go organic. As for smoking plants that's really not my cup of tea, so use your own noggin when it comes to that one!

Now I know this chapter might bring about some negativity. Shock horror how can a health professional drink let alone say it's okay for me to do! Just being honest and open with you, that's all. Life is about balance. If it has brought about some negative feelings towards me, I'll show you how to get over them in the next chapter and how always to be positive no matter what is happening in the world around you. For now, it's time to take some action and bring about those lifestyle changes.

Resources

Go to **www.TomBroadwell.com/resources** to see;

- A video of my *Almost* Alkaline Bloody Mary recipe.

Action Steps

If you drink more than three times per week cut down by one night over the next seven days, then repeat after that one night per week until you reach 2-3x a week.

- Next time you go out, ask for the local beer or wine.

- Change the coffee you drink at home to organic.

- Change all food treats such as chocolate, cookies and ice cream to organic.

- Next time you are buying alcohol in a store look for an organic choice and/or one from a small, local brewery/winery.

- Next time you have a big night, do either a fast or juice cleanse the next day.

Chapter Fourteen
Negativity Kills Longevity

"If you are depressed you are living in the past. If you are anxious you are living in the future. If you are at peace you are living in the present."– **Lao Tzu**

As the elderly American couple slowly shuffled hand-in-hand on the sandy path heading down to the beautiful Okinawa beach,

The lady pointed to a stone carving and laughed,

"I certainly don't feel youthful; this short walk has made me feel anything but!"

At eighty-four they were doing better than most their age,

For people from the USA at least,

The carving read;

'At seventy you are but a child,

At eighty you are merely a youth,

and at ninety if the ancestors invite you into heaven,

ask them to wait until you are one hundred,

and then you might consider it.'

Is this an accident do you think?

Centenarians

The place with the highest percentage of centenarians (people living to 100 or more) in the world (Okinawa) has a proverb showing their positive mindset around ageing. A lifestyle based around physical activity, healthy nutrition, little exposure to toxic chemicals, low-stress levels and a positive mental attitude has them also living the longest disability-free expectancy of any people around the world. In another place that has high life expectancy the area of Nova Scotia of Canada, a medical study of why so many people lived to become a centenarian revealed that half never suffer any serious or chronic diseases. They actually have a saying;

"It's not true that the older you get, the sicker you become. It's the older you get, the healthier you have been."

These are the types of people that first inspired the title of this book. Not because I imagine living to 100 years old in a nursing home after years of stress, most of it in a dead-end job I hated, riddled with disease and disability. No, because I imagine my later years still fishing on my boat, working in my vegetable garden and walking hand-in-hand down the beach with the love of my life, full of energy and vigour with a zest for life just like the Okinawan's do! Maybe even writing books like this one, but obviously with more wisdom and intellect than now.

Research conducted by Bradley Wilcox of Harvard Medical School attributed working into their 80's and 90's to why the Okinawan's live so long. Basically not sitting down for long periods of time watching shite on TV like my grandparents used to do. Other reasons are an active social life, low-stress levels, a strong sense of community, and a respect for older people. This positive mindset is kept up through the entirety of their lives, the oldest man at the time of the research in both Japan and Okinawa, Genkan Tonaki, only gave up proposing to nurses at the age of 108! Cheeky bugger. He worked in sugar cane fields until he retired at the age of 85 and would drink six bottles of beer a day. Go on Genkan sir! Thank you for proving my reason for writing the previous chapter perfectly!

Okinawan's show good health well into older age, with heart disease, strokes, dementia, clogged arteries, and high cholesterol a rarity.

Cancer rates are low, and they suffer 80 per cent fewer heart attacks than North Americans and are twice as likely to survive if they have one. They have a fourth of the breast cancer and prostate cancer rates and one third less dementia than Americans.

Bradley Wilcox showed once again genes have little to do with your health and life-expectancy as he showed that younger Okinawan's who frequent fast-food restaurants around US Military bases are now the fattest people in Japan, and Okinawan men under 55 years old have the highest mortality rate. He showed that Okinawan's who moved to both the US and Brazil adopted the disease rate and life expectancy of that country. Oh, and some individual Okinawan's attributed their longevity to drinking a concoction of garlic, honey, turmeric, aloe and awamori liquor before they go to bed. Hang on! Is that an almost all alkaline mixture and a little bit of alcohol?...I might be onto something here!

Positive Mental Attitude

Science is now proving a Positive Mental Attitude (PMA) goes a long way to achieving optimal health and a good long life. Researchers at the Department of Psychology, at the University of Michigan, showed that experiencing frequent positive emotions, paying attention to the positives rather than the negatives, being more socially integrated and having a sense of life purpose leads to a better quality of life.

Dr Lisa Yanek from the Johns Hopkins Bloomberg School of Public Health showed that even people with a family history of certain diseases could avoid what some might think is inevitable if they have a positive mindset. Her research showed that positive people with a family history of heart disease were one-third less likely to have a heart attack or other cardiovascular event than those with a more negative outlook. Again, showing it's not all about genes. If you have a more positive outlook on life, you are far more likely to live a longer healthier life than your family member who is a Negative Nancy. That my friends is a scientific term, *Negative Nancy*.

Placebos

Research done on placebos seriously backs up just how powerful the mind is. Placebos work somewhere between 18-80% of the time depending on which research you look at. But the fact is, they *work*. They work on diseases that are thought 'incurable' in Western medicine, yet the mind cures them with nothing but a sugar pill, a saline injection, or fake surgery.

In 2008, researchers at Chicago University did an anonymous web-based survey of 231 physicians, and ninety-six per cent of the respondents believed that placebos could have therapeutic effects. 96%, by the way, makes room for the 4% of doctors who are stuck in the tiniest box in which only what they got taught at school can possibly be true (we've covered this before).

The response to placebos seems to be only getting stronger. Researchers at McGill University in Montreal stated, 'We were absolutely floored when we found out.' The group examined 84 clinical trials of drugs for the treatment of chronic neuropathic pain over 23 years and found the response to the drug in question was the same, but the placebos had become more powerful. In 1996, patients in clinical trials reported that drugs relieved their pain by 27% more than a placebo did. By 2013, it was down to just 9% more.

I believe in the Information Age that we are currently in, people are becoming far more aware of the power of the mind and positive thinking, and so this could potentially increase the effectiveness of placebos. It's not only taking sugar pills that have proven incredibly effective either. A group of researchers in Finland took a group of 146 people aged 35-65 who needed knee surgery and found that there was no difference in the patients regardless of if they had had the surgery or simply *thought* they had had it. After 12 months patients who had had the sham surgery were back to normal activities with far less or no pain, even doing such things as playing basketball! Now that truly is the power of the mind!

Nocebos

The opposite of a placebo is the nocebo effect and can be just as powerful. A nocebo is when someone is put into a negative frame of mind before given medicine or treatment such as surgery, and it harms their health. Some of the case studies that come up are truly remarkable. As per the NewScientist magazine; 'In the 1970s, for example, doctors diagnosed a man with end-stage liver cancer and told him he had just a few months to live. Though the patient died in the predicted time, an autopsy showed the doctors had been mistaken. There was a tiny tumour, but it had not spread. It seemed the doctors' prognosis had been a death curse.'

An astonishing case first reported in the Herald Tribune in 1966 talks of three sisters who were born on Friday 13th, the midwife delivering them said because of the day they were born on they were all cursed. The first, she announced, would die before her 16th birthday. The second would not survive her 21st. The third was told she would die before her 23rd birthday. The third sister turned up at the hospital three days before her 23rd birthday, saying she was going to die in the next two days. She claimed her two sisters had died as predicted and she believed she would too. She died the day before her birthday, after an episode of "severe apprehension and profuse sweating," doctors reported.

Dr John C. Harvey was researching the case, a professor of medicine at Johns Hopkins Medical School pointed out that physicians have demonstrated that the body can translate a patient's state of mind into physiological disorders. Dr Harvey studied native voodoo practices in Nigeria and said the woman's case had all the elements of a voodoo death. Dr Harvey said there is no doubt that people in Africa die as a result of voodoo curses.

These are obviously two extreme cases, but most people know of someone who had, had cancer for months on end without knowing it, but when they got told they were dead within days or a few weeks at most. This shows that we can live with a disease sometimes for years at a time without knowing it. However, especially in the case of cancer, there is such hysteria around it, that it has a devastating physical impact on most people once it is diagnosed. Some people, like in the case of Tom Dennis who was one of the most positive people I've ever met, take a completely different approach mentally to the whole situation and is living proof you don't have to be scared to death once a doctor tells you some bad news.

The Subconscious vs Conscious Mind

Now we can see the power of the mind in all its glory, how does one become more positive? You first need to know your subconscious mind stores everything that has ever happened to you, every experience, every thought, every sight, every smell, every sound, every taste, everything you touch and say is stored away. Its capacity is virtually infinite, and by the time you're 21 years old, you will have stored more information than 100 editions of the Encyclopaedia Britannica! This is why when people are under hypnosis, they can recall events from decades earlier with perfect clarity. It's your conscious mind that is the one that has trouble remembering things.

Your subconscious is just like a farmers field; what you plant there is what will grow. If you plant poison ivy, then expect poison ivy to grow. If you plant a field full of delicious organic vegetables, then you can fully expect delicious organic vegetables to grow.

Around 95% of your behaviours and reactions happen at the subconscious level.

The subconscious is how we can learn habits and skills and recall on them whenever we want without really thinking about it; everything we need is stored in the subconscious mind. How many times have you driven home from work and arrived in the driveway without remembering how you got there? It is how musicians put on masterful performances without thinking about where to put each finger when playing their instrument. The subconscious mind is also what keeps your heart beating, your lungs breathing and billions of cells in your body functioning in complete harmony.

Your subconscious is subjective. It doesn't think for itself, it doesn't judge, nor does it question. It is unaware of what is real and what is your imagination. Its job is to store and retrieve the data you have planted. It does this so it can make sure you react to any situation in the way you have programmed it to do so. And that is the most important thing to remember.

You are in control of how your subconscious mind is programmed.

Your subconscious will work hard to keep you comfortable. It wants homeostasis for both body and mind. Whenever you feel uncomfortable doing something new, this is because your subconscious mind made those patterns a long time ago from the information you input throughout your entire life. You feel those feelings of discomfort and fear because you are now out of your comfort zone and potential harm to the homeostasis of your mind. Whatever the situation was and how you reacted to it at that time will be stored and called upon again in the future. One thing we need to change is your thought process in certain situations. Rather than reacting, let's make it, so you *respond*. I'd much prefer a doctor saying I am responding to my medication rather than reacting to it, wouldn't you? For your health, it is much better to respond to events in your day rather than constantly reacting in fight or flight mode.

However;

Nothing will change in your life if you don't first change something.

Breaking old habits is difficult because you've now got to go against 10, 20, 30 or even 70 years of the old you. Once we go outside of your comfort zones, that's where the magic lays. That is where you want to put yourself—*every day*. Keep giving your subconscious diamonds to grow, and expanding your comfort zones, until new behaviours are developed, and new habits are formed. Then new skills are made, and things that were uncomfortable beforehand (or even caused you fear) are now easier. You may have felt uncomfortable with a lot of the Action Steps in this book so far, but if you've been doing some of them from the beginning, they will now feel much more comfortable to you. And if you skipped over some, go back and start doing the one you feel is the absolute worst, every day. Once you've eaten that frog, then the others will feel easier!

How do we forge new habits and patterns of behaviour and become a more positive person? The first factor comes down to, what are you filling your subconscious with?

If you are filling your subconscious with massive amounts of negativity, your reactions to circumstances will be negative, as will your thoughts, your words, your actions and then your entire outlook on life!

If you are putting in positivity on a regular basis, then you will be responding more, and your thoughts, words, actions, perspective and experience will be positive.

The second factor is all about your conscious mind, which is very different from the subconscious. It is objective, has no memory and is responsible for how you react to the world around you. It can only think one thought at a time and will delve into your subconscious to know whether it should react (or respond) positively or negatively to a particular situation. It can't do both at the same time! With a more mindful way of thinking, we can control what we think, feel and do, so our future responses and behaviours can be more positive. Over time we can use our conscious mind to reprogram our subconscious to develop better thoughts, attitudes and habits.

Why So Negative?

Your mind is much like your muscles; your skeletal muscles, your heart and your liver. Ha! Just joking about the liver, in case you skipped over the last chapter! Just like muscles, your mind needs training to become stronger. Meaning, it takes work to become positive; it doesn't just happen overnight. This is because from your very first days on Earth you've been surrounded by negativity. As a toddler, you were told the word *no* far more than you ever heard the word yes. In fact, you were told no an astonishing *400 times* per day on average! No, you can't do this, and no, you can't do that. Jimmy no. Jimmy stop. Jimmy behave. Jimmy no, stop it, Jimmy, don't do that. In school, you're told to be realistic, and if you're anything like me, you were told off for your actions more than you were praised! Man, if I did that today (act like a child naturally should, staring out of the window, bored with the stuff they were teaching, as I'd figured out I wouldn't need 90% of it when I left), I'd have been doped up on all sorts of ADHD medications and the like. Poor little fuckers today.

While sitting through an unbearably boring algebra class, kids can't even stare out of a window, day dreaming of running around outside in the sunshine without getting prescribed pills.

Throughout life, everyone around you from your caring parents, to school teachers, to close friends tell you not to aim too high in life to avoid disappointment. Any aspirations outside of those achieved through an expensive university degree are shot down. The idea of the rich only being wealthy because they are bad people is drilled into you if you are from the working class. The rich get richer - you need to aim lower, get a 9-5 job and maybe, just maybe you can work up from there.

The entire idea of the education system is for you to conform, work hard and get a 'normal' job. The very first mission statement of the General Education Board in 1906 which was funded by J.D. Rockafella should give you an idea of what you have been up against since your earliest days;

'In our dreams, people yield themselves with perfect docility to our molding hands. The present education conventions of intellectual and character education fade from their minds and unhampered by tradition we work our own good will upon a grateful and responsive folk. We shall not try to make these people or any of their children into men of learning or philosophers, or men of science. We have not to raise up from them authors, educators, poets or men of letters, great artists, painters, musicians, nor lawyers, doctors, statesmen, politicians, creatures of whom we have ample supply. The task is simple. We will organize children and teach them in a perfect way the things their fathers and mothers are doing in an imperfect way.'

The modern schooling system is based on factories, where the working class were meant to go and work. Now it's an office cubicle with hundreds of other people who 'did well in school'. The positions of politicians, CEO's of large corporations and top levels of journalism are held for those who went through private schooling and to top universities. The people who mould our society go through an entirely different education system. The masses leave school without learning anything about starting a business, investing money, creative thinking or even how to cook a healthy meal!

Instead, you wear a uniform to look the same as everyone else, don't you *dare* have your individual personality shining through. When you hear the bell, you do the same thing as everyone else, just like in a factory. Don't dare be late or you'll face detention to write lines about how you should *conform*. Do well in your tests, which is literally a memory test of what they taught you. How well do you remember what everyone was taught? How well do you conform? Do well, and you can work 40+ hours per week in a cubicle.

Be 'normal'; don't be anything else unless you want to face ridicule. Negativity breeds negativity, and it's all around you, every day, in school and then at work; people continually complaining about the job that they hate. Life is all about fleeting moments of happiness like Friday afternoons that is quickly followed by hating Monday mornings. One or two weeks away in Spain or the Caribbean once per year, and then back to the hard slog that is life. Wow, I feel depressed just typing all that. But for most people it's true, and so you have to train your mind to get to a positive state because from the get-go it's been drowned in negativity. Don't worry, though! There are solutions. First, we need to limit the negativity coming in.

Reducing Negativity

Muting The Mainstream Media

Where else is that constant negativity hitting you hard? Television, especially the news. My word, have you ever seen a positive news report? Very few and far between. It's all about war, murder, economy crashes and fear. Fear this race of people, fear that religion, fear that weather report, fear this financial crisis, fear that virus or that terrorist group. Besides that, there are endless hours of absolute garbage on TV. Reality TV and shows about stealing, corruption, horror films, and TV programming that tears apart traditional family values and shoves sex, violence, adultery and divorces down your throat. I know some of you may be thinking, hang on the bad language throughout this book is against my personal values. In my personal opinion (and it's only my opinion!) I think the odd four-letter word simply portrays passion and allows one to express oneself. I'm writing about things in this book and the behaviours of governments and corporations that should offend you a lot more than a swear word. I'm hopefully not hurting anyone swearing as that is never my intention. I believe in the notion that if someone is not hurting someone else (physically, mentally, spiritually, financially), then go ahead and do your thing. Being offended doesn't count, as I see that we are getting our freedom of speech brought continuously into question because someone or some group of people got offended. Which means books like this and others I will be recommending will not be allowed in future, and so the only narrative people will have to go by is the mainstream media, which in my opinion, absolutely sucks!

Now, onto one of the most profound health tips that I already gave all the way back in Chapter 2: Stress Less, which can be done for absolutely nothing, is not to watch the evening news and go for a walk instead. Hopefully, you're already regularly walking with your partner, your family, your pet or yourself and your building up to somewhere near one hour a day. If you can watch junk on TV for two or three hours a night, you can find the time to walk for an hour! Do yourself the favour of not filling your brain with negative images of babies being blown up by bombs just before you fall asleep in front of the TV and do your health the justice it deserves and move your body on a daily basis. Going for a walk in safe sunshine (early morning or the late afternoon/evening depending on where you live in the world) has been shown to be as effective for depression as antidepressants.

In fact, according to Dr Stephen Ilardi a respected psychologist and university professor, antidepressants only have about a 50% success rate with half of the patients relapsing, taking the actual recovery rate down to 25%. The side effects are well known, and for me easy to spot, I can usually spot someone on antidepressants who sit down with me for a consultation because there is a lost look in their eyes which is a sign of emotional blunting. Then there's the weight gain and sexual dysfunction. Dr Ilardi says,

"Our Stone Age brains just weren't designed to handle the sedentary, isolated, indoor, sleep-deprived, fast-food-laden, stressed-out pace of twenty-first-century life."

On the flip side to antidepressants researchers at the Department of Psychiatry, University of North Carolina showed that light therapy gave a significant reduction in depression symptom severity. As far as exercise goes, Duke University researchers reported in a study of 156 older patients diagnosed with major depression that 16 weeks of regular exercise had a significant impact on symptoms comparable to that as those who took medication. In a follow-up study, it was found those who continued exercising were far less likely to have their depression return.

How does all this work? Lack of sunlight has a proven negative impact on serotonin levels; hence why seasonal affective disorder (SAD) is so common in colder parts of the world when winter sets in. Exercise and sunlight both increase the production of serotonin, which is the exact neurochemical targeted by antidepressants, just without the terrible side effects. Obviously being depressed means it's going to be much more difficult to start exercising and as such, simply start with walking outside and do as much as you can on that given day.

After my first contract on cruise ships, I had travelled to parts of the world I had never been and was exposed to cultures and people I had never encountered. It was an amazing experience that I will always remember. I would urge everyone both younger and older to travel. It expands the mind so much it made me a completely different person. I like to think for the better.

However, when I say travel, I don't mean just to go away for a week or two on a beach holiday. I mean to go and fully submerge yourself in someone else's country or culture. Possibly by living somewhere new, at least for a short while, somewhere with a different culture to your own. If you have children, urge them to travel, as scary as it may seem it is nothing like what you think or what you've seen on television. The world is a far less dangerous place than what the mainstream media has conditioned you to believe.

Travel helped me grow so much as a person and is a massive part of why I'm writing this book today.

Beyond that, the reason I was telling you is because when I got home after travelling the world while working on a cruise ship, I did what I did almost every day after school or work up until that point, I sat down and turned on the TV. I flipped through the channels and found a show I used to love. I remember sitting there and thinking, *'What am I doing? I feel like I'm wasting my life.'* After not watching TV for ten months on the ship I realised I didn't need or even want to anymore. I turned it off, and to this day, 12 years later I have never watched television. I have watched the odd film don't get me wrong, but I have not watched any of the reality shows people waste their lives watching, and I've certainly watched no news. In fact, I haven't read a newspaper, a magazine or checked the news online once in the last 12 years and I am pretty certain I will *never* do again. Before anyone points it out, yes I clicked on the odd article usually from years ago when researching for this book. But I've never in my life gone onto a news website to find out 'what's happening in the world today'.

People are often shocked by this. "Well, how do you stay informed!?!" What I've found is that if it's important enough, someone tells me about it! Honestly, nothing important (or apparently important in someone else mind) escapes me. I know, for example, who both the President of the USA and the Prime Minister of the United Kingdom are. Me not watching the news or opening a newspaper in the last 12 years has me both well enough informed for me to be able to write this book and made sure I've not had the negative images of people being blown up, news of famine, war or murder enter my mind. And as sad as war and famine are, the fact is me seeing on television helps nobody. The images I'm seeing have already happened, and I can easily donate either money or time without being exposed to this negative imagery on a daily basis like most people are!

Oh, and when I mean news, I mean all the news. Local news is even worse, talking about fires that have killed entire families or a woman being raped in the park. Writing both of them things makes me feel sick to the stomach, but the sad fact is they've already happened, and I can't do anything about it if I'm hearing it on the television now. Other news to avoid like the plague is all the celebrity crap they pump out on television, in magazines and on the internet today. Really, who gives a shit if Kim Kardashian farted this week? *Yes*, I know who she is because someone told me about her. The conversation went something like this, "Oh, what does she do, is she a singer or an actress?" "No". "Why's she famous then?" "Don't know she just is. She's got her own reality TV show." "*Holy fuck* what has this world come to?"

I remember stories from many years ago flicking through crappy tabloid papers and celebrity gossip magazines while on holiday with my friends by the pool. So much body shaming. A female celebrity, I can't remember who, but it doesn't matter, had a full-page spread, with a magnifying glass type closeup on her upper leg, claiming she had cellulite. I imagined a fat journalist sat behind a desk typing this trash. Why did it matter? Who cares? Why are you making young girls feel crap about their body? Just awful journalism, but obviously it sells. This is why we have today's major, unhealthy problem of people feeling inadequate and so, so many eating disorders. It's disgraceful, to be honest. I am hoping I don't come across that way. I am simply offering truths, followed by facts, followed by solutions. That sort of journalism offers zero solutions—just body shaming.

Do this one thing for yourself. Give up all forms of news for one week. You will soon see; you will know everything you need to know. The world will have gone on without you watching, and you will be far happier for it. Don't knock it until you try it! Do it. Now. Once you've done that, can you do no television for one month? This one thing could change your life, with more time to spend on things that matter, such as family, friends and your health, for example.

Limit Social Media

Another far more modern technology that is affecting peoples mental health mostly in a terrible way is Social Media. Study after study show the negative effects of spending too much time on Social Media. I have to say I felt this myself long before reading any such studies and as such, for at least the last five years, I have only used Social Media platforms for business. I also use Messenger for keeping in contact with friends and family while I'm away, and for both of these uses, they are brilliant tools.

However, years ago, I found myself needlessly scrolling through my Facebook newsfeed. I was bored out of my head without really realising until I snapped out of it, looking aimlessly at pictures of people's dinner or getting annoyed at couples *pretending* to be perfect when deep down I knew it was all bullshit. I'd catch myself wasting an hour of my time doing this and felt depressed. Then I thought, *why* am I doing this? As such, I've never posted on Twitter or Instagram, only making a profile for business use. The only platform I was using at the time was Facebook, and so I deleted the easy to use app and forced myself to sign out each time, meaning I had to go on the internet and login each time I wanted to use it. Even though that's seemingly not the hardest thing in the world to do, it stopped me simply logging in and wasting countless hours that added up over the course of a week.

Deleting my app has since been proven to work in marketing. Amazon calculated that a page load slowdown of just *one second* could cost it $1.6 *billion* in sales each year. Google calculated if a search slowed down by just four-tenths of a second, they could lose 8 million searches per day. Holy smokes, I was correct in my thinking I reckon, me having to login in on the internet rather than just simply tapping on a Facebook app icon saved me endless hours of boredom, anger and depression. Brilliant news!

Researchers at Washington State University reported that anxiety and depressive symptoms were highest among adolescents with the most social media accounts. Researchers at the University of Glasgow, School of Psychology, found in a study of 467 adolescents that social media use is associated with poor sleep quality, anxiety, depression and low self-esteem.

If you have teens or children of any age, do your best to protect them from this modern problem. Especially young children, don't make it normal for them to have a phone or a tablet in their hands from a young age, as this is shown to severely limit creativity amongst other problems. Much more on this in Chapter 17: Smart Technology, Dumb Humans. No child should have a social media profile. The amount of bullying that goes on is a testimony to this.

For now, let's stay on topic, with one more study done at the University of Pennsylvania found that people who use less social media are less depressed and less lonely. Which is quite ironic isn't it! So, start limiting your time on social media, if it's a case of mindlessly scrolling through looking at stuff you don't need to know, then you can always use my technique and delete the apps. If you have depression, give up all Social Media platforms for one month and see how much better you feel. *Do it.* You can even post something like, *'I'm doing a Social Media Detox. If you need to contact me, please do so via email or phone. See you in 1 month.'* Done. There's also the added benefit of being held accountable since you've announced it to everyone!

Letting Go Of Negative People

The final piece of our limiting negativity is getting rid of negative *people*. Now that sounds harsh! But it is one of the most profound things you can do. I mentioned this briefly all the way back in Chapter 1: Mindset Mastery Matters Most. Stop eating with people who put you down about the way you look or comment negatively on what you eat. I mentioned this because the way you think will affect *everything*, and so if you have done this and stopped hanging around those negative people, you'll have realised just how good it feels to not have the negativity while you eat. Now it's time to implement this in *every* avenue of your life.

What I realised after travelling the first time on cruise ships and spending time with people from all over the world, with different cultures to mine, was that I didn't want to go back to what most people consider a 'normal' way of life in England. I stood back and realised most of my friends from school had settled down with a girl they met from the same town and bitched about them constantly, they moaned about going to work on Monday and were in jobs simply to make money and not because of the love of it. Their only fleeting moment of happiness was finishing work on a Friday and their holidays which came around once or twice per year, the rest of the time they bitched and moaned. I realised I didn't want that life.

Beyond that, I realised that when I talked about travel or health as I am doing now, they didn't want to hear it. They simply wanted to talk about football or women or rubbish they'd watched on TV. I realised that they were negative people, to me at least and that I had outgrown them. I realised, which was the hardest realisation and thing I'd ever had to do at that time was that I had to stop hanging around with (most) of them. Some grew with me, talked about things other than sport and women, and I consider friends for life. Most of them though had to go, and now I am better off for it.

You may be thinking about a couple of people who you feel the same about, people who are stopping your growth as a person or you simply don't like hanging around but feel you *have* to because they are old friends or even family. My advice to you would be to let go of those people or at least limit your time with them. If you don't feel comfortable talking about things outside of the mainstream with someone, for fear of ridicule, then you have to look at what they are bringing into your life. They might be kind and loving, and so the positives outweigh the negative, but for those people who bring nothing more than negativity into your life, it's best to let them go.

Increasing Positivity

Reading Books

Okay, so now we've reduced the negativity coming in, in some pretty dramatic and life-changing fashion! Now it's time to start putting more positivity in. Which can be a lot of fun and will be easy now you've given up watching hours upon hours of crap on TV! Firstly, start reading more. Yes, I know, you are currently reading this book, so that might not be a problem for you. If this is the first book you've read in a while, I would like to thank you for giving me that pleasure to reintroduce you into the wonderful world of books, but just know it is a habit you need to continue.

"Reading a book is like re-writing it for yourself." – Angela Carter

Whereas television *programming* is exactly that, telling you what to think, reading a book allows you to think for yourself and interpret what the author is saying in your own mind. The world of books is not tightly controlled like the world of TV, hence why you are currently reading these controversial words. This means you are going to go deep into the minds of people who do not follow the mainstream line and will actually teach you some amazing things that the schooling system and TV have never bothered to teach you. And because they have an entire book to do so, rather than an hour or so on TV, deep truly is the right word.

You can delve deep into subjects that will fill your mind with amazing possibilities and give you skills that you can only dream of. I'm often asked, how do I know so much stuff, on so many subjects and the answer is, because I read. How did I find the time (often working 14 hours a day) to write a book and the answer is because I write. Sounds simple, but put it this way;

While you're watching crap on TV, I'm reading. While you're watching crap on TV, I'm writing. Get it?

The more you read books about having a positive mindset and ones that give you the tools to change your life, the more positive thoughts you are putting into your mind. And so, whenever faced with a circumstance that most people might have a negative *reaction* to, you are far more likely to *respond* positively and come up with a solution. And therefore, you will stop the old adage 'negativity breeds negativity' and be the positive change that people need in their life. And as mentioned if that person just keeps on wanting to be negative, and navigates towards bitching and complaining or seeking out others who they'd rather be negative with, maybe you've outgrown that person and it's time to stop hanging around with them so much...

As also mentioned, the best way to get the most out of *this* book is to reread and apply the Action Steps you didn't already, but once you're done with that, it's time to fill your brain with other ideas from different people. I'll be giving you a list of books that helped me know what I know today in the Resources section if that tickles your interest. But finish this book first! As much of the gold is in the following chapters.

Seminars And Events

An amazing experience had by all is events that are organised by leaders in the positive mindset industry. Or indeed any industry that you'd like to hone your skills at. People who attend these events are often on their own journey of self-discovery and so have a much more open mind than maybe some for the people in your home town. It's a great way to meet new friends and surround yourself with like-minded, positive people! Plus you are opening up the opportunity to learn from the very best, keep this in mind for when you read Chapter 21...I won't tell you what it is yet, and don't look! It will spoil the surprise. And don't worry, I'll remind you of this conversation when you get there!

Hang Around Positive People

"You are the average of the five people you spend the most time with." - Jim Rohn

This is absolutely a true statement when you really think about it. You start to develop the same attitudes and behaviours as those around you. As mentioned when I came home from travelling, I realised I had outgrown old friends with limiting beliefs, which showed me I needed to surround myself with different people. People who were on the same wavelength and path as I. For me at the time I wanted to succeed in business and not rely on a 9-5 job for income, so I started hanging around with successful Personal Training clients of mine. I say hanging around; really we just gravitated towards each other because of the conversations we had while we had our workout sessions. From there, I learned a lot of new life skills that I would never have learned hanging around with old friends stuck in there 9-5 jobs.

I also wanted to learn more about health, and so as life happened I made friends with people like Jane from Chapter 12: ...You Are Also What You Don't Excrete and Mariesa from Chapter 11: Alternative Therapies, and would hang out with them and chat all about subjects that I never felt comfortable talking to my friends and family about. I didn't feel comfortable then, but now I openly talk about different subjects and still get ridiculed, but because I've expanded my comforts zones, I really don't give a shit what people say or think. If only one person benefits from what I'm saying then it's worth it in the end.

And so, what do you want in life? To begin with, maybe you read this book purely for health & fitness reasons, but now maybe you want more! So, start choosing the people you hang around with carefully. Find people with the same goals as you, or even better, people who have already achieved what you want to achieve. A mix of the two is always good. Now that you are letting go of the negative people, this is the perfect time to start filling those voids with new, positive, successful, healthy, happy friends. Maybe it could be from the events you are planning on going to...

Social Media

Whoa, hang on now! How can this be both negative and positive!?! Look, if you are going to use Social Media, start picking and choosing who is coming up in your newsfeeds. There are lots of wonderful, positive pages out there that only share positive thoughts and memes and the like. Some pages also share useful information which is great!

The same goes for people, some share only positive thoughts and offer different spins and opinions on events that maybe you want to see. Then there are people who are utterly obsessed with the mainstream narrative and only sharing depressing, fear-driven news stories, so unfriend them! Or if you are sick to death of seeing pictures of their dinner or the perfect life they are portraying untruthfully, and it annoys you, at least block them from showing up in newsfeeds.

Positive Affirmations

One thing that is very powerful that you can start right away for free is Positive Affirmations. As long as the rest of your lifestyle is geared towards being more positive by following the above advice, then these will work a treat to help you not only to have a more positive outlook on life but also to *love yourself*. Loving yourself is absolutely essential for creating the healthy, vibrant, toned and sexy body that you desire so much.

Start your day by looking in the mirror and saying an affirmation ten times. Starting your day with this positive self-talk will set your mind on the right track straight away. You can say your affirmations numerous times throughout the day, whenever you need a little boost, that is absolutely fine too. For any affirmations in any area of your life that you are struggling to believe you can repeat the same affirmation every day for a month until it is fully ingrained in your subconscious. Remember, your subconscious mind does not know the difference between what is real and what is in your imagination. It will eventually change your beliefs to match those of your new thoughts if given enough time. To really hammer home a new belief, write down your affirmation ten times at any point in the day. Writing with a pen and paper is a potent tool, as discussed in Chapter 3: Sweet Dreams.

Positive Affirmations do not need to just be about health. They can be about any area of your life where you feel like you need to reprogram your subconscious. However, since this is a book predominantly about health, start with the following;

Positive Affirmation: 'I am happy. I am healthy. I am whole'

Gratitude Journal

As mentioned in Chapter 3: Sweet Dreams, you should be writing down 20 things that you are grateful for before you go to sleep. If you didn't already start keeping this list in a separate Gratitude Journal, now is the time. You can add anything and everything you are grateful for into your Gratitude Journal at any time, it doesn't have to be just before bed. You can then go back and reread all the amazing things, people and experiences you've had in your life to flood your subconscious mind with positive thoughts, and it will remind you, even in the bleakest of times, that life is great.

Goal Setting

Everyone I've ever met with a Positive Mental Attitude always has goals. They are going somewhere in life. They get up on a morning with purpose. To have goals will help you maintain a vigour for life which in turn will help you stay healthy. Having set goals will also help you achieve what you want to achieve. If for example, you simply state you want to be fitter and healthier, that's like jumping in a boat without a specific destination. You'll just be floating around the ocean with no direction, docking in any place that you come across, which more than likely will lead to a lot of disappointments unless you get very, very lucky on your first shot.

To get your goals achieved, they want to be written down and put in a place you can see them every day. Dr Gail Matthews, at the Dominican University in California, led a study on goal setting and found you are 42% more likely to achieve your goals if they are written down. A good place to write short term goals is on post-it notes that are put on the bathroom mirror. Staring you in the face at the start of your day as you read out your Positive Affirmations aloud. Go over your goals, making sure you are on track. Once a goal has been achieved take it down and place it on the mirror you look into as you leave the house, the one where you make sure you're looking at your best. Right there staring you in the face as you leave for the day ahead are your successfully achieved goals, pumping your subconscious with positive vibes. Make sure to celebrate *every* goal you achieve. It could mean buying yourself a coffee or having a piece of dark chocolate. It could even be something more material like a new watch for completing 15 short terms goals, new clothes for reaching a certain weight or maybe just celebrating by cheering in the mirror to yourself.

I urge you to write out all your medium to long term goals in each specific area of your life in detail. Write down your health, spiritual, family, work, financial, and social goals. Looking at health, rather than just saying, "I want to lose weight," or "I want to be healthy" let's look at specific goals you can achieve. Where do you want to be in terms of health? What does that look like to you? Are you off of your medications, dropping 50 lbs or looking like Angelina Jolie? Do you want to run a marathon or simply want to walk up a flight of stairs without getting out of breath? *When* do you want that? Do you want to be able to bend over and tie your shoelace in the next 30 days but in 1 year you want to look like Brad Pitt? *Who* will help you achieve that? What new *skills, knowledge* and *information* do you need to acquire to achieve your goals?

List every single step you can currently think of (maybe looking back at Action Steps in this book) that you need to do to achieve your goal. If new actions, people, skills etc. become apparent on your journey, add them to your list later. Once you see your goal listed out, it becomes far more achievable. Now put it into a *detailed plan* with timeframes. Break it down into *daily, weekly* and *monthly* goals. Put the daily and weekly goals on your bathroom mirror. Say Positive Affirmations daily to go with your goals and your plan.

Vision Board

Around 65% of people are visual learners, with 90% of the information you gather coming visually, and 40% of all the nerve fibres coming from the brain are linked to the retina. So, having your goals written down is one thing, but a fun activity that you can do with (or without) the kids is creating a Vision Board. And remember, your subconscious mind does not know the difference between reality and what is in your imagination, so giving it constant visuals to work with is extremely powerful. It will help you expand your comfort zones and help you achieve more.

Taking a corkboard, start cutting out pictures from magazines or that you've found on the internet and pinning them to your board. Again, making it an art and crafts activity rather than building one on a computer is far more powerful and rewarding. Choose pictures that make you feel good, of all the goals you have written out. Add pictures of how you want your business, your body, and your home to look, places you want to travel and the new car that you want. Be creative and have fun. You can cut out words that describe the person you'd like to become. Put your Vision Board in a place where you will look at it multiple times per day. Whether that's opposite your desk or at the foot of your bed where your TV used to be...

Meditation

Here it is again if you didn't start already, now is the time! One of the best ways to get control of your subconscious mind is meditation, which is once again proven in science. In 1983, neuroscientist Benjamin Libet showed that it took 200 milliseconds on average for a person's finger to move after them feeling like they decided to make that movement. However, the subjects subconscious mind made the decision a further 350 milliseconds before the subject felt like they had decided to move the finger. He did this looking at electrical activity in subjects brains when asked to press a button whenever they felt like it. Showing that the subconscious was making the decisions before the conscious mind.

A more recent study was done at the University of Sussex in Brighton, UK. Taking the same test of pressing a button, the researchers compared people who regularly meditate versus those who didn't. The meditators had a longer gap in between when they felt like pressing the button and their finger moving, 149 compared with 68 milliseconds for the other group. Showing they were more in tune with their subconscious mind and internal body processes.

Researchers at Carnegie Mellon University, Pittsburg also showed that stressed-out adults significantly reduced a key inflammation marker that is linked to cancer, Alzheimer's and autoimmune diseases after four months of meditation—showing the highly important connection between body and mind. As you work on your positive mindset, which is not easy especially if you already have a health complaint that plagues every area of your life. I assure you I know exactly how you feel. In the next chapter we are going to learn all about an area of my body that constantly wanted to pull me back to negative thoughts, from the way it looked, the way it felt and the pain it caused me. That area is right there for the world to see and just happens to be the largest organ of the body. We will now learn what we need to do to love the skin that you are in...Before that it's time to take action. Don't put this off, get the hard work done now and the world will be your oyster.

Resources

Go to **www.TomBroadwell.com/resources** to see;

- A link to my Social Media pages for more positive mindset stuff than you can shake a stick at! Positive Affirmations, quotes, health tips, recipes and more...

- A list of books, events and people I recommend to get you to where you want to go.

Action Steps

- Here's a challenge for you. Go without TV for the next seven days. See how much happier, healthier and more productive you feel. I can tell you right now one thing; I would never have had the time to write this book if I watched reality TV shows or endless hours of sport on TV.

- If you want a really big challenge, try doing a 7-day Social Media Detox at the same time as not watching TV. If this is all too much at once, then do them separately. Make sure to sign out of all Social Media platforms while doing your detox. No cheating whatsoever, and if you find yourself scrolling any Newsfeed on any platform, you need to start the seven days again. Do this to break the habit of mindlessly scrolling with no aim whatsoever.

- Start meditation daily if you don't already do that.

- Call a (true) friend you've not spoken to in a while. Meet up and have a coffee, tea or a couple of drinks together. Start to socialise more if you've been a hermit for a while. (i.e. stop watching garbage on TV and go spend time with friends or family), there's a pattern emerging here...

- Look online to see if any events are going on that would either build your PMA or hone your skills. Book in to go, now.

- Write out your favourite Positive Affirmation ten times and put it on your bathroom mirror.

- Write out your medium and long term goals in detail with a plan broken down into timeframes.

- Take the short term goals and put them onto sticky notes that you can put onto your bathroom mirror.

- Say your Positive Affirmation ten times and go over your short term goals every morning.

- Make sure to put your completed goals on the mirror you use when leaving the house.

- Celebrate your completed goals every day.

- Have an arts and crafts day and have everyone build vision boards.

- If there is anyone in your life who you feel you've outgrown or you simply don't like hanging around with because they are negative, start to limit your time with them at the very least. If you are brave enough, look to break ties completely with that person.

Chapter Fifteen
Nourish The Skin You're In

"Be good to your skin. You'll wear it every day for the rest of your life."– **Renee Rouleau**

He sprayed on the deodorant just like he'd seen a thousand times on TV,

Walked out of the door,

Without a care on his face,

Except,

He worried a little about the lump under his arm,

As he headed to the gym, he decided to ask his Personal Trainer, who just so happened to be his son about it,

It was getting difficult to perform the lat pulldown exercise he had prescribed him,

He arrived and asked his son who was walking the gym floor,

"Am I doing this, right?"

"Sure, but why is your left arm not going up the same level as your right arm?"

"I don't know, there's been a lump there for a while, and I can't move it very well anymore, but the doctor has told me two visits in a row that it's nothing to worry about."

"Dad, tell him you want to see a specialist, it seems like it could be something serious."

"I already did the last time..."

True story and one that is repeated over and over every day in the UK. A know-it-all General Practitioner who doesn't refer someone for months on end either because the specialist is too expensive on the NHS or it would hurt his ego to be wrong about something. The latter is true about the GP in the example, the same GP who sent me to my busy, city hospital on Christmas Eve with so much pain in right testicle it hurt to walk, and a wrong step had me shouting out loud in pain.

He sent me to get checked to see if it was a twisted testicle, all because I walked into his office and declared I had mumps, going on the fact my brother currently had the highly contagious mumps and lived in the same house as me. That along with the flu-like symptoms I was displaying. He looked me up and down and said; "Another Internet diagnosis." I told him no and presented the above evidence.

The doctor was obviously pissed off that day and seemed to take delight in studying and playing with my right bollock, which was one of the most painful experiences of my life. He declared I must have twisted the testicle and got flu on the same day, even though I had, had flu-like symptoms for four days and as such if my testicle were twisted it would have gone black and fallen off by then. But still, he wielded his power and sent me off to the hospital, on Christmas *fucking* Eve to get checked. The Urologist walked in, and I told him the same evidence as above, he didn't even do anything but laugh and said; "Go home to bed you have mumps."

The reason I'm telling you this is not to bash doctors, but because by the time my father had seen a specialist *six months* later, the quite obvious cancerous lump that had grown in his armpit had spread into his lung and his bones. As I mentioned before, doctors are humans, and so some are kind, some are amazing, some are good, some are bad, some have huge egos, and some are assholes.

Everything a doctor tells you is an *opinion*, and as such, you should get second and third opinions if something is worrying you, and they are not supporting you in the best way possible.

This was again just proven to me as my girlfriend May went to get some lumps in her breasts checked. They turned out to be cysts that were not dangerous. The doctor on the ship said she must get checked every six months. The doctor who gave the diagnosis at the hospital said, "Please don't come back, as some of my peers will perform the surgery when you really don't need it. Instead of spoiling the look of your breasts with surgery, try Vitamin E. I'm not sure it will really work, but it's worth a try, and these are not dangerous, so there is no need whatsoever for surgery." That proves doctors can be fantastic at their job and caring people. It also proves through him not trusting other doctors that everything a doctor says is an opinion and by no means the last word. We did get some **Raw Organic Vitamin E** and some **Evening Primrose Oil** which is proven to be good for both cysts and hormones, and the cysts entirely disappeared within a month.

Now on to how this relates to the largest, living, breathing organ in the body - the skin. My father was eventually diagnosed with lymphoma and went to see a couple of different specialists, to find out what the best way forward was. Of course, the doctor specialising in radiation recommended just that, radiation. The doctor whom specialised in chemotherapy recommended chemotherapy, and I have no doubt whatsoever, if surgery was remotely an option the surgeon would have recommended surgery...

Deodorant

A few days went by, and I was in my father's bathroom and noticed that there was a can of spray-on deodorant on the side. I took it down to confront him about why he was being so silly and defying his specialist's orders by using spray-on deodorant while having lymphoma in his armpit. He told me he didn't know what I was talking about, as nobody had mentioned anything about deodorant in any of the meetings. In fact, no one had talked about the possible dangers of *anything*, just the treatment that they could do. Throughout his entire treatment, no one mentioned anything about the possible causes of his cancer, and so with an apparent genetic weakness there, cancer would likely come back unless I took charge and taught him some lifestyle changes.

Luckily (luck he created) he has made changes and has been cancer-free for over twelve years. The first thing I started with was to throw his deodorant in the dustbin and went to buy him a deodorant stick made out of salt crystals. He still uses it to this day and has never smelled of body odour. As well as lymphoma being linked to spray-on deodorants, breast cancer has also. Researchers at The University of Reading in the UK found that everything from deodorants to body lotions and suncream is applied to the area around the breast, on an ever more frequent basis to ever younger people. Again it is stated that no one really knows what this exposure to toxic chemicals will have as the skin continuously absorbs anything that is put on it.

Amazing to me is the fact that only two studies have ever been conducted showing the relationship between spray-on deodorant and cancer. The reason I find this amazing is that it is the one thing that most people seem to know and nod along to when I present my health seminars. The first one published in The Journal of the National Cancer Institute found that there was no relationship between the two. However, the second paper published in the European Journal of Cancer Prevention found that the more the products that are used by someone, there was a direct correlation with how young they were diagnosed with breast cancer. But wait, there's more! As the first study was *extremely* limited, by the reliance on self-reported information from the study group, by the lack of a nonuser population (so how can you know what caused anything?), and by the lack of consideration to historical usage. And the second study was far more in-depth and far more credible with *none* of the above limitations.

Now even more amazing than all of this, if you were to search the internet for yourself and type in, 'spray-on deodorant and cancer' the internet is awash with naysayers who say it is a *myth*. The websites promoting this the most is that of different cancer *charities*, who quote only the first, extremely limited, research. Whoa, wait! Cancer charities who make *billions* of dollars off of people *having* cancer might not show the *whole* truth when it comes to cancer prevention...hmm *serious* food for thought...

Skin Absorption

Looking back at the research done in Reading, UK, not a lot of people know that the skin absorbs almost everything that is put onto it.

Many people take good care of what goes in their mouth but don't even *think* about what goes on their skin.

When in reality, it all goes to the same place, which is into the bloodstream and lymphatic system and then the liver, or worse the fat cells or vital organs like your brain. There are many studies proving that chemicals from cosmetics absorb through the skin. Way back in 1988, Mortician's Mystery which was published in the New England Journal of Medicine demonstrated that long-term topical exposure of hands to embalming creams could result in endocrine disruption to the *whole* human body.

Lead acetate, which is used in hair dyes, has shown to be readily absorbed through the skin and was banned in 2018 by the FDA. The Environmental Working Group says it has been linked to developmental issues in children, reduced fertility, organ system toxicity, cancer, and other problems. The problem was it was banned in Canada in *2005* and even before that in Europe, but it took way more than a *decade* and the pressure of a petition by more than a *dozen* consumer watchdog groups to be banned in the US. Why? Because the FDA only ever checks chemicals in cosmetics for safety when there is a clear problem with a chemical, which can then take years to get around to the testing. That's astonishing when you consider that it all ends up in the same place as if you'd eaten it...

Consider that The European Union has banned over 1300 chemicals found in cosmetics. The FDA has only banned *eight*!

The average woman now puts 515 chemicals per day onto her skin, of which 60% is absorbed into her body. Let's take a look at some of the most toxic ingredients you need to be avoiding in cosmetics:

- **Phthalates** are used in children's toys, shower curtains and vinyl flooring, but are also found in shampoo, perfume, aftershave, deodorant and hairspray. The National Institute of Health have linked at least one phthalate with cancer, and they have been linked to problems with reproduction and child development.

- **Parabens** are designed to preserve the shelf-life of cosmetics and are one of the most widely used preservatives in the world. They're found in shampoos, hair gels, shaving gels and body lotions. However, with their use becoming more controversial due to links with them accumulating in the body and causing cancer, many companies are going 'paraben-free' on their label. However, what they are switching over to is not a lot better, and it's something I'm going to struggle to pronounce in my audiobook! **Methylchloroisothiazolinone** is a known sensitising allergen that is linked with causing contact dermatitis more and more frequently. It will be interesting to find what other diseases this synthetic chemical is linked to in the future.

A point I need to make is that methylisothiazolinone which is from the same happy family of chemicals is often found in baby products such as baby wipes and has been linked to serious allergic reactions, especially in children. As we can see from the use of baby powder (talcum powder), the manufacturers don't suddenly make the products pure and healthy just because it's for a baby! And so once again you have to always take note of the ingredients before applying anything to your children's skin as well! Interestingly, The American Contact Dermatitis Society named methylisothiazolinone its "allergen of the year" in 2013.

- **Sodium Lauryl Sulfate (SLS)** is common in shower gels, face wash, shampoos and toothpaste. SLS can be contaminated with **ethylene oxide**, which is known as a human carcinogen. SLS, along with other sulfates, can irritate the skin and eyes as they are pretty darn harsh soaps.

- **Polyethene Glycols (PEGs)** are petroleum-based compounds that are used to increase the absorption of the product they are in, namely moisturisers and different anti-ageing products. This means that if the product you are more rapidly absorbing does not contain great ingredients, then you are causing yourself more trouble than it's worth! PEGs are regularly contaminated with **1,4 dioxane**, which is very toxic and according to the FDA is a potential human carcinogen. A group of US researchers found it was in 46 out of 100 products tested. It can be gotten rid of with a vacuuming process as recommended by the FDA, but it appears most manufacturers just don't bother...

I could go on, but there are thousands, and so I recommend to keep reading the labels and continue educating yourself. However, as with your supplements and food, remember if the brand says it is 'natural' on the label or that it's in a health food store that it is *not* necessarily a good product. One area I've been burned in the past, and so a word of warning, is thinking that if the brand has other pure products that the product you are looking at is the same quality. It sometimes is, but a lot of the time it isn't. So, check the labels!

Also, something else to think about when it comes to anti-ageing products and if they are more readily absorbed into your skin. When they contain synthetic chemicals, rather ironically and hilariously (or sadly depending on how you look at it) they will *speed up* the ageing process. Why? Well, as mentioned, when toxic chemicals reach a cell, in this case, the skin cells, the cells will either mutate which will develop into a disease or they will die, which is the ageing. This is again why there are lawsuits aplenty surrounding synthetic anti-ageing products because they don't actually work!

Chemical Sunscreen

When looking at chemicals absorbing into the bloodstream, we can't ignore sunscreen, suncream or sunblock. A recent study performed in January 2020 and published in JAMA showed that six active ingredients (**avobenzone**, **oxybenzone**, **octocrylene**, **homosalate**, **octisalate**, and **octinoxate**) often used in sunscreen are absorbed into the bloodstream at higher levels than is recommended safe by the FDA after a *single-use*. From there it was applied again on days 2-4 at the recommended four times per day, but not thereafter and was still at levels that are deemed unsafe on day *twenty one*! The study stopped there but just imagine after an average holiday lasting one week or a fortnight, the levels at which we are exposing ourselves to, or if you live in hotter parts of the world and regularly apply this synthetic concoction on a daily basis.

What's the problem you might say. Well amazingly (perhaps not so amazing at this point in the book) the ingredients have barely been tested. From the tests done, we can see the usual neurotoxic effects and massive hormonal disruption. We also see mothers who are exposed during pregnancy having shorter than normal pregnancies and adverse effects on birth weight. Oxybenzone, for example, was found in 96% of Americans by the FDA and is consistently found in mothers breast milk.

"Is my super necessary sunscreen to blame!" I hear you cry. A study published in 2015 in the journal Environmental Research found levels of oxybenzone were higher in those who reported regular sunscreen use, but also in those who used it infrequently compared with those who did not. Again, showing that it absorbs with a single-use, but not only that, once it's in your bloodstream it's in there to stay and wreak havoc on all of your bodily systems.

And not only is it us the humans that pay the dire consequences of people slapping on sunscreen day in, day out. On beaches around the world, people go for an innocent swim in the ocean not realising the damage they are doing to the coral reefs and marine wildlife in that area. Of the chemicals that don't get pulled into your bloodstream are then leached into the water. This has been *proven* not only to cause massive damage to coral but also the crustaceans and fish start to develop the same birth defects and hormonal disruptions that we humans do. It has even been shown to be absorbed by dolphins and then passed onto their young.

My question is...

Do you want to cause birth defects and a life of misery in baby dolphins?

I didn't think so, so stop using these chemical sunscreens! (By the way it's okay if you didn't know you were maiming baby dolphins so don't be too upset, but now you know it's a good time to stop).

One more thing I need to address before I give you the solution. The elephant in the room, *skin cancer*...Well, in epidemiologic studies, sunscreen use is associated with increased risk of cutaneous melanoma and basal cell skin cancer. *Hmmm.* Now, how this is usually explained off in medical circles is that people who wear a higher factor sunscreen stay out in the sun longer and therefore get skin cancer. Again *hmmm.* I have some major problems with this theory and a straightforward explanation of why I believe in most cases; it's not the sun causing skin cancer, but the chemicals within the sunscreen itself.

Firstly, in my experience at least, the people laying out in the sun too long have the lowest possible factor on because they want to get a tan and wouldn't be using SPF 50+ to achieve that goal. They are laying there all day and trying to get away with something around SPF 15 or 20, usually with more frequent applications, because if they get sunburnt, then goodbye suntan as it will peel off. But let's just imagine its true, people with higher factor sunscreen are staying out for longer but still getting skin cancer. Sort of means it doesn't work that well does it?

I mean, we are now using more sunscreen than at any other point in history, but the incidence of skin cancer is at an all-time high...I don't know about you, but it's not making all that much sense to me. I then try to look at things from a different but in my mind, logical standpoint and ask you this question. Do you agree that smoking a shitstorm of chemicals can cause lung cancer? So then, why can lathering your skin in a shitstorm of chemicals not cause skin cancer?

What to do? Well, as mentioned, it's best to go out in the safer sun of the early morning, late afternoon and evening without sunscreen and sunglasses on. Whenever it is best for you, depending on where you are in the world. However, if you must go out in the midday sun, there are more natural sunscreens available, which I will cover in the very next section.

For me when living in Sydney, Australia, which is seen as a hotspot for skin cancer (where 56% of people use sunscreen at least five days per week mind you! And yeah, I know about the ozone layer but still...) I would sunbathe in shorts on my balcony starting at 5 minutes in the latter stages of winter. Winter in Australia for an Englishman is not all that bad by the way! Heading into spring, I had built that up to around 30 minutes and so by the time we went to the beach I wouldn't need sunscreen. My skins natural defences were ready for the sun. I would rarely go out between 10 am-2 pm or look for shade at that time. Anytime I would find myself in the hot sun for prolonged periods I would use the mineral sunscreen I am about to discuss now and wear loose-fitting clothing to cover up.

Natural Cosmetics

So, what am I saying? Treat your cosmetics exactly as you'd treat your food up to this point in our journey.

Use products that are as close to as nature intended and go organic as much as possible.

Mineral Sunscreen

As far as sunscreen goes, there are mineral-based sunscreens that use zinc oxide and titanium dioxide. You may recognise titanium dioxide as been listed as toxic from Chapter 9: SupplementNation, which it is if it gets into your body. However, when applied to your skin, both zinc and titanium oxide have been shown to enter your bloodstream either not at all or in tiny, tiny amounts. For example, a 2010 study published in the journal Toxicological Sciences found that volunteers who applied mineral sunscreen twice per day for five days had 1/1000th that of total zinc in the blood after the fifth day of application. Compare that if you will with oxybenzone, and an FDA study that found blood levels 438 times above the cutoff for systemic exposure. Quite a difference I think you'd agree.

Having said that, be aware that zinc or titanium dioxide can get in your body in different ways. For example, if you apply sunscreen and then start eating food with the same hand; it can be ingested. The other way is to use sunscreen spray and inhale it, which can cause damage to your lungs. This is the same for all the sunscreens mentioned, so only use lotion. And again, not only is it you that you are affecting. The number of times while laid on the beach on my time off that I have had to endure breathing in massive amounts of someone's toxic sunscreen because entire families are spraying each other being either completely unaware or not giving a shit about those around them. Don't be that person! Seriously if someone has severe asthma, it's not going to end well for them.

Toothpaste

Other things to think about is to change your toothpaste immediately. I've already presented evidence of how harmful and what a scam fluoride is, so hopefully, you don't want that in your toothpaste. There are fluoride-free toothpaste and mouthwashes available at health food stores. I switched my toothpaste to fluoride-free twelve years ago, and as mentioned never drink tap water and have had far, far *fewer* dental problems than I did versus when I was using a toothpaste that contains fluoride. Now for that stunning piece of evidence, I mentioned all the way back in Chapter 4: Life Begins With Water about whether fluoride is even good at preventing tooth decay.

The Cochrane Collaboration is a group of doctors and researchers who are widely regarded as the *gold standard* of the assessment in the effectiveness of public health policies. In 2015 they reviewed *every single* study done on fluoridation that they could find. They concluded;

'There is very little contemporary evidence, meeting the review's inclusion criteria, that has evaluated the effectiveness of water fluoridation for the prevention of caries.'

Some brave scientists who face the wrath of science bloggers are openly now discussing the fact that fluoride not only doesn't protect against dental problems but as in my personal experience it could be the other way round. Researchers at The University of British Columbia, Vancouver, Canada compared communities that still fluoridate and those who ended it. They found that incidents of dental caries went down for those with no fluoride in the water, but the still fluoridated stayed the same!

Besides all that, it still comes back to needing to discuss the overall effects on your health and whether even if it does work on reducing dental cavities, even with the severe lack of credible evidence, is it worth it? Let's hear it from the horse's mouth, shall we? The Guardian newspaper quotes Northumbrian Water manager David McDermott as saying, "It's an extremely corrosive chemical in neat form. Without a protective suit and boots, I am not permitted to step within 10ft of the three 10,000-litre tanks that hold the acid."

Digesting something every day that in its purest form requires a body suit to go within 10ft of does not sound too good for your health in the longterm.

Skincare, Haircare And The Rest

With me having severe eczema, I very quickly learned exactly what was good for my skin and what wasn't, because the chemical-laden cosmetics felt like I was being set on fire. Whereas the organic products, in general, didn't feel like they were burning me. Some would see this as a rather painful blessing. So, I now only use organic deodorant, face cream, body moisturiser, shampoo and shower gel. Basically, everything that goes onto my skin is as natural as can be.

Makeup

The thing I find females are most attached to is their brand of makeup. However, I've taken even the most loyal customers to different large brands and converted them to organic makeup, while watching their skin magically clear up and breakouts becoming a thing of the past. All you have to do is find one that works with your skin. I'm not saying all organic brands are good and will work well with your skin, but there is absolutely something out there for you, you just have to go out there and find it!

Just to gently remind you can easily inhale things like powder makeup, and even when mineral it is not a good thing to have entering your lungs. Hence, using liquid is best, and being incredibly careful about what the ingredients are for anything you put on your lips (which can obviously be ingested) is of utmost importance.

Homemade Cosmetics

Other than that, the absolute best option is to make your own cosmetics! Then you know precisely what is going in them, onto your skin and into your bloodstream. This is obviously more time consuming than buying them in a store, but as well as being healthier, it can be a more cost-effective way of doing things too. On my website, there is a section based around creating not only your own skincare but also cleaning products too. As you will soon learn in the next chapter, household cleaning products can be some of the most toxic things in your home. Choosing wisely on which ones you buy (or make) can not only contribute hugely to you and your family's health but also Mother Nature's wellbeing too. If you have children or grandchildren, let's work together on leaving them as beautiful a place to live as we have had up until this point.

We are heading into the next section of our health house, which contains chapters on subjects that are rarely thought about from a health perspective. Maybe because the naked eye cannot see most of the dangers or health benefits of the topics discussed, but it doesn't mean they don't exist. Once again, we will look to science prove what I present is a very real thing, but I will also ask you to consider what you feel on an energetic and physical level when it comes to believing. First, we must put what we have learned thus far into action.

Resources

Go to **www.TomBroadwell.com/resources** to see;

- The brands and products of cosmetics I recommend and use.

Action Steps

- Check online or head down to your health food store to buy organic fluoride-free toothpaste and natural roll-on deodorant. Start there if you are on a tight budget.

- Now start changing your shampoo, conditioner, shower gel and body moisturiser.

- Now it's time to change your expensive chemical-laden face creams, night creams, and serums.

- Test as many brands of organic makeup as possible and start choosing the right products for you.

- There are organic hair products available, even hair dyes that some hairdressers offer. Search your local area for someone who does this if you like getting your hair coloured at the salon.

- Start researching into how to make your own cosmetics and start with simple things like body wash and toothpaste, or you can always head over to my website to find some great videos on how to do this.

The Doors and Windows of Your Health House

"Look on every exit as being an entrance somewhere else."
– Tom Stoppard

Chapter Sixteen

Green Mean Cleaning Machine

*"Anything else you're interested in is not going to happen if you can't breathe the air and drink the water. Don't sit this one out. Do something."– **Carl Sagan***

I walked in on my mother in the shower,

Luckily, she was fully clothed!

She was simply cleaning the shower,

I asked her what was wrong,

As she had tears streaming down her face,

"Oh, it always happens,

I think because of the chemicals in the cleaning products in such an enclosed space",

I was like,

"Holy fuck mother,

Don't you see that maybe there is something wrong here?"

"Oh, I thought it must be normal,

What else can I do...?"

I have obviously hung around a lot of health-conscious people and people who care for the environment. People who eat organic food, vegetarians and vegans, holistic health practitioners, people who religiously recycle and more and the surprising thing is that not a lot think about the *cleaning products* they use.

They don't realise the negative impact on the Earth they are having when using the standard cleaning products from a supermarket and the massive affect they are having on their own, their families and their pet's health.

Most people actually think that the only way to properly clean is to buy heavily toxic, extremely harsh synthetic cleaning products containing bleach and other chemicals when nothing could be further from the truth. I only used eco-friendly, all-natural cleaning products while living in Australia and was not sick once in 4 years. The only day off I had from work was when I had eaten egg, which I have been allergic to since birth. Which by the way, I didn't do on purpose, some cafes and restaurants do not take allergies at all serious and will feed you whatever you are allergic to regardless of if you have told them you might die or not!

Natural Cleaning Products

Anyway, back on topic, as mentioned, there are lots of natural cleaning products available which means you don't need to be breathing in toxic chemicals anymore. Or your pets and toddlers alike don't have to crawl about in them. Nor do they need to ingest them when they are chewing on furniture or sleeping, drooling into their pillows.

One of the most profound things that happened on my journey to healing eczema was changing my washing powder to an organic detergent, which made a life-changing difference to my skin.

When my clothes were washed in big brands detergent, I would itch and scratch all day. As soon as I changed to an organic detergent, my itching practically stopped. Realise that just because you might not have sensitive skin, doesn't mean the chemicals that you can't feel in the way I did are not being absorbed through the skin, into your bloodstream and affecting your health in some other way. Or that it won't do down the line, and when you go to your doctor with complaints, there are very few doctors on the face of the Earth that will link your chronic health issue with the chemical-laden washing detergent that you use.

I use natural cleaning sprays for the bathroom, kitchen and windows. Everywhere, in fact. I've not found a single synthetic cleaning product that's not available as an eco-friendly, natural counterpart. I even go as far as to use eco-friendly toilet cleaner, partly because I don't want any chemicals in my home, but more so for the environment and of course what is reentering into our water supply. As mentioned in Chapter 4: Life Begins With Water, when we discussed what is found in the water supply today. A lot of that is coming from what has gone down the drains from our very own home. As the quote below the title of this chapter suggests, *do your bit*, even when no one is looking!

"Integrity is doing the right thing even when no one is watching." - C.S. Lewis

In the paper titled, 'Getting Up to Speed: Ground Water Contamination' we once again we have a government agency, this time the Environmental Protection Agency (EPA) admitting that there are *hundreds* of chemicals in our drinking water that are *not regulated* and the health effects are *not known or understood*. They regulate the volume of chemicals such as benzene, which is a known carcinogen and has many adverse health effects, including birth defects, kidney and liver problems and learning difficulties in children. Which means, it's still in there! Along with hundreds of other chemicals!

Just from that one paper, there is a lot of evidence to back up what I've already said in this book. At a risk of repeating myself, it mentions lead which we just talked about in the previous chapter and the need to avoid large brand cosmetics. It backs up what I said about not drinking tap water, and it again shows the need to detoxify your body. It also backs up the fact you shouldn't blindly follow what your government says and to do your own research, as they have just openly admitted to not regulating hundreds of chemicals that they know nothing about!

Beyond that, research done in 2010 for the American Academy of Pediatrics found that from 1990-2006 an estimated 267'269 children □under five years of age were treated in US emergency departments for household cleaning product-related injuries. Bleach was the leading source.

If you have small children or pets and want to keep them safe, ditch the bleach and synthetic household cleaning products.

Homemade Cleaning Products

Even better than buying expensive natural cleaning products, why not make your own for next to nothing!? There are hundreds of uses for **white vinegar**, one of which is using it as a multipurpose cleaner.

All Natural Scented Multipurpose Cleaner

Ingredients

- One part white vinegar

- One part filtered water

- Lemon rind

- Rosemary sprigs

Method

1. Combine the ingredients in a spray bottle.

2. Shake and let infuse for one week before using.

Another amazing cleaner is **baking soda**. Use the following mixture to clean your kitchen and give stainless steel appliances an extra shine.

All Natural Kitchen Cleaner

Ingredients

- Four tablespoons baking soda

- 1-litre warm filtered water

Method

1. Mix ingredients in a bowl.

2. Use the mixture with a clean sponge.

Videos for how to make these and other homemade all-natural cleaning products will be added to my website. Now, just as the Chemical Age brought about some truly fantastic benefits, such as initially doing a great job of cleaning up bacteria which up until that point had killed hundreds of millions of people around Earth in events such as The Bubonic Plague. You can add to that the invention of plastic which brought about many amazing creations such as the laptop I'm typing on now. However, as we can see with both of those things, if we go too far, we end up with the very chemicals we loved at first causing havoc to our health and to the world that we live on. Our next chapter covers a subject which has some wonderful benefits for mankind but ends up in the same bracket as chemicals and plastic, which is something we need to protect ourself from when the human race goes *too far*.

For now, let's put some of the stuff we have learned into *action*.

Resources

Go to **www.TomBroadwell.com/resources** to see;

- The brands of natural cleaning products I recommend and use.

Action Steps

- Start changing cleaning products to at least the eco-friendly brands, if at all possible, go for all-natural or organic.

- Try making the homemade cleaning products above to see how quick, easy and cheap it is!

Chapter Seventeen
Smart Technology, Dumb Humans

"Sensitivity to electromagnetic radiation is the emerging health problem of the 21st century. It is imperative health practitioners, governments, schools and parents learn more about it. The human health stakes are significant."– **William Rea**

I looked out across the restaurant,

I seemed to be the only person not staring at my phone,

Young couples staring at their screen almost like they were possessed,

Opposite them, their partner did the same,

Seemingly not caring about what their partner did that day,

Or what they made of the meal so far,

Or indeed anything at all,

One guy put the phone back in his pocket instead of leaving it on the table,

Polite in a way,

I guess,

But did his balls need that dose of radiation...

Another thing people rarely think about when it comes to health is the radiation coming from their phones, laptops, and basically every electronic device in their homes and on their person. The worst offenders of which are wireless devices. Different types of radiation can be known under different names. There's electromagnetic frequency

(EMF), radio-frequency radiation (RFR), and radio-frequency electromagnetic radiation (RF-EMR).

Radiation

People don't think about it mainly because they can't see it. That doesn't mean it's not there and it doesn't mean it's not harmful. In the whole scheme of things, mobile phones, tablets, laptops and other wireless devices are fairly recent technology that once again has not been properly tested for the effects on human health. Only now are people coming to realise what a massive impact it is having on people's health, but still, it is often ignored by both government and the companies that make the products - surprise, surprise.

Not all governments, though. France made history in 2015 when it became the first country to ban WiFi in nursery schools and limit WiFi in schools in a bid to limit public exposure to electromagnetic fields generated by wireless technology. You have to ask yourself the question, why would they do this? It's because time and again, studies are showing that EMF exposure increases your risk of many diseases, including cancer. The more you are exposed, the higher the risk. That's why way back in Chapter 3: Sweet Dreams I told you to charge your phone at night in another room to start to limit your exposure.

Researchers based in Canada, USA and Israel, came to the conclusion that RFR (radio-frequency radiation) should be classified as 'Carcinogenic to Humans'.

They refer to nine studies (2011–2017) that report increased risk of brain cancer from mobile phone use. However when you type into search engines the first page it is littered with government reports and cancer charities (again) claiming there is 'no scientific evidence' linking EMFs, RFRs and cancer together, however, all these reports are from before 2011. The same researchers found an increased risk of brain, vestibular nerve and salivary gland tumours with mobile phone use. They had a concern for other cancers as well, such as breast, testicular, leukaemia, and thyroid.

The largest collection of studies and data on RF-EMR has been put together by the Oceania Radiofrequency Scientific Advisory Association Inc. (ORSAA), which is a nonprofit, independent scientific organisation. Their goal is to provide an independent perspective on the subject of radiation and the effects it has on humans, animals, and the environment. Which is great to have access to, because as we've seen, when there is money involved, and companies are doing their *own* research into the safety of *their* products, there can be some major conflicts of interest.

The ORSAA recently evaluated 2266 studies on RF-EMRs and found that 68.2% have demonstrated *significant* biological or health effects associated with exposure to manmade electromagnetic fields. In a paper published in The Lancet, researchers found that 89% of the 242 papers studied, showed the oxidative stress caused was significant.

This massive amount of scientific evidence completely goes against the prominent claim that wireless technologies pose no health risks and should be taken very seriously by everyone.

Researchers at Assam Agricultural University, in India, found that radiation is not only affecting human health, but also the health of animals in seriously dramatic fashion. The animal they were looking at could, in turn, bring an extremely bleak future as it is seen as *essential* to human life, the honey bee. They found that the bee colonies in close proximity to mobile phones towers were most affected by the electromagnetic radiation emitted by the tower. And the negative effects on wildlife carry on across a huge array of different species. The scariest thought of all is to lose *all* insects.

If the insects go, we go too!

A paper published in the journal Biological Conservation in 2019 showed that over 40% of insect species are threatened with extinction. The total mass of insects is falling by a frightening 2.5% per year, which means they could *vanish* within a century. Other animals such as birds and whales rely on the Earth's magnetic field for direction. That is how they navigate the world, knowing how to travel south for winter, for example. Research is showing that they are having their inner compass disrupted with manmade electromagnetic fields, and that is one of the reasons we are having whales wash up on beaches and huge flocks of birds suddenly dying.

Whether it's radiation, pollution or pesticides, we are not treating Mother Earth with a great deal of respect, and something needs to change soon. As mentioned, *you* can make a *huge* difference by choosing where to spend your money. Buying organic food, cosmetics, and natural cleaning products is one way to do this. Choosing to vote against things that affect the whole of humanity is another. Vote against the coming mass introduction of 5G, which is looking likely to impact our wildlife and the health of humanity in no way that *any other* form of radiation has done before it in *history*.

In an appeal to the European Union, more than 360 scientists and doctors from more than 40 countries have so far warned about the danger of 5G, which will lead to a *massive* increase in involuntary exposure to electromagnetic radiation. The expansion of the 5G network, which is intended to enable faster wireless transmission of larger amounts of data, requires the installation of many more antennas in urban areas. An estimated *10 to 20 billion* 5G-transmitters will be within housing, shops and in hospitals, connected to refrigerators, washing machines, surveillance cameras etc. this will make up what they are calling the Internet of Things. So, there will no longer be a way of escaping the harmful effects of radiation. In my mind, a frightening dystopian future awaits where you also won't be able to escape the ever watching eye of big brother. Everything and everyone will be tracked. This is being rolled out now, with no thought for anyone's wellbeing and most certainly nobody's privacy.

The consequences for the health of humans, plants and animals have not been discussed anywhere near enough.

So far there has been no scientific study that proves 5G is safe, but it's been rolled out nonetheless!

Boobs And Balls

I've mentioned balls a few times so far and will come back to that important subject in a moment, but something far more dear to my heart even more so than my testicles is boobs, or breasts if you want to talk scientifically. Please, ladies, protect these wonderful things. Every time I see a lady with a mobile phone in her bra, I wince and ask her to remove it immediately. My point is 100% proven in a paper published in Case Reports in Medicine. Researchers based in California found that ladies who carried their mobile phones in their bra developed tumours in that same exact area where they most regularly placed it, with none of the participants having any family history of breast cancer, and no other breast cancer risks.

Back to the sensitive subject of testicles where researchers at Technion University in Haifa found that sperm levels of men who kept their phones in their pocket during the day were seriously affected in 47 per cent of cases compared to just 11 per cent in the general population. Professor Gedis Grudzinskas, a fertility consultant at St George's Hospital London put it correctly when she said of the study: "Men need to think about their wellbeing and try to stop being addicted to their phones. Do you need to keep the phone right next to you on the bedside table? Some men keep their mobile in their shorts or pyjamas in bed. Is that really necessary?" Thank you for backing up my original thoughts, doctor.

Limiting Exposure

So, limiting your exposure is a huge thing. Here is a list of ways to limit your exposure to radiation that I recommend you do straight away.

- Don't go getting a **Smart Meter** in your home as these are shown to have very high levels of radiation causing headaches, fatigue, dizziness and insomnia in a study done in Victoria, Australia.

- **Energy Saver Lightbulbs** were shown to release cancer-causing chemicals phenol, naphthalene, and styrene when switched on by researchers at Alab Laboratory in Berlin. Phenol was the chemical of choice for the Nazi's to execute prisoners in war camps. Lovely job on saving the world there guys!

- If you have **Wi-Fi** turn it off at night when nobody is using it and get a low-radiation Wi-Fi transmitter. (Yes, they really exist!)

- Charge your phone on aeroplane mode in another room.

Expert scientists at the ORSAA also recommend the following;

- The use of **hands-free** for mobile phone calls where possible.

- Do not store against the body when switched on (non-aeroplane mode).

- Do not use wireless devices on your lap for long periods.

- Use mobile phones like answering machines for those employed in non-emergency roles rather than keeping them on.

- Use **wired connections** rather than Wi-Fi connections in your home.

- Do not leave active wireless devices near to where you sleep.

All these are ways to limit your exposure. There are also different ways to block radiation in your home and from your mobile devices

Blocking Radiation

In a paper published in the International Journal of Advances in Agricultural & Environmental Engineering, it was proven that **orgonite** has the capability to absorb harmful radiation being emitted into the environment by technology. Orgonite can be purchased online, from some health food stores, or you can even make it cheaply and easily at home. I place my orgonite pyramids on my modem and others on my bedside table. There are also phone cases and other technologies available which block EMF radiation. Some are better than others, so I advise you to do your research.

Lowering IQ

Now don't get me wrong, I love technology and how easy it has made it for me to contact home when I'm away and to write this book and do the research I need to back up what I'm saying. However, there comes a time when we need to step back and see that it has gone too far. As stated in the opening story, people connect more with their phones now than people, even when out to dinner in a social setting. *That is so freaking sad.* It truly is making us dumber too. Your mind is exactly like a muscle, if you don't use it, you lose it. We now simply search for answers on a search engine rather than trying to figure the answer out.

As a young boy I knew the telephone numbers of all of my friends, now I can't even recite my *own* number. We used to have to add up using our brain because we didn't carry a calculator around with us, now it's literally *all* there at the press of a button.

One thing I urge all parents and grandparents to do is to stop giving little kids phones and tablets to play with; it is seriously crushing their creativity.

Give them a pencil and paper and let them draw, not watch absolute garbage on YouTube or mindlessly press their finger on a screen. It just seems so lazy to give the kid a phone to shut them up, rather than interacting with them and helping them nurture their developing brain's. With kids staring at a tablet from such a young age stops it using their *imagination* and also developing their *social skills*. Kids don't talk to each other anymore; they all just sit on their own individual tablets, even when there's a group of them at a family party.

In the next chapter we are discussing one of the most toxic industries on Earth. Voting with your dollar and choosing which companies you will give your hard-earned cash to goes a long way to changing the world, and where some of the most disgusting atrocities committed against humanity are made is in the fashion industry. Before we find out who makes your clothes, complete the following Action Steps to make sure you are protecting you and your family against the toxic effects of radiation.

Resources

Go to **www.TomBroadwell.com/resources** to see;

- A link to the EMF blocking technology I use and recommend.

- A link to the low-radiation Wi-Fi transmitter I recommend.

Action Steps

- Immediately change out all Energy Saver Lightbulbs.

- Start charging your phone in a different room if you didn't already.

- Turn off your Wi-Fi at night.

- Buy some orgonite and place it around the house.

- Immediately stop putting your phone in your bra if you do that, ladies.

- Guys stop carrying your phone around in your pocket so much, either put it in a bag if you take one with you or leave it on your desk or any surface when at home - you don't need it with you 24/7.

- Practice leaving your phone at home when going out for something to eat or drink with someone so you can actually talk to that person.

- Stop giving small children phones and tablets to play with.

- I would also question if anyone under the age of 16 actually *needs* a phone? And if anyone under 12 years old should own a tablet?

Chapter Eighteen
Conscious Clothing

"There is no beauty in the finest cloth if it makes hunger and unhappiness."– **Mahatma Gandhi**

The little girl, no more than six years old,

Feeling light-headed in the sweltering conditions,

Looked out over the factory floor as her best friend passed out,

The air was thick with dust from cotton,

Making it hard to breathe,

Yesterday she'd seen a boy lose his hand in the heavy machinery,

Now she was watching as her friend was dragged away to the back,

Hoping she was okay,

But not stopping what she was doing for fear of another brutal beating,

She had her quota to meet,

It seemed impossible to do,

Feeling so tired from so little sleep,

Working 19 hours per day,

She had to meet her quota though,

Wondering if she'd ever get to go home,

Was this it?

Seven days per week,

One meal per day,

Eat, sleep, wake up and do it again,

No time to go home,

Her parents seemed to believe it was for the best,

They were promised she'd be given her full pay when she was old enough to get married,

For now,

She'd be given three nutritious meals per day,

And a full education,

It was the dream opportunity to get ahead in life that her parents never had...

One hundred and seventy *million* children are child labourers today, although that is likely to be a conservative number. Most are in the fashion industry.

Modern-Day Slavery

The story above is commonplace. Children are taken away from families with promises of a brighter future, only to endure horrific work conditions which is basically modern-day slavery, with little or no pay. Working in and amongst heavily toxic chemicals such as pesticides in the cotton fields, and then formaldehyde, acids and dyes in the factories. Children either get severely ill or are injured working with the heavy machinery and are cast aside, left to beg on the streets, only to create another generation of poverty.

You've got the child slaves, but then the adults don't fare much better. Looking at the Rana Plaza building collapse in Dhaka really shows the true colours of most large clothing manufacturers and fashion brands. Adults were working for as little as $38 *per month* in terrible conditions, and huge clothing corporations were dragging their feet on signing for improved work conditions and better pay. Many brands *continued* not signing even after more than 1100 people died when the poorly maintained building collapsed in 2013. Something that could have been *prevented* if large corporations *invested* in the people who make their branded clothing.

That's the price of fast fashion, and just like fast food, it may look good in the moment, but it always ends up leaving a bad taste in your mouth.

Environmental Issues

Not only are atrocities committed against the humans that work in the industry, but the fashion industry is also one of the most polluting industries on Earth. The clothing industry is accountable for over 20% of industrial water pollution in the world. Just for the production of **polyester**, there are over 70 million barrels of oil used per year. Polyester is a by-product of petroleum, which is a long and extremely toxic process, which is done by many of the children labourers which suffer debilitating diseases as a consequence. Polyester being another hormone disruptor and breast cancer causer.

On average, a person buys around 60lbs of new clothes per year and throws away more than 50 pounds. This then goes into landfills of which two-thirds of the materials are synthetic chemicals that will take more than 300 years to break down.

Human Health

That's the *human beings* behind the making of your clothes and what the industry is doing to the environment. But what are the clothes you wear doing to you, and your health? As mentioned, your skin is the largest organ of elimination and absorption.

Whatever you put *on* your body, goes *in* the body.

At the turn of the 20th century, our clothes were made up of purely natural materials. Now clothing contains a large variety of synthetic fibres such as **rayon**, **acrylic**, **polyester**, **spandex** and **olefin**, and there are over 8000 synthetic chemicals that are used in the manufacturing process.

"The use of manmade chemicals [in clothing] is increasing," says Dr Richard Dixon, Head of the World Wildlife Federation (WWF) Scotland, "and at the same time we have warning signals that a variety of wildlife and human health problems are becoming more prevalent."

We've already mentioned the toxicity of flame retardants, which are used in children's pyjamas. Then we have chlorine bleach, formaldehyde, VOCs (volatile organic compounds), PFCs (perfluorinated chemicals), and ammonia that is on your skin almost 24/7, making its way into your body. The toxic pesticides used on non-organic cotton persists in the material even after manufacturing. There is all-natural, ethically made clothing available.

Look for clothes made with organic cotton, hemp, flax, and bamboo.

Do some research into *who* (meaning the human beings behind the scenes) makes that brands clothing and accessories. I've done a lot of that research for you, and you can find links in the Resources section.

Skin Issues

Just like synthetic cosmetics, I know full and well what synthetic clothing does to my skin as I am very sensitive. Contact dermatitis and other skin problems are regularly discussed when looking at synthetic materials used in clothing. My skin always feels better in natural materials. Unfortunately, the line of work I'm in means that my uniform is always made up of synthetic materials. While on time-off, I only wear natural materials, and I am on the lookout for more natural sportswear which I will be using for my own workout videos.

I have been *very* naive in the past, thinking the *only* sportswear available is from the huge brands in the high street stores that everybody knows. Part of this is because I've *never* shopped for clothes online, only in the stores on the high street. It never even occurred to me that there were alternative brands available! Although in my defence, while living in Sydney, I did stick to my only shopping local rule. I bought all of my casual clothes exclusively at a store that only had one single store which was in my suburb, which was designed by the guy who owned the store, and I never even entered in a big brand store unless it was for workout clothes (which he didn't design). As I say, I'm also on a continuous journey of learning and will hold my hands up when I've been either wrong about things or completely blind to the truth! As I always say, you don't know what you don't know! So please forgive me, a lot of my videos are me wearing brands that have unethical practices and toxic clothing, which I was unaware of at the time. Going forward, I will be looking at only ethical sportswear too.

Underwire Bras

Another culprit of causing skin conditions but one I don't have too much experience in wearing, *ahem*, is tight-fitting underwire bras, worn over and over for years on end. The tightness of the wire and straps can also cause neck, shoulder and back pain, leading to headaches. Another concern is ladies having their breasts constantly strapped down against the body, because of their higher temperature. Much like testicles, they are supposed to hang free, somewhat away from the body to maintain their correct temperature. It's been known for some time that men who wear tight underwear can end up struggling with fertility and testosterone production because of the high temperature of the testicles. Certain cancers also like warmer environments.

The wire cutting into the body has also been shown to cut off the lymphatic drainage from the breast to the armpit leading to an accumulation of toxins, which can lead to breast cancer. This was first presented in 1995 by scientists Sydney Ross Singer and Soma Grismaijer in their book *Dressed to Kill*. Through their research with 5,000 women between 1991 and 1993, they discovered that breast cancer risk dramatically increased in women who wore bras over 12 hours per day and women who wear their bras 24 hours per day having a three out four chance of getting breast cancer. Those who barely ever wore a bra having the same chance to develop it as men.

Now this study did get a lot of detractors because it was an epidemiological study rather than the traditional double-blind study. Meaning it took a broad look at lots of information but didn't isolate one factor. So, for example, the study didn't take into account family history, weight, nutrition etc. However, even if an epidemiological study doesn't find the smoking gun, it can bring about some extremely strong correlations between two factors. From the number of women studied to the fact that the correlation was between *4-12 times* stronger than smoking and lung cancer, if you are any reasonable human being without a certain agenda, you'd have to say there was definitely *something* there! I mean you're not going to go from 3 out of 4 ladies wearing a bra 24/7 getting cancer to 1 in 152 if you wear your bra less than 12 hours per day if it hasn't got something to do with it!

Since then, there have been other studies showing very similar results. A study performed at the Guangdong Women and Children Hospital, Guangzhou, China in 2009 found that ladies not sleeping in their bras reduced risk by 60%. In 2011, a study by the Department of Public Health in Venezuela found that underwire bras and pushup bras, or indeed any bra that leaves an indent or red mark increases the risk for both fibrocystic breast disease and breast cancer. And finally back on home soil in the UK, research carried out at the Western General Hospital in Edinburgh compared 2,500 cases of cancer in women diagnosed 40 years apart and found that bra fit and length of wear was connected to increases in breast cancer rates.

However! As always, there is one study that goes to disprove this evidence completely. The National Cancer Institute (NCI) released data from its study in September 2014, which was conducted by The Fred Hutchinson Cancer Research Center in Seattle. When examining 1500 women who had both had and hadn't had cancer, they found zero evidence that bras had any connection to breast cancer. Ignoring almost every other study ever done remotely around the subject, they said they'd found literally nothing. It didn't matter the type of bra, the length of time you wore it or if it was correctly fitted, the size, the age in which one started wearing a bra, *nothing*. They only took into account one Harvard study from 1991 that found breast cancer rates were 100% higher in younger women who wore bras when compared with those who did not. But the Hutchinson team said it was flawed, however, *without any explanation* as to why they thought so. When mainstream media outlet USA Today, as part of a "myth-busting" segment, interviewed one of the researchers and asked about the link between bras and breast cancer, he simply responded, "There's just nothing there." That was it! Haha, you couldn't make this shit up. But wait! There's more!

The study had 1500 women who all wore bras their *entire* adult life. This means, once again with these studies around the *lucrative* breast cancer industry, there was no control group to compare to, so it's *impossible* to make any assumptions about any data collected. Ironically it almost proves the bra and cancer connection as a lot of the women had had breast cancer. *Also*, something else to consider, The Fred Hutchinson Cancer Research Center get monetary donations every year in an event called the Bra Dash. Much like in England, where we have the Race for Life; both are a 5km run. At the Bra Dash, all the ladies wear a pink bra on the outside of their clothes. Some might say that's a conflict of interest...

As for the Race for Life, over the past 20 years, more than 8 million people have taken part in raising over £547 million for charity. That is a lot of money! I honestly wonder where more than half a *BILLION* pounds in the UK alone has gone? Very little (if *anything*) has gone into studying any of the subjects I've covered in this book. Every time I've seen a news article while researching for this book, connecting for example bras to cancer, the final word is from a representative at a large charity. They send us a warning (not joking, they hammer the word Warning! down our throats) us not to jump to a conclusion about things like antiperspirants, bras, and shaving creams causing cancer. Why? *Every freaking time.* Why not let us come to our own conclusions about stopping spraying our armpits with heavy metals? They always say the only true way to prevent cancer is to keep your weight down and exercise regularly (without ever telling you how to do it *properly*). I'm talking to you now, big charities. Why don't *you* not jump to conclusions and spend some of the billions on researching heavily toxic chemicals and how the body *actually* works?

Sorry rant over. Oh no, not quite. By the way, again, you will always see the word myth thrown about when it comes down to bras and breast cancer, and again it's always on cancer charities, medical and so-called science websites. Guess which one of the studies they all choose to quote...Yep, you got it, The Fred Hutchinson Cancer Research Center...

Oh, and by the way, what *is* a myth is that not wearing a bra makes your breasts droopy. In fact, it's more likely they will sag because your chest muscles are not doing the work of holding your breasts up, and so the muscle will atrophy quicker over time. Consider making some changes to your wardrobe. **Wireless bras** are available, and you can easily remove the wire in your current bras. Never wear a bra to bed and consider going braless when you get home from work. If your bra is leaving red marks, it's too tight.

Bedtime

On an evening, I only sleep in **organic sheets**. At home (when not on a cruise ship), I have a **mattress made of natural materials**. Both of these things are something to seriously consider, especially if you still struggle to sleep at night. It's going to be difficult to sleep while breathing in flame retardant from your mattress and synthetic chemicals from your sheets! I sleep on an **organic buckwheat pillow** which is a fantastic purchase. It keeps you cool even in the warmest climates and moulds to fit the perfect shape of your head and neck area leading to the most wonderful night's sleep. Takes a little getting used to, but my gosh is it worth it.

And there you have it; you need to be thinking about what is on your skin at all times if you truly want perfect health or to heal any health issues you might be having at the moment. Hopefully, you can now see the massive difference to the world you can make by voting with your dollar. Think before you buy anything from a large manufacturer in any industry to help other humans live a half-decent life and to help save Mother Earth for future generations.

"Every time you spend money, you're casting a vote for the kind of world you want." - Anne Lappe

The next chapter goes the other way completely and does not talk about the dangers of anything, but the almost magical health benefits of Mother Nature. Before we get to connect you to your wild side, go ahead and take action to make some changes.

Resources

Go to **www.TomBroadwell.com/resources** to see;

- The brands of ethical clothing I recommend and use.

- The brands of natural bedding and buckwheat pillow I recommend and use.

Action Steps

- Most people only wear 20% of their wardrobe, so give the other 80% away to someone who will wear it; friends, family or people in need and then stay *minimalistic*.

- Only buy clothes that you *love* and actually *need*.

- Buy ethical, 100% natural clothing from now on.

- Change your bras to wireless and wear them less!

- Change your bedding and mattress to natural.

- Purchase an organic buckwheat pillow; you won't regret it!

- Think before you buy anything from a large company. I'm not saying *all* are bad, but it's okay to ask. Who makes this? Who loses out? Is there a better, more ethical way?

Chapter Nineteen

Eco-Therapy

"Nature's peace will flow into you as sunshine flows into trees. The winds will blow their own freshness into you, and the storms their energy, while cares will drop off like autumn leaves."— **John Muir**

Surrounded by the tall trees,

In all their grounding glory,

The smell of flowers and herbs triggering feelings of warmth and comfort,

The sunlight peeping through the branches,

He knew deep down that he felt right at home,

Now the short but beautifully fulfilling walk down to the beach,

He slipped his flip-flops off as his feet touched the sand,

That feeling felt so...right,

Just like walking barefoot in the grass at home,

This place was magical,

Filled with so many of nature's wonders,

So much of nature's beauty,

He felt his worries melt away,

His illness felt like it was fading away too,

To be at one with nature,

Was to be whole again...

This is our vision. My partner May and I are creating our retreat to be a place for people to reconnect with nature and their true self. Away from the craziness that is modern life and the busyness of the city. For those who are suffering from illnesses or not. An eco-therapy getaway with extensive herb and vegetable gardens. Organic food, juice cleanses, detox programs, health seminars, group meditations, yoga on the beach, a holistic spa where you get to choose herbs from the gardens for your treatment and much, much more. For those who would like the idea but also want a more 'normal' type of holiday, we will also have a beach bar serving organic cocktails, wine and beer as per Chapter 13: Your Liver Is A Muscle... ;)

Spending Time In Nature

Moving on from the almost shameless plug and a friendly reminder of our retreat to what exactly is 'eco-therapy'? Studies have shown nature is indeed the great healer it has always thought to have been throughout history. I've shown you evidence of plants and herbs and their healing powers and that of saltwater and the ocean, but what about simply spending time in nature? All you have to do to understand me is to *trust yourself* and your own *feelings*.

That feeling of walking barefoot in the grass or on the sand at the beach. That feeling of swimming in a lake or the ocean. That feeling does not lie. It truly is both magical and healing to spend time in nature.

Researchers at UEA's Norwich Medical School looked at 140 studies involving more than 290 *million* people around the world. They found spending time in or living close to nature has significant health benefits. These include reducing the risk of diabetes and cardiovascular disease, as well as significantly reducing levels of cortisol which of course is the nasty stress hormone we want to avoid as much as possible.

In a study done of 20'000 mobile phone users in the UK, participants were asked to fill out a questionnaire stating their current mental health. Researchers used satellite positioning (GPS) to determine the participant's geographical coordinates. The group contributed over *one million* geo-located data points. Talking about making technology and GPS useful for the future of the human race rather than constantly imposing on our privacy! Anyway *personal* opinion over...In the study marine and coastal margins were comfortably the happiest locations, and participants were significantly and substantially happier outdoors in all green or natural habitats, far more so than urban areas. The researchers equated it to "the difference between attending an exhibition and doing housework".

I seemed to have always known the power of nature, partly because I have always dreamed of living on a beach. I came oh so close as I worked ungodly hours when living in Syndey, as to be able to afford to live at Balmoral Beach. But the huge expense of even living *close* to the beach brought about stress I was trying to alleviate by living there in the first place! Mosman is the name of the suburb in which I was situated, which is damn near the most expensive place to live on Earth! My two-bedroom apartment was A$850 *per week*, and I couldn't even see the sea. I was simply close to it.

Then as I came back to work on Cruise Ships, I realised I could have everything for a lot less. I travelled the world, spending time on the most beautiful beaches, in places where the cost of living was far less than Australia, or England where I grew up. I thought to myself, why not earn the US Dollar or the Great British Pound and live somewhere far cheaper? Get out of the rat race. Even though I earned a decent amount of money as a Personal Trainer while living in Australia, I was always under pressure to find the money for paying rent and bills because of the extremely high cost of living. Then I moved to the Philippines, and someone offered to sell me a beach, my *own* beach, with a small wooded area as a backdrop...how could I say no? So now I am lucky (luck I created) enough to live in nature every day.

This all ties into the next chapter and truly living the life you want. But spending time in nature is hugely beneficial for your health. If you currently live in a concrete jungle of a city, make sure to plan weekends away that incorporate either mountains or beaches or lakes or countryside of any type. Get out there and explore. Show your family how beautiful Earth is, breathe the fresh air and feel the wonders of nature.

Forest Therapy

An activity known as forest bathing is already very popular in Japan. Participants spend time in the forest, either sitting, lying down or just walking around. Researchers in Japan found, 'that phytoncides -- organic compounds with antibacterial properties -- released by trees could explain the health-boosting properties of forest bathing.' In a paper published in the journal Evidence-Based Complementary and Alternative Medicine, researchers compared walking in the forest and urban environments. The group walking in the forest had a significantly lower heart rate and anxiety levels. They also reported walking in the forest significantly reduced negative emotions compared with walking in the urban environment.

In a study of 585 participants published in 2018 conducted in Japan, researchers found that 'walking through forest areas decreased the negative moods of depression-dejection, tension-anxiety, anger-hostility, fatigue, and confusion and improved the participants' positive mood of vigour compared with walking through city areas.'

If you have troubled youngsters, my advice would be to take them for regular walks in the forest, or along the beach. Science is constantly proving the undeniable positive effects on both physical and mental health of being in nature. If they are struggling in school, nature has also proven to be great for many cognitive functions, including creative thinking. In a paper published in PLOS One, researchers found that people who spent time in nature were able to solve puzzles that needed creative thinking 47% more of the time than those who did not.

Grounding

As I write these words once again, I'm on a plane, 14 hours from Manila to London. I know after travelling such a huge distance that once I land I need 'grounding'. One of the best ways I've found to do this, and it sounds funny, I know, is to hug a tree. Trees are quite often centuries old and (literally) have deep roots to the long history and origins of Earth. To reconnect with Earths past is something I feel we all need to do, and hugging a tree is one of the easiest and best ways to do this. This again is backed by science, with even reports for The UK

Parliament stating, 'safe, green spaces may be effective in treating some forms of mental illnesses.'

It has now been proven that everything is made up of *energy* that vibrates. *Everything* has a vibrational pattern.

You and I are made up of energy that vibrates, the food you eat, the music you listen to and the water that you drink.

Some vibrations are good for human health, and others are bad. Amazingly researchers at Universidade do Estado do Rio de Janeiro found that when drinking water that is treated with a 10Hz vibration blood coagulation rates will change immediately. They found that white blood cells increased significantly, and LDL (bad cholesterol) decreased.

When touching a tree, its vibrational pattern will affect various biological behaviours within your body. It has been shown to improve many health issues such as; mental illnesses, Attention Deficit Hyperactivity Disorder (ADHD), depression and can alleviate headaches. Speaking of vibration, that's another reason why natural spring water that is bottled at the source beats filtered tap water all day long. As the natural spring water winds its way through rocks picking up minerals along the way it develops very different *energy* to the water that has been chemically treated and wound its way through miles of metal pipes.

Even living *near* trees is massively beneficial for your health. In a 2015 paper published in the journal Scientific Reports researchers concluded, 'having 10 more trees in a city block, on average, improves health perception in ways comparable to an increase in annual personal income of $10,000 and moving to a neighborhood with $10,000 higher median income or being 7 years younger.'

Clearly, there's something healing about trees.

Energy is also why eating as close to as nature intended is so important. You need to limit the intake of food that is changed from its natural state by the hand of man. For movie fans out there, I hope you realise Avatar was trying to teach you something about *reconnecting* with

Mother Earth and her wondrous, magical ways. The next chapter will scare the bejesus out of most people so take this opportunity to go outside and spend some time in nature to calm down and alleviate stress. Take the next Action Steps, and I will see you at our resort sometime soon...

Resources

Go to **www.TomBroadwell.com/resources** to see;

- A link to our resorts website if you haven't checked it out yet.

Action Steps

- Go and hug a tree!

- Plan to spend more time in nature if it is something you don't do regularly.

- Start by going for a daily walk in nature or at least a park with lots of grass and trees.

- Plan weekends away at the ocean, a lake or a forest.

- Book a holiday that submerges you in nature.

Section Five

The Chimney of
Your Health House

*"Life is like a chimney - you sometimes have to get through the dark before you see the light." — **Matt Haig***

Chapter Twenty
Quit Your Job

"Never get so busy making a living that you forget to make a life." —
Dolly Parton

Shattered from another long day at work,

The 40-year-old man threw down his bag,

He didn't even bother hanging his coat up,

He wearily lowered himself into his favourite chair,

He knew what was next,

His two young children ran in,

"Daddy, daddy!" they excitedly shouted,

He barely had the energy to answer,

He felt terrible, but he desperately needed some alone time,

Work had been particularly tiring that day,

He felt his blood pressure rising again,

Counting down the weeks to his much-needed vacation,

Wondering where the time had gone,

It seemed like yesterday that he left school,

A fit, young man so full of life and ambition,

Now a middle-aged man with declining health and a potbelly,

Stuck in a job he went to,

8-12 hours a day,

5-6 days a week,

If he was ever asked why he went to work,

His answer was nothing other than,

"To make money.",

Now he didn't even have the energy to play with his young children,

Whom he worked so hard for,

So, they could have a brighter future,

He then thought to himself,

'Can I continue working in a job that I hate for another 30 years'...

This is how life is for the majority of people I speak to; most people wake up every single day, crawl their ass out of bed and go to work because they *have* to. Not because they want to. But because they need money to survive. If this is not you, and you love what you do for work, then feel free to skip this chapter and move on, but even you still might find some gold in this short chapter.

Of the people who go to work because they have to, a small amount still has some ambition. In my experience it's usually the corporate type, who have a carrot dangled in front of them for decades, saying that they could become a director one day and earn great money. They are told *every* director worked their ass off, working inhumane hours and gave *everything*. So, they pursue that life, through all the hard work, the blood, sweat, and tears. You probably won't hear of the ones who tried but failed due to mounting health problems...

Doing What You Love

I know, it sounds crazy. *Quit your job.* Because in today's world *money* rules all and we *need* it to survive. My point here is a couple of things. Number one, we need to start looking at life as maybe our one and only because no matter what our beliefs are, there is no *guarantee* of another life. (And hey, I believe *this* is not just it but still I want to make this life as great as possible). And so, it should be your mission to have as greater life as possible and working 40+ hours per week in a job that you hate is not the way to do that. All I'm saying is, how would you feel if you could do something you *love* every single day? Now *that* would be a great life!

I'm not saying quit your job *tomorrow*, but when you have saved enough to go out there and do something you love. To do that, as my story suggests, needs much less money than you think. You can live like a freaking *king* in a lot of countries on very little, or by earning a stronger currency than the one in the country you want to live. If you love the country you currently live in, there are many ways to start creating the life that you want and doing what you love. Start building your dream line of work on the side while still working in your job.

The second point here is most people don't do things because of fear. "Oh no, what if I never, ever get another job." That sounds crazy I know, but that's what a close friend of mine's excuse was for not quitting a job he hated so much it kept him awake at night, who by the way, is incredible at his line of work. If you have skills in your area of expertise, you'll get another job. Others don't do things like going after their dreams because of what others might think if they fail. Excuse the language for a moment but who gives a *flying fuck* what others think? Seriously, get out of the prison cell of other people's *opinions*. One of my favourite quotes comes to mind right now, and that is;

"Care about what other people think and you will always be their prisoner." - Lao Tzu

Let me tell you through experience, you'll have a fair few people telling you can't do certain things and that you'll fail. Imagine how many times I've heard this after doing such things as making and starring in a movie with no prior acting experience (that's had over 40 *million* views on YouTube). I've lived and successfully built businesses on three different continents. And then everything else I've set out to do like buying my very own beach, to setting up a website, to writing this book and many other 'not normal' things I've done. Were they all a success? Absolutely not. Did I learn valuable lessons from each failure that lead me to be the person I am today? Yes. Do I regret anything I've done that was out of the ordinary? No.

The first type of person who will tell you that you might fail are people who actually care about you and are looking out for you. People like close friends and family, who are telling you it's not possible because of *their* past experiences and *their* insecurities, which is coming from a position of love. The second type of person is like *poison* to your dreams, and so, in my opinion, you need to classify them as negative people who you should have got rid of already. They are coming from a position of jealously—people who want to piss on your bonfire because they have no bonfire of their own. Neither type of person is worth listening to a whole lot. Yes, you might learn some things from relatives or friends, but if their advice is coming from a place of fear, you're best blocking out pretty much all of it.

The people you need to listen to are people who have succeeded at what you are trying to do.

I don't mean to be rude, but I find it a little bit funny when I see overweight people passionately giving out nutrition and exercise advice in the gym. Or more often than not, the people giving relationship advice are those who *don't* have a partner and have a history of broken relationships. The people I most often see giving advice on how to make money and build businesses are *broke*. Why follow the advice of people who have failed? Hey, I'm far from perfect in lots of areas, I've had my fair share of failed relationships and never been a millionaire, so I won't I be handing out tons of advice there.

Would you ever read the biography of someone who came second in the Olympics? I doubt it. Usually you would search out the winners, the champions in their chosen discipline. And look, I just mentioned someone who got a *silver medal* in the Olympic Games! I didn't even mention the person who came last. I bet you can't name *one* athlete who came last in the 100-metre sprint final at the Olympics in any year...And at the time that was the 8th fastest person on Earth! An *astonishing* feat. So why would you listen to the average Joe who completely failed at what they are trying to give you advice for...?

Basically put, when it comes to going out and chasing your dreams, you'll come up against *a lot* of resistance and have to jump over a *massive* amount of hurdles. As scary as it is, you have to ask yourself one question, 'If I do this, what's the *worst* that can happen?' If the answer is not death or serious injury, *then you should do it*. In most situations, if you somehow fail, you *will* bounce back, and after a little struggle, life will look pretty darn okay, plus you will have a lesson or two to *learn* from. If you do fail, yes people will say things, and you might not have your dream life...just yet, but you're not dead. So pick yourself up, brush yourself down and carry on.

On the flip side if you don't try, then you'll work the next few decades in a job that you don't like (if you don't like it) and maybe, possibly have some stress-related illnesses. And you'll without a doubt regret not trying...

"In the end...We only regret the chances we didn't take, the relationships we were afraid to have, and the decisions we waited too long to make." - Lewis Carroll

Age Is Just A Number

So, there you have it. Stop messing around, stop with the excuses and go out there and live your dreams. How does this relate to health? As mentioned, stress is one of, if not the biggest killer in the world. Doing what you love can be stressful, however, if you jump out of bed on a morning excited for your day, that is *far* less of a burden on your health than waking up every day hating the fact you have to go to work. Working on something you have *passion* for and *love* doing, leads to far more positive thoughts which we know now is the one thing that most centenarians claim is the secret to their longevity.

"Stress less, don't worry and be happy." - Every old and wise person ever.

I can tell you now, on an almost daily basis I meet people who have given *everything*, including their *health* to a career where all in all they made *someone else* rich and someone's else's dreams come true.

Now I know what the most common objection to this chapter will be for most of my readers, and that is age. I'm *too old* to start something new, most will claim. Even those in their *forties* might be thinking this. In a bit of irony here in this book all about health, I'm going to use

Colonel Sanders as a perfect example that you are never too old to try. The Colonel is the man who started Kentucky Fried Chicken, a man who didn't become a professional cook until he was 40 years old when he developed his famous chicken recipe. From there, he only started franchising his restaurants at the age of 62 and became a world-famous icon at the age of 75 years old when he sold the rights to KFC. And there will be a *million and one* examples out there, so use this and others as your inspiration to build the life of your dreams at any age.

Now I'm not going to go *too* deep in how to build the life of your dreams, as I haven't quite done it yet and so it's not my place to do that...just yet. But I've been on that journey since high school when I realised there was more to life than going to university, getting a degree and then working a dead-end job you hate. It's been an epic journey of ups and downs, and *many* expensive lessons. However, it's a journey in which I have not regretted one moment, and one day I might write a how-to book on building the life of your dreams, detailing all of my lessons and achievements, ups and downs, and greatest highs and most epic lows. That will happen once I *know* that I have achieved what I am currently going out to achieve. For now, my expertise lays in the health field, which is a huge part of living that dream life for anyone.

If you're not healthy, then you can't enjoy the fruits of your labour.

Finding Your Passion

The one thing I can tell you though, is this, the reason that my expertise is health is it is my *passion*. I yearn to learn more every day, and I *love* writing about it and I love how it makes me feel every day. Happy, healthy, positive and full of vitality. Once you find your passion, you *know* that this is your *calling*. That's what you should be doing with your life, at least in a bit part. So, I urge you to *right now*, write down what makes you passionate.

What would make you get up every morning full of excitement?

Once you find your passion, ask yourself, what does your dream life look like in 5 years? What do your health, spirituality, love life, family life, work life, finances, and social life look like? Blue sky thinking, meaning if *nothing* could go wrong. Write it all out in detail. Keep it somewhere you can look at it every day. *Knowing* whether you are on track or need to focus more on a particular area.

Then you need a why. *Why* do you want those things? Once you have your passion and your why you now have what you need, to start to get shit done. From there it's onto business plans and the like, which is not what this book is about, so we won't be going into it here. However, check out the Resources section for some links to books and people that I've used to great success on my journey so far.

This is the chapter I was referring to in Chapter 14: Negativity Kills Longevity in the Seminars and Events section. These sorts of events will be taught by the people you need to be listening to, successful people who have achieved what you want to achieve. They will be attended by (generally) happy people who are on the same path as you, whom you can share ideas with, people who in general will help you get what you want if you are willing to help them get what they want too. One thing I do know is to be successful in business you want to be creating a lot of win-win situations.

"You will get all you want in life, if you help enough other people get what they want." - Zig Ziglar

These events will help you build the knowledge and skills you need to succeed. So, if you haven't booked onto one already, do so now. Find your passion and search for events based around that. Or if you want something that will teach you from a broader perspective on how to be successful in general, there are loads of 'gurus' that run events based around everything from developing a Positive Mental Attitude to building a profitable business, investing money, increasing sales and the like.

Being happy at work is one thing, but what we discuss in the next chapter has the potential to bring about abundant joy throughout your *entire* life with *pure* love and affection that only one thing on Earth can give. Okay well, two, one is a baby (which then turns into an adult and all the baggage that they bring). However, the second is pure and innocent for its entire life... Not only will I show the health benefits that *you* will feel from owning a furry little friend, but I am going to show you how to take care of your little critter to improve *its* health and wellbeing. Before we get to that take the following Action Steps to bring about clarity if you are struggling with what you want to do in life.

Resources

Go to **www.TomBroadwell.com/resources** to see;

- A link to books and people who can get you on the right path to the life of your dreams.

- Just for some fun, a link to the film I starred in and co-produced.

Action Steps

- Write down a list of things which you are passionate about.

- Write out what *your* dream life looks like in five years.

- Find your *why*.

- *Start* (straight away) writing out a plan on how you are going to achieve this.

- Head to the Resources page to find more information on what to do next, but don't stop reading this book yet, you're almost at the end!

Chapter Twenty-One

Get A Pet

"Animals are reliable, many full of love, true in their affections, predictable in their actions, grateful and loyal. Difficult standards for people to live up to." – **Alfred Armand Montapert**

Driving home from what seemed like the longest day ever at work,

Drained from the constant human interaction I'd had that day,

People constantly on at me for things out of my control,

Which they were adamant were in my control,

Not knowing anything of what goes on behind the scenes,

Telling me how shit the company I worked for was,

As if after a horrible day in that particular moment I gave a shit about their opinion,

Not stopping when I was politely telling them to fuck off in my mind,

Man, what a day,

I just needed to be secluded and not see another human that I don't love for at least the next 12 hours,

I pull up in the drive,

Exhausted,

I rush to close the door behind me to shut out the rest of the world,

As I enter both my cat and my dog are sat waiting for me,

My dog jumps excitedly when he sees me,

As no human has,

Ever,

My cat purrs and strokes herself up against me,

Ahh, the true unconditional love made me feel immediately better...

A lot of people know the pleasure of owning a pet, but the healing abilities of animals can be often overlooked.

Health Benefits Of Pets

Anthrozoology is the study of the interaction between humans and other animals and has been growing for the last 35 years. Studies have shown a massive amount of health benefits to owning a pet which includes;

- Lowered stress levels

- Decreased blood pressure

- Decreased cholesterol levels

- Decreased triglyceride levels

- Decreased feelings of loneliness

- Increased opportunities for exercise and outdoor activities

- Increased opportunities for socialisation

In children there are also benefits that go beyond just having a friend to always play with;

- Cognitive stimulation

- Improved behaviour in children

- A heightened understanding of others

- Increased immunity

- Lower anxiety levels

Caring For Your Pet

The health benefits are truly amazing and all the more reason to get a pet if you don't have one already. As we can see, the positive effect of animals on humans stretch even beyond the pure love that a pet can bring. But now we need to be asking, how should we be caring for our pet's health? Just like us, pets need regular exercise and to eat well. Once again, there is a *real* problem, with one-third of cats and dogs in the US being overweight. Just like a child, we think we are being nice giving a dog scraps from the table, believing it's a treat. When really, we are lowering its quality of life and increasing its risk of many diseases that only domesticated animals seem to get, such as diabetes, heart disease and cancer.

When a pet is overweight, it is far likelier to develop bone issues and breathing problems. Smaller breeds of dogs have their life expectancy lowered by over two years according to research done by The University of Liverpool and WALTHAM Petcare Science Institute. Portion control is absolutely necessary, but studies show 87% of pet owners simply *guess* at how much their pets need when it comes to feeding them.

However, once again for me at least, it's not how much we are feeding our pets that is the main problem, it's *what* we're feeding them. Now if you thought what they get away with feeding to *humans* is bad, be prepared to be *shocked* to your very core when it comes to what we are feeding our pets! I'm going to look at cats and dogs as our main focus in this section; however, for *any* other pet, all the basic principles of what you need to implement are the same.

The first thing we need to learn is that just like with human food, it's all about clever labelling and advertising, and a few huge corporations own most of the brands.

Most of the 'premium' products are made from *exactly* the same ingredients as the cheap stuff and are in *no way* better for your pet's health.

The second thing is, in the wild, dogs are mainly carnivores and cats are pure meat-eaters. If we look at the main ingredients in pet foods from the leading manufacturers, the most common ingredient by far is *corn*. I'm going to teach you how to read labels throughout this chapter, of which most of what I say, including the next part, is true for *humans* too. On pet and human food labels, ingredients are listed in order of weight. The heaviest ingredient being first and the lightest in weight listed last. This can be *very* misleading, as you might see chicken meal listed as the first ingredient and then ground corn as the second, then corn gluten meal as the third. Followed by rice meal somewhere further down the list, and so the combination means *starch* is by far the main ingredient in a *carnivore's* meal. That will *not* lead to good health and vitality.

In the wild, our pets eat *zero* starches and so are not designed to break down enormous amounts of carbohydrates.

But that's only the *start* when it comes to what's in your pet food. Pet food is bunched in with animal feed when it comes to laws, which we briefly touched on in Chapter 10: Grown By Nature. Cattle are fed cats and dogs that are killed by euthanasia in pet homes, and so are cats and dogs... I'll let that sink in for a moment...Little Rex over there is an unwitting *cannibal*. Sodium pentobarbital, the drug that is used to kill pets by euthanasia, is regularly found in pet food and will obviously wreak havoc with your critter's health. In the so-called food 'laws', your cats and dogs can be fed animals that die from causes other than slaughter, such as disease or drug contamination while on a farm. But it doesn't stop there. Roadkill comes under what is allowed in pet food. The carcasses of all the different animals are rendered at very high temperatures in order to extract proteins, fats, and other usable parts while killing the bacteria. The high temperatures at which rendering occurs destroys the DNA of the animal, so no one can ever truly tell what is in the final product. It might contain some chicken, but also some cats and dogs. Then a dead skunk may have been thrown in for good measure.

Something Else To Consider...

Beyond that, we have all the synthetic chemical additives to deal with. Most of these are in processed human food too, along with supplements and cosmetics, so you can learn some *more* ingredients to add to what you have already learned, that are definitely worth avoiding when buying products for the kids and yourself.

Carrageenan is one to avoid. It's used as a thickener, stabiliser and emulsifier not only in pet food but also dairy products, soy milk, sandwich meats and infant formula. It is not only used as a food additive, but it is also used to induce inflammation in laboratory animals. Excellent work, whoever decided to put that in food for a newborn baby!

Butylated hydroxyanisole (BHA) and **butylated hydroxytoluene (BHT)**, **propyl gallate**, and **propylene glycol** are all harsh synthetic preservatives that are all allowed in pet food. This concoction of synthetic wonders makes pet food last more than 25 years, outlasting the pet it was designed for! The food industry uses BHA and BHT for humans by the way and they are listed as carcinogenic by The National Institute of Health. **Vitamin E** is a much better alternative to look out for on the label.

Amazingly propylene glycol was banned for use in *cat food* because it was causing blood disorders but is still allowed in *human* and dog food! That is even though The Environmental Working Group has ranked it at the highest level of concern in regard to its effects on blood. I'd avoid this one if I were you! Even if that cake and ice cream looks too good to resist. Guys and gals, if you are *still* regularly eating nonorganic processed foods with the amount of evidence presented up until now, I'm struggling for words to say...

Propyl gallate is also used in human food, mainly in processed meats like sausages. In some studies, it's been shown to cause cancer, even though a lot of manufacturers claim its safe. In 2014 The European Food Safety Authority concluded that the available studies showing it to be safe are outdated and poorly described. So again, I wouldn't take my governments word, or your governments word for what is safe and what is not.

Protect yourself, your family and your pet and follow every Action Step in this book.

There are organic pet foods available that will avoid most of these toxic ingredients; however, just be careful of clever labelling again. Some companies' name has the word organic in (or something close to it) or natural, when they are, in fact, not organic and have synthetic ingredients in. So please still read the labels. As I always say, just because it's in a health food store does not mean it's healthy!

Homemade Pet Food

A great way of giving your pet exactly the right nutrients it needs, without all the nasties, while saving tons of cash, is to prepare its food, with love, at home! Just focusing on cats and dogs for a moment here, but if you have another type of pet, do the same research I'm going to recommend for cats and dogs, and you will be able to feed your pet, whatever it is, a healthy, nutritious, balanced diet.

Please consult your veterinarian so you can transition your pet to homemade food safely without it getting sick.

This is a must! Ask them for advice about ratios for your particular pet too. However, please be advised, just as it is with our own doctors, veterinarians barely cover nutrition while studying and are sometimes incentivised to sell certain brands of pet food. Meaning, just like my advice was to you about doctors, if they are unwilling or unable to help you with your pet's nutrition, find a new vet.

To get you started, the best balance of ingredients for dogs is 75% meat, organs, and bones, and 25% vegetables and fruits. For cats, the best balance of ingredients is 88% meat, organs and bone, and 12% vegetables and fruit. This is more fruits and vegetables than either would eat in the wild, but the extra fibre, vitamins and other nutrients have shown to be good for their health. Some ingredients should be avoided entirely, including garlic and onions (for cats), macadamia nuts, grapes/raisins, avocados, spinach, chocolate, caffeine, milk, and salt for both cats and dogs. Please consult your veterinarian and web sources for complete lists. Please note as well, just like us, your pets can become addicted to their processed food, so if it doesn't work straight away *don't give up*, they may need to be weaned off their favourite 'treats'.

And there we go. As we head into the final section, and the final chapter, all I have to say is it was a pleasure going on this journey with you. I hope there are many more experiences we can have together in the future. The final chapter will tie this all together and give you some more useful tools you can add to make sure you continue achieving your goals. Before you head there, complete this set of Action Steps and I will see you on the other side.

Resources

Go to **www.TomBroadwell.com/resources** to see;

- The brands of pet food I recommend.

Action Steps

- Buy a pet if you don't already have one! Make a smart choice with what pet would be best for you, regarding work schedule, family etc.

- Start either exercising with your pet daily, taking them for walks or letting them have a workout by opening the cage door.

- Practice portion control with your pet too. Research how much food it actually needs.

- Change your pet's food to either organic or even better yet start transitioning into homemade pet food.

- Make sure your pet is getting the same quality of water that you are!

Section Six

The Garden Path of Your Health House

"No one saves us but ourselves. No one can and no one may. We ourselves must walk the path." – **Buddha**

Chapter Twenty-Two
Summary & Implementation
"The great aim of education is not knowledge but action." – ***Herbert Spencer***

I stood there at reception,

Awaiting my next client,

Drinking my beetroot and ginger juice,

My mid-afternoon boost,

I could hear someone coming up the stairs,

I thought it must be my next client and so I put down my juice readying myself to put them through the latest workout I had created,

But no - it was a lady who felt familiar but was no client of mine,

She said, "Tom, you still work here!"

I was slightly taken aback that she knew my name,

Trying not to look like I didn't know who she was, I replied, "Yes, I do..."

The lady knew it was clear I might not know who she was and so clarified,

"I was here a few years ago, maybe it was three or four years.

Anyway, I came in and had a session and as great as you were, I temporarily declined, and said I'd think about it...

Well, here I am.

I've thought about it, and I'm 10kgs (22lbs) heavier and have just been diagnosed as prediabetic."

"Okay, so you're ready now?" I cheekily asked, knowing if she'd had a session with me, she knew I'd be at least a little bit cheeky.

"Yep." she said.

"One thing I'll tell you Tom is this,

I wish I had started sooner."

True story. The final sentence she said I will never forget. This event has happened and will continue to happen repeatedly the world over.

People don't realise how important their health is until it's *gone.*

It's a condition that *plagues* the human race. People push their health and their body to the *limit*, thinking that it won't happen to them: the cancers, the heart attacks and the type 2 diabetes. Modern day life taxes our body more than at any other time in history, and it shows the world over.

Don't become a statistic!

Take care of your one and only body while it functions to the best of its ability. Now, I'm not saying you need me after reading this book, but if you do, I'm here for you. The number one reason people struggle with their weight and their health is *consistency*. Crash diets, Biggest Loser TV shows, celebrity gossip magazines and 21-day detoxes create an *illusion* that you can achieve your dream body and optimal health in a short period of time. You've lost a ton of weight on your latest diet, and then what? If this sounds like you, I can help *you* on an ongoing basis.

"Your goals and dreams desperately need your consistent actions right at this very moment, and the future will surely judge and reward you based on how often and well you attend to them." - Edmond Mbiaka

If you need *truly* healthy recipes that are based on the information in this book and not the huge amounts of recipes based on counting calories, low-fat and high-protein that will only lead to ill health then come see me.

If you want fun 20-minute workouts, video series on how not to get injured, stretching, creating the perfect posture, and more health tips than you can shake a stick at all designed by me; but best of all a *community* of people that is on the same journey as *you* then come and join me at **www.TomBroadwell.com** - have a free trial and see if;

1. You take action and use it as you should. (Hopefully, this book motivated you enough to do so!).

2. You *LOVE* it. Many others do, and the results are nothing short of amazing. You'll potentially find the most complete health program available on the world wide web. It's not just about working out, it all about living the *holistic*, healthy lifestyle everyone should.

If you can achieve your goals on your *own*, then go for it! I'm simply stating that in my experience, *more than* 90% of the people I've met *needed* Personal Training. This was because they had no idea what they were doing (often when they thought they did), because they lacked the motivation to exercise 3 times per week, or they needed someone to push them to get maximal results in each session.

I'll be honest, I *always* train with a partner, because I'm not an idiot and will stop at any sign of pain unless someone is motivating me not to do so. The painful reps, unfortunately, are the ones that bring about the best results. That's one of the reasons there are more gyms than ever before, but so many people are either overweight or don't have a 'beach body'. 'No Pain, No Gain' and all that jazz.

Finding a Personal Trainer you can trust is an excellent way to go, however, and I'm not just saying this to scare you, but most are *fantastic* at being completely *average*. I truly think it's the same in *any* profession. Most people are completely average or below average. You need to be seeking out the *best of the best* if you want the results that lead you to reading this book. I've seen Personal Trainers who are doing rather well for themselves who are good looking, charming, talk the talk but don't even know how to perform a simple exercise like a squat correctly. Let alone speak about nutrition other than advising clients to add a protein shake here and there.

The other option is to come over to a Personal Trainer who so far you've trusted enough to read this *entire* book. One that goes *way* beyond exercise (crappy Personal Trainers only focus on this) and nutrition (better ones will *include* this but usually with minimal knowledge) and has a simple, fun and holistic approach that can get you to where you want to go.

Me offering training online is my way of reaching out to more clients. Because the fact is when I was doing 100 sessions per week, I had to turn people away because I couldn't physically train anyone else. This upset me, as I knew I was the best trainer in town if not far further reaching than that and the ones I turned away had to go away and more than likely train in mediocrity. That's not me blowing my own trumpet, but as far as I could see in my 19 years in the industry, it's the truth. So, me being able to train people no matter *where* they are in the world is a great privilege in today's modern world. I'm excited to offer this service and hope you will let me continue to support you on your continuing journey.

In reading this book to the very end, you have taken a monumental first step towards a happier, healthier, new *you*. Now I challenge you to take the next step towards consistency and *permanent* change.

The *Final* Action Step

- If you haven't already done so, come and see me over at my website **www.TomBroadwell.com** for your *free* trial. Come and join an ever growing community of people who are on the same path as *you*, a health and fitness tribe that can support you every step of the way on your journey to achieving your goals. It takes two minutes to do, and you literally have *nothing* to lose. Take that action and sign up *now...*

References

Chapter 1: Mindset Matters Most

"Impact of a stress management program on weight loss, mental health and lifestyle in adults with obesity: a randomized controlled trial," Niovi Xenaki et al. *The Journal of Molecular Biochemistry*. Springer. 2018

"Stress management can facilitate weight loss in Greek overweight and obese women: a pilot study," Christaki E et al. *Journal of Human Nutrition and Dietetics*. Wiley. 2013

"Mindfulness Intervention for Stress Eating to Reduce Cortisol and Abdominal Fat among Overweight and Obese Women: An Exploratory Randomized Controlled Study." Jennifer Daubenmier et al. *Journal of Obesity*. Nature Research. 2011

"The Mind Made Flesh," Nicholas Humhprey. Oxford University Press. 2002

"Magic or Medicine: An Investigation of Healing and Healers," Robert Buckman, and Karl Sabbagh. Prometheus. 1993

"Positive Attitude Towards Life, Emotional Expression, self-rated health, and depressive symptoms among centenarians and near-centenarians," Kaori Kato et al. *Aging and Mental Health*. Routledge. 2016

"Centenarians' Positive Attitude Linked to Long Life," Kim Carrollo. (www.abcnews.go.com) June 5, 2012

Chapter 2: Stress Less

"Deaths: Leading Causes," Melonie Heron, Ph.D. National Vital Statistics Reports, Vol. 68, No. 6, (https://www.cdc.gov) June 24, 2019

"2019 Heart Disease & Stroke Statistical Update Fact Sheet Older Americans & Cardiovascular Diseases" American Heart Association, Inc. (https://www.heart.org) 2019

"The Relationship Between Workplace Stressors and Mortality and Health Costs in the United States" Joel Goh, Jeffrey Pfeffer, Stefanos Zenios. *Management Science*. Vol. 62. INFORMS. March 2016

"Stress: Concepts, Definition and History" G Fink, *Neuroscience and Biobehavioral Psychology*. Elsevier. 2017

"Everest College's 2013 Work Stress Survey" by Harris Interactive, United States. (https://everestcollege.wordpress.com) 2013

"Seasonal Affective Disorder: An Overview of Assessment and Treatment Approaches." Melrose S. *Depression Research and Treatment*. Hindawi. 2015

"Clinical Practice Guidelines on the Use of Integrative Therapies as Supportive Care in Patients Treated for Breast Cancer" Heather Greenlee et al. *CA: A Cancer Journal for Clinicians*. Wiley. 2017

"Beyond Medications and Diet: Alternative Approaches to Lowering Blood Pressure: A Scientific Statement From the American Heart Association." Brook, Robert D. *Hypertension*. AHA Journals. June 2013

"The effects of relaxation response meditation on the symptoms of irritable bowel syndrome: results of a controlled treatment study." Laurie Keefer, and Edward B Blanchard. Behaviour Research and Therapy Volume 39, Issue 7. Elsevier. July 2001

"Elevated resting heart rate, physical fitness and all-cause mortality: a 16-year follow-up in the Copenhagen Male Study" Magnus Thorsten Jensen et al. *Heart*. BMJ Journals. 2013

"The Four Stages of Competence" Martin M. Broadwell. (http://www.mccc.edu/~lyncha/documents/stagesofcompetence.pdf) 1969

"Health and Light" John Ott. Devin-Adair. 1973

"The Influence of Ocular Light Perception on Metabolism in Man and in Animal" Fritz Hollwich. Springer-Verlag, 1979

"Role of emotional factors in adults with atopic dermatitis." Iona H. Ginsburg et al. *International Journal of Dermatology*. Wiley-Blackwell 1993

"Expressive writing and wound healing in older adults: a randomized controlled trial." Koschwanez HE et al. *Psychosomatic Medicine*. July/August. Lippincott Williams & Wilkins. 2013

"Hypotheses on the Development of Psychoemotional Tearing" Juan Murube. *The Ocular Surface*. Elsevier. 2009

'Is crying a self-soothing behavior?' Asmir Gračanin, Lauren M. Bylsma, and Ad J. J. M. Vingerhoets. *Frontiers in Psychology*. Frontiers. 2014

Chapter 3: Sweet Dreams

"The effects of handwriting experience on functional brain development in pre-literate children" Karin H. James, and Laura Engelhardt. *Trends in Neuroscience and Education*. Elsevier. 2012

"The Effects of 884 MHz GSM Wireless Communication Signals on Self-reported Symptom and Sleep (EEG)" Bengt Arnetz et al. *Progress in Electromagnetics Research Symposium*. PIER 2008

"Does Television Kill Your Sex Life? Microeconometric Evidence from 80 Countries" Adrienne M. Lucas, and Nicholas L. Wilson. *The B.E. Journal of Economic Analysis & Policy*. De Gruyter. 2019

"Fiber and Saturated Fat Are Associated with Sleep Arousals and Slow Wave Sleep" Marie-Pierre St-Onge et al. *The Journal of Clinical Sleep Medicine*. AASM. 2016

"Caffeine Effects on Sleep Taken 0, 3, or 6 Hours before Going to Bed" Christopher L. Drake. *The Journal of Clinical Sleep Medicine*. AASM. 2013

"Effects of caffeine on the human circadian clock in vivo and in vitro" Tina M. Burke et al. *Science Translational Medicine*. AAAS. 2015

"The health benefits of nose breathing" Dr Alan Ruth. *Nursing in General Practice*. Nursing in General Practice. 2016

Chapter 4: Life Begins With Water

"Water-Induced Thermogenesis" Michael Boschmann et al. *The Journal of Clinical Endocrinology & Metabolism*. The Endocrine Society. 2003

"Using Chlorine In Water Raises Risk of Cancer" Joanne Omang. (https://www.washingtonpost.com) December 18, 1980

"Water Fluoridation: A Critical Review of the Physiological Effects of Ingested Fluoride as a Public Health Intervention" Stephen Peckham, and Niyi Awofeso. *The Scientific World Journal*. Hindawi. 2014

"Fluoridation Revisited" Dr. Murray N. Rothbard. *The Rothbard-Rockwell Report*. 14 December 1992

"Are fluoride levels in drinking water associated with hypothyroidism prevalence in England? A large observational study of GP practice data and fluoride levels in drinking water." Peckham S, Lowery D, and Spencer S. *The Journal of Epidemiology and Community Health*. BMJ. 2015

"Mapping the PFAS Contamination Crisis: New Data Show 610 Sites in 43 States" Monica Amarelo. Environmental Working Group, and Northeastern University. (https://www.ewg.org) May 6, 2019

"Per- and Polyfluorinated Substances (PFAS) Factsheet" Centers for Disease Control and Prevention. (https://www.cdc.gov) 2017

"A Review of the Carcinogenic Potential of Bisphenol A" Darcie D Seachrist et al. *Reproductive Toxicology*. Elsevier. 2015

"Estrogenic chemicals often leach from BPA-free plastic products that are replacements for BPA-containing polycarbonate products" George D Bittner et al. *Environmental Health*. BioMed Central 2014

Chapter 5: You Are What You Eat...

"The Hidden Dangers of Fast and Processed Food" Joel Fuhrman. *American Journal of Lifestyle Medicine*. SAGE. 2018

"What does sugar do to our health?" Emma Luxton. *World Economic Forum*. (https://www.weforum.org) 22 Feb 2016

"Potential role of sugar (fructose) in the epidemic of hypertension, obesity and the metabolic syndrome, diabetes, kidney disease, and cardiovascular disease" Richard J Johnson et al. The *American Journal of Clinical Nutrition*. Nutrition Press. 2007

"Long-term Trends in Diabetes" Centers for Disease Control and Prevention. (https://www.cdc.gov) April 2017

"The National Diabetes Statistics Report. Estimates of Diabetes and Its Burden in the United States" Centers for Disease Control and Prevention. (https://www.cdc.gov) 2020

"CYP2E1 and oxidant stress in alcoholic and non-alcoholic fatty liver disease." Leung TM, and Nieto N. *European Association for the Study of the Liver*. Elsevier. 2013

"The toxic truth about sugar" Robert H. Lustig et al. *Nature*. Nature Research. 2012

"Sugar addiction: is it real? A narrative review" James J DiNicolantonio, James H O'Keefe, and William L Wilson. *British Journal of Sports Medicine*. BMJ. 2018

"Food Additives: Do They Hurt?" Jane E. Brody. (https://www.nytimes.com). July 12, 1978

"We are what we eat: Regulatory gaps in the United States that put our health at risk" Maricel V. Maffini et al. *PLOS Biology*. Public Library of Science. 2017

"Iceland's Last McDonald's Order Just Turned Ten" Jelena Ćirić. (https://www.icelandreview.com) November 2, 2019

"Food and drug cues activate similar brain regions: A meta-analysis of functional MRI studies" D.W. Tang et al. *Physiology & Behavior*. Elsevier. 2012

"The Neural Correlates of "Food Addiction"" Ashley N. Gearhardt et al. *Archives Of General Psychiatry*. JAMA Psychiatry. 2011

"Donald Rumsfeld and the Strange History of Aspartame" Robbie Gennet. (https://www.huffpost.com) May 25, 2011

"Increasing brain tumor rates: is there a link to aspartame?" Olney JW et al. *Journal of Neuropathology & Experimental Neurology*. Oxford University Press. 1996

"Testing Needed for Acesulfame Potassium, an Artificial Sweetener" Myra L. Karstadt. *Environmental Health Perspectives*. NIEHS. 2006

"Acesulfame Potassium: Soffritti Responds" Morando Soffritti. *Environmental Health Perspectives*. NIEHS. 2006

"Sucralose, A Synthetic Organochlorine Sweetener: Overview of Biological Issues" Susan S. Schiffman, and Kristina I. Rother. *Journal of Toxicology and Environmental Health, Part B: Critical Reviews*. Taylor & Francis. 2013

"Why Mouse Matters" National Human Genome Research Institute. (https://www.genome.gov) 2010

"Stevia, Nature's Zero-Calorie Sustainable Sweetener. A New Player in the Fight Against Obesity" Margaret Ashwell. *Nutrition Today*. Lippincott Williams & Wilkins Ltd. 2015

"Intake of saturated and trans unsaturated fatty acids and risk of all cause mortality, cardiovascular disease, and type 2 diabetes: systematic review and meta-analysis of observational studies." de Souza RJ et al. *The BMJ*. BMJ. 2015

"How the Nurses' Health Study Helped Americans Take the Trans Fat Out" Christine J. Curtis et al. *The American Journal of Public Health*. The American Public Health Association. 2016

"New data on harmful effects of trans-fatty acids" Ginter E, and Simko V. *Bratislava Medical Journal*. Comenius University, Faculty of Medicine. 2016

"Long-Term Consumption of Sugar-Sweetened and Artificially Sweetened Beverages and Risk of Mortality in US Adults" Vasanti S. Malik et al. *Circulation*. AHA Journals. 2019

"Short-term exposure to a diet high in fat and sugar, or liquid sugar, selectively impairs hippocampal-dependent memory, with differential impacts on inflammation" J.E.Beilharz et al. *Behavioural Brain Research*. Elsevier. 2016

"Effects of carbohydrates on satiety: differences between liquid and solid food." Pan A, and Hu FB. *Current Opinion in Clinical Nutrition and Metabolic Care*. Wolters Kluwer. 2011

"Sugar Content of Popular Sweetened Beverages Based on Objective Laboratory Analysis: Focus on Fructose Content" Emily E. Ventura, Jaimie N. Davis, and Michael I. Goran. *Obesity*. Wiley. 2011

"Fructose content in popular beverages made with and without high-fructose corn syrup" Michael I. Goran et al. *Nutrition*. Elsevier. 2014

"Colas, but not other carbonated beverages, are associated with low bone mineral density in older women: The Framingham Osteoporosis Study" Katherine L Tucker et al. *The American Journal of Clinical Nutrition*. Nutrition Press. 2006

"Association Between Soft Drink Consumption and Mortality in 10 European Countries" Amy Mullee et al. *The Journal of the American Medical Association*. American Medical Association. 2019

"Sugar- and Artificially Sweetened Beverages and the Risks of Incident Stroke and Dementia" Matthew P. Pase et al. *Stroke*. American Heart Association. 2017

"Sugar-sweetened beverage and diet soda consumption and the 7-year risk for type 2 diabetes mellitus in middle-aged Japanese men" M. Sakurai et al. *The European Journal of Nutrition*. Springer. 2013

"Artificial sweeteners induce glucose intolerance by altering the gut microbiota." Suez J et al. *Nature*. Nature Research. 2014

"Altered processing of sweet taste in the brain of diet soda drinkers" Erin Green, and Claire Murphy. *Physiology & Behavior*. Elsevier. 2012

"Update on Emergency Department Visits Involving Energy Drinks: A Continuing Public Health Concern." Mattson ME. *The CBHSQ Report*. Substance Abuse and Mental Health Services Administration. 2013

"Impact of High Volume Energy Drink Consumption on Electrocardiographic and Blood Pressure Parameters: A Randomized Trial" Sachin A. Shah et al. *Journal of the American Heart Association*. John Wiley & Sons. 2019

"Energy drink consumption, health complaints and late bedtime among young adolescents" Leena Koivusilta, Heini Kuoppamäki, and Arja Rimpelä. *International Journal of Public Health*. Springer. 2016

"Health Effects and Public Health Concerns of Energy Drink Consumption in the United States: A Mini-Review" Laila Al-Shaar et al. *Frontiers in Public Health*. Frontiers. 2017

"Is This Common Kitchen Appliance Harming Your Health?" Joesph Mercola. (https://www.huffpost.com) 2010

"Phenolic compound contents in edible part of broccoli inflorescences after domestic cooking" F. Vallejo, F. A. Tomás-Barberán, and Cristina García-Viguera. *Journal of the Science of Food and Agriculture*. Wiley. 2003

"Most Plastic Products Release Estrogenic Chemicals: A Potential Health Problem That Can Be Solved" Chun Z. Yang et al. *Environmental Health Perspectives*. NIEHS. 2011

"Unhealthy eating and physical inactivity are leading causes of death in the U.S." The Center for Science in the Public Interest. (https://www.cspinet.org) 2016

"Endotoxemia of metabolic syndrome: a pivotal mediator of meta-inflammation." Jialal I, and Rajamani U. *Metabolic Syndrome and Related Disorders*. Mary Ann Liebert, Inc. 2014

"Role of the gut microbiota in health and chronic gastrointestinal disease: understanding a hidden metabolic organ" Caitriona M. Guinane, and Paul D. Cotter. *Therapeutic Advances in Gastroenterology*. SAGE. 2013

"Leaky Gut As a Danger Signal for Autoimmune Diseases" Qinghui Mu et al. *Frontiers in Immunology*. Lausanne : Frontiers Research Foundation. 2017

"Leaky Gut, Leaky Brain?" Mark E. M. Obrenovich. *Microorganisms*. MDPI. 2018

"Modulation of immune function by dietary lectins in rheumatoid arthritis" Loren Cordain et al. *British Journal of Nutrition*. Cambridge University Press. 2007

"Cardiovascular disease resulting from a diet and lifestyle at odds with our Paleolithic genome: how to become a 21st-century hunter-gatherer." O'Keefe JH Jr, and Cordain L. *Mayo Clinic Proceedings*. Elsevier. 2004

"Phytic acid in health and disease." Zhou JR, and Erdman JW Jr. *Critical Reviews in Food Science and Nutrition*. Taylor & Francis. 1995

"Food Combining" Dr. Kaslow.
(http://www.drkaslow.com/html/food_combining.html) 2017

"Oral Delivery of Proteins and Peptides" Gaurang Patel, and Ambikanandan Misra. *Challenges in Delivery of Therapeutic Genomics and Proteomics*. Elsevier 2011

"What Is the Optimum pH for Human Stomach Enzyme Activity?" Emily Updegraff. (https://sciencing.com) 2018

Chapter 6: Move It Or Lose It

"Relationship of Leisure-Time Physical Activity and Mortality: The Finnish Twin Cohort" U M Kujala, J Kaprio, S Sarna, and M Koskenvuo. *JAMA*. American Medical Association. 1998

"Physical Activity and Coronary Heart Disease in Men" Howard D. Sesso , Ralph S. PaffenbargerJr , and I-Min Lee. *Circulation*. AHA Journals. 2000

"Effect of an acute period of resistance exercise on excess post-exercise oxygen consumption: implications for body mass management" Mark D. Schuenke, Richard P. Mikat, and Jeffrey M. McBride. *European Journal of Applied Physiology*. Springer. 2002

"Effect of strength training on resting metabolic rate and physical activity: age and gender comparisons." Lemmer JT et al. *Medicine & Science in Sports & Exercise.* Lippincott. 2001

"Exploring the therapeutic effects of yoga and its ability to increase quality of life" Catherine Woodyard. *International Journal of Yoga.* S-VYASA University. 2011

"Is high-intensity interval training a time-efficient exercise strategy to improve health and fitness?" Gillen JB1, and Gibala MJ. *Applied Physiology, Nutrition, and Metabolism.* NRC Research Press. 2014

"Pilates: how does it work and who needs it?" June Kloubec. *Muscle, Ligaments and Tendons Journal.* CIC Edizioni Internazionali. 2011

Chapter 7: The perfectHealth Scale

"The Nobel Prize in Physiology or Medicine 1931" (https://www.nobelprize.org). Nobel Media. 2020

"Otto Heinrich Warburg, 1883-1970" Hans Adolf Krebs. *Biographical Memoirs of Fellows of the Royal Society.* Royal Society 1972

"On the Origin of Cancer Cells" Otto Warburg. *Science.* American Association for the Advancement of Science. 1956

"Cancer as a metabolic disease: implications for novel therapeutics" Thomas N. Seyfried, Roberto E. Flores, Angela M. Poff, and Dominic P. D'Agostino. *Carcinogenesis.* Oxford University Press. 2014

"Cancer as a mitochondrial metabolic disease" Thomas N. Seyfried. *Frontiers in Cell and Developmental Biology.* Frontiers. 2015

"The Prime Cause and Prevention of Cancer" Otto Warburg. *Second Revised German Edition of the Lindau Lecture (delivered June 30, 1966).* Konrad Triltsch. 1969

"Diet-induced acidosis: is it real and clinically relevant?" Pizzorno J, Frassetto LA, and Katzinger J. *The British Journal of Nutrition.* Cambridge University Press. 2010

"Diet-Induced Low-Grade Metabolic Acidosis and Clinical Outcomes: A Review." Carnauba RA et al. *Nutrients.* MDPI. 2017

"J. Craig Venter—The Human Genome Project" Marc A. Shampo, and Robert A. Kyle. *Mayo Clinic Proceedings.* Elsevier. 2011

"Prevention" Alzheimers Association. (https://www.alz.org) 2020

"Cancer is a Preventable Disease that Requires Major Lifestyle Changes" Preetha Anand et al. *Pharmaceutical Research.* Springer. 2008

"Puberty and Genetic Susceptibility to Breast Cancer in a Case–Control Study in Twins" Ann S. Hamilton, and Thomas M. Mack. *The New England Journal of Medicine.* Massachusetts Medical Society. 2003

"Higher diet-dependent acid load is associated with risk of breast cancer: Findings from the sister study." Park YM et al. *The International Journal of Cancer.* Wiley. 2019

"The Sister Study" The National Institute of Environmental Health Sciences. (https://sisterstudy.niehs.nih.gov) 2020

"The Alkaline Diet: Is There Evidence That an Alkaline pH Diet Benefits Health?" Gerry K. Schwalfenberg. *The International Journal of Environmental Research and Public Health.* MDPI. 2012

"Homogenized Milk: Rocket Fuel for Cancer" Robert Cohen. (http://health101.org/art_milk_cancer_fuel.htm) 2007

"Health Benefits of Culinary Herbs and Spices." Jiang TA. *The Journal of AOAC International.* AOAC International. 2019

"Cytotoxicity and genotoxicity of lipid-oxidation products." Esterbauer H. *The American Journal of Clinical Nutrition.* Nutrition Press. 1993

"Acrolein induced DNA damage, mutagenicity and effect on DNA repair." Tang MS et al. *Molecular Nutrition & Food Research.* Wiley-Blackwell. 2011

"Profitability of Large Pharmaceutical Companies Compared With Other Large Public Companies" Fred D. Ledley et al. *JAMA.* American Medical Association. 2020

Chapter 8: Trust Me I'm *Not* A Doctor

"The truth about drug companies: How they deceive us and what to do about it." Marcia Angell. Random House. 2004

"Excess in the pharmaceutical industry" Marcia Angell. T*he Canadian Medical Association Journal.* Canadian Medical Association. 2004

"The Genome Revolution" Salveen Richter (https://www.goldmansachs.com/insights/pages/genome-revolution.html) 2018

"Association of Patient Out-of-Pocket Costs With Prescription Abandonment and Delay in Fills of Novel Oral Anticancer Agents" Jalpa A. Doshi et al. *Journal of Clinical Oncology.* American Society of Clinical Oncology. 2018

"Luxturna: FDA documents reveal the value of a costly gene therapy" Jonathan J.Darrow. *Drug Discovery Today.* Elsevier. 2019

"Taking Financial Relationships into Account When Assessing Research" David B. Resnik, and Kevin C. Elliott. *Accountability in Research.* Taylor & Francis. 2013

"Conflict of interest in the debate over calcium-channel antagonists." Stelfox HT et al. *The New England Journal of Medicine.* Massachusetts Medical Society. 1998

"Evaluation of conflict of interest in economic analyses of new drugs used in oncology." Friedberg M et al. *JAMA.* American Medical Association. 1999

"Pharmaceutical industry sponsorship and research outcome and quality: systematic review." Lexchin J. *The BMJ.* BMJ. 2003

"Scope and impact of financial conflicts of interest in biomedical research: a systematic review." Bekelman JE, Li Y, and Gross CP. *JAMA.* American Medical Association. 2003

"Pharmaceutical company funding and its consequences: a qualitative systematic review." Sismondo S. *Contemporary Clinical Trials.* Elsevier. 2008

"Rofecoxib (Vioxx) voluntarily withdrawn from market" Barbara Sibbald. *The Canadian Medical Association Journal.* Canadian Medical Association. 2004

"Vioxx Lawsuits" Kristin Compton, and Kevin Connolly. (https://www.drugwatch.com/vioxx/lawsuits/) 2020

"Guest authorship and ghostwriting in publications related to rofecoxib: a case study of industry documents from rofecoxib litigation." Ross JS et al. *JAMA.* American Medical Association. 2008

"Reporting mortality findings in trials of rofecoxib for Alzheimer disease or cognitive impairment: a case study based on documents from rofecoxib litigation." Psaty BM, and Kronmal RA. *JAMA.* American Medical Association. 2008

"Research and Development Spending to Bring a Single Cancer Drug to Market and Revenues After Approval" Vinay Prasad, and Sham Mailankody. *JAMA Internal Medicine.* American Medical Association. 2017

"Curbing Unfair Drug Prices: A Primer for States by the Global Health Justice Partnership" Aaron Berman et al. *Yale Law School, Yale School of Public Health, National Physicians Alliance, and Universal Health Care Foundation of Connecticut.* 2017

"The World Factbook' Central Intelligence Agency. (*https://www.cia.gov*) 2017

"Health Care Spending in the United States and Other High-Income Countries." Papanicolas I, Woskie LR, and Jha AK. *JAMA.* American Medical Association. 2018

"Worries About Autism Link Still Hang Over Vaccines" Scott Hensley. *National Public Radio (NPR).* Houston Public Media. (*https://www.npr.org*) September 29, 2011

"AUTISM AND VACCINES AROUND THE WORLD: Vaccine Schedules, Autism Rates, and Under 5 Mortality" *Generation Rescue, Inc.* April 2009

"National Vaccine Injury Compensation Program" Health Resources & Services Administration (https://www.hrsa.gov) 2013

"Infant mortality rates regressed against number of vaccine doses routinely given: Is there a biochemical or synergistic toxicity?" Neil Z Miller, and Gary S Goldman. *Human & Experimental Toxicology.* Sage. 2011

"Truth Will Prevail" Dr Alan Palmer. Version 2.5. (http://www.chiropractic.org/1200studies/) 2020

"Limiting Infant Exposure to Thimerosal in Vaccines and Other Sources of Mercury" Neal A. Halsey. *JAMA.* American Medical Association. 1999

"Vaccine Excipient Summary Excipients Included in U.S. Vaccines, by Vaccine" CDC. (https://www.cdc.gov/vaccines/pubs/pinkbook/downloads/appendices/b/excipient-table-2.pdf) 2020

"Metal-Sulfate Induced Generation of ROS in Human Brain Cells: Detection Using an Isomeric Mixture of 5- and 6-Carboxy-2',7'-Dichlorofluorescein Diacetate (Carboxy-DCFDA) as a Cell Permeant Tracer" Aileen I. Pogue et al. *The International Journal of Molecular Sciences.* MDPI. 2012

"Aluminum vaccine adjuvants: are they safe?" Tomljenovic L, and Shaw CA. *Current Medicinal Chemistry.* Bentham Science Publishers. 2011

"Medical Management Guidelines for Formaldehyde" Agency for Toxic Substances and Disease Registry. CDC (https://www.atsdr.cdc.gov) 2014

"Excitotoxic cell death." Choi DW. *Journal of Neurobiology.* Wiley. 1992

"Use of Aborted Fetal Tissue in Vaccines and Medical Research Obscures the Value of All Human Life" Kyle Christopher McKenna. *The Linacre Quarterly.* SAGE. 2018

"Impact of environmental factors on the prevalence of autistic disorder after 1979" Theresa A. Deisher et al. *Journal of Public Health and Epidemiology.* Academic Journals. 2014

"5 of 7 vaccines analyzed are not compliant" Corvelva Staff. (https://www.corvelva.it/en/) NOVEMBER 15, 2018

"New Quality-Control Investigations on Vaccines: Micro- and Nanocontamination" Antonietta M Gatti, and Stefano Montanari. *International Journal of Vaccines & Vaccination.* OMICS. 2017

"Traffic in Metro Manila" *Wikipedia* (https://en.wikipedia.org/wiki/Traffic_in_Metro_Manila) 2020

"Biological activities and medicinal properties of *Cajanus cajan* (L) Millsp." Dilipkumar Pal et al. *Journal of Advanced Pharmaceutical Technology & Research.* Society of Pharmaceutical Education & Research. 2011

"A systematic review of Calendula officinalis extract for wound healing." Givol O et al. *Wound Repair and Regeneration.* Wiley. 2019

"Management of Diabetes and Its Complications with Banaba (*Lagerstroemia speciosa* L.) and Corosolic Acid" Toshihiro Miura, Satoshi Takagi, and Torao Ishida. Evidence-Based Complementary and Alternative Medicine. Hindawi. 2012

"[The antibacterial activity of oregano essential oil (Origanum heracleoticum L.) against clinical strains of Escherichia coli and Pseudomonas aeruginosa]." Sienkiewicz M, Wasiela M, and Głowacka A. *Medycyna Doswiadczalna I Mikrobiologia.* Panstwowy Zaklad Higieny. 2012

"Essential oil composition and antibacterial activity of Origanum vulgare subsp. glandulosum Desf. at different phenological stages." Béjaoui A et al. *Journal of Medicinal Food.* Mary Ann Liebert. 2013

"Antiviral activity of the *Lippia graveolens* (Mexican oregano) essential oil and its main compound carvacrol against human and animal viruses" Marciele Ribas Pilau et al. Brazilian Journal of Microbiology. Springer. 2011

"A Trial of Wound Irrigation in the Initial Management of Open Fracture Wounds" The FLOW Investigators. *The New England Journal of Medicine.* Massachusetts Medical Society. 2015

"Chemical composition and antioxidant activities of essential oils from different parts of the oregano" Fei Han et al. *The Journal of Zhejiang University Science B: Biomedicine & Biotechnology.* Zhejiang University Press and Springer. 2017

"Quorum Quenching and Antimicrobial Activity of Goldenseal (*Hydrastis canadensis*) against Methicillin-Resistant *Staphylococcus aureus* (MRSA)" Nadja B. Cech et al. *Planta Medica.* Thieme Medical Publishers 2012

"The Antiviral Activities of Artemisinin and Artesunate" Thomas Efferth et al. *Clinical Infectious Diseases.* Oxford University Press. 2008

Chapter 9: SupplementNation

"Historical changes in the mineral content of fruits and vegetables" Anne-Marie Mayer. *British Food Journal*. Emerald. 1997

"Changes in USDA food composition data for 43 garden crops, 1950 to 1999." Davis DR, Epp MD, and Riordan HD. *Journal of the American College of Nutrition*. Taylor & Francis. 2004

"What You Don't Know Might Kill You" David Epstein. Sports Illustrated. (https://vault.si.com) ABG-SI LLC. May 18, 2009

"Comparative bioavailability to humans of ascorbic acid alone or in a citrus extract." Vinson JA, and Bose P. *The American Journal of Clinical Nutrition*. American Society for Nutrition. 1988

"Milestones" Eastman Kodak Company. (https://www.kodak.com) 2020

"Natural vitamins may be superior to synthetic ones." Thiel RJ. *Medical Hypotheses*. Elsevier. 2000

"How Much Is Too Much? Excess Vitamins and Minerals in Food Can Harm Kids' Health" Olga Naidenko, and Renee Sharp et al. *Environmental Working Group*. (https://static.ewg.org) June 2014

"Coke to change Vitaminwater labels to settle U.S. consumer lawsuit" Jonathan Stempel. *Reuters*. (https://www.reuters.com) October 1, 2015

"*Eat Your Heart Out: Why the food business is bad for the planet*" Felicity Lawrence. Penguin. 2008

"Dietary Supplement Labeling Guide: Chapter IV. Nutrition Labeling" *Food and Drug Administration* (https://www.fda.gov) 2005

"Food Dyes: A Rainbow of Risks" Sarah Kobylewski, and Michael F. Jacobson. *Center for Science in the Public Interest*. (https://cspinet.org) 2010

"Diet And Nutrition: The Artificial Food Dye Blues" Carol Potera. *Environmental Health Perspectives*. ISEE. 2010

"The Effects of Hydrogenation on Soybean Oil" Fred A. Kummerow. *Soybean - Bio-Active Compounds*. IntechOpen. 2013

"Talcum Powder Lawsuits" Michelle Llamas. *drugwatch* (https://www.drugwatch.com) 2019

"Carcinogenicity of carbon black, titanium dioxide, and talc." Baan R et al. The Lancet Oncology. Elsevier. 2006

"Talc-coated rice as a risk factor for stomach cancer" G N Stemmermann, and L N Kolonel. *The American Journal of Clinical Nutrition*. Nutrition Press. 1978

"Titanium Dioxide Exposure Induces Acute Eosinophilic Lung Inflammation in Rabbits" Gil-Soon Choi et al. *Industrial Health*. National Institute of Occupational Safety and Health. 2013

"Effects of Th1 and Th2 cells balance in pulmonary injury induced by nano titanium dioxide." Chang X et al. *Environmental Toxicology and Pharmacology*. Elsevier. 2013

"Effect of a novel dietary supplement on pH levels of healthy volunteers: a pilot study." Anton SD et al. Journal of Integrative Medicine. Science Press & Elsevier (China). 2013

"An Increase in the Omega-6/Omega-3 Fatty Acid Ratio Increases the Risk for Obesity" Artemis P. Simopoulos. *Nutrients*. MDPI. 2016

"Omega-6 and omega-3 polyunsaturated fatty acids and allergic diseases in infancy and childhood." Miles EA, and Calder PC. *Current Pharmaceutical Design*. Bentham Science Publishers. 2014

"Can Early Omega-3 Fatty Acid Exposure Reduce Risk of Childhood Allergic Disease?" Elizabeth A. Miles, and Philip C. Calder. *Nutrients*. MDPI. 2017

"Omega-3 fatty acids: An update emphasizing clinical use" David Kiefer, and Traci Pantuso. *Agro Food Industry Hi Tech*. Tekno Scienze Publisher. 2012

"Antifungal Activity of Palmatine against Strains of Candida spp. Resistant to Azoles in Planktonic Cells and Biofilm" Rosana de Sousa Campos et al. *International Journal of Current Microbiology and Applied Sciences*. IJCMAS. 2018

"Disruption of the Gut Ecosystem by Antibiotics" Mi Young Yoon, and Sang Sun Yoon. *Yonsei Medical Journal*. Yonsei University. 2018

"The hidden dangers of protein powders" *Harvard Health Letter*. (https://www.health.harvard.edu) Harvard Health Publishing. September 2018

"Calcium supplements: an additional source of lead contamination." Rehman S et al. *Biological Trace Element Research*. Springer. 2011

Chapter 10: Grown By Nature

"A Growing Problem Selective Breeding In The Chicken Industry: The Case For Slower Growth." *ASPCA*. (https://www.aspca.org) 2014

"Pulmonary arterial hypertension (ascites syndrome) in broilers: a review." Wideman RF et al. *Poultry Science*. Elsevier. 2013

"Super-size problem" Karen Lange. *The Humane Society of the United States*. (https://www.humanesociety.org) March 1, 2017

"What is Organic?" *CCOF Foundation*. (https://www.ccof.org) 2018

"Omega-3 fatty acids in inflammation and autoimmune diseases." Simopoulos AP. *Journal of the American College of Nutrition*. ACN. 2002

"Global Assessment of Polybrominated Diphenyl Ethers in Farmed and Wild Salmon" Ronald Hites et al. *Environmental Science & Technology*. ACS. 2004

"Policy and Guidance for Polychlorinated Biphenyl (PCBs)" *United States Environmental Protection Agency*. (https://www.epa.gov) 2020

"[Sexual maturation of children and adolescents in Germany. Results of the German Health Interview and Examination Survey for Children and Adolescents (KiGGS)]." Kahl H et al. *Bundesgesundheitsblatt – Gesundheitsforschung – Gesundheitsschutz*. Springer. 2007

"Reexamination of the Age Limit for Defining When Puberty Is Precocious in Girls in the United States: Implications for Evaluation and Treatment" Paul B. Kaplowitz, and Sharon E. Oberfield. *Pediatrics*. American Academy of Pediatrics. 1999

"Insecticide Uptake from Soils, Absorption of Insecticidal Residues from Contaminated Soils into Five Carrot Varieties" E. P. Lichtenstein, G. R. MyrdalK, and R. Schulz. *Journal of Agricultural and Food Chemistry*. ACS. 1965

"A Comparison of the Nutritional Value, Sensory Qualities, and Food Safety of Organically and Conventionally Produced Foods" Diane Bourn, and John Prescott. *Critical Reviews in Food Science and Nutrition*. Taylor & Francis. 2002

"Genetically Engineered Crops in the United States" Jorge Fernandez-Cornejo, Seth Wechsler, Mike Livingston, and Lorraine Mitchell. *United States Department of Agriculture*. (https://www.ers.usda.gov) February 2014

"What GM crops are currently being grown and where?" *The Royal Society*. (https://royalsociety.org) 2016

"Health risks of genetically modified foods." Dona A, Arvanitoyannis IS. *Critical Reviews in Food Science and Nutrition*. Taylor & Francis. 2009

"IARC Monograph on Glyphosate" International Agency for Research on Cancer. (https://www.iarc.fr) 2016

"Genetic diversity and disease control in rice." Zhu Y et al. *Nature*. Nature Research. 2000

"Traitor Technology: How Suicide Seeds Work / Where They are Being Patented" *ETC Group*. (http://www.etcgroup.org) January 14, 1999

Chapter 12: ...You Are Also What You Don't Excrete

"Meaning of toxin in English" *Cambridge Dictionary* (https://dictionary.cambridge.org/dictionary/english/toxin) 2020

"Meaning of toxic in English" *Cambridge Dictionary* (https://dictionary.cambridge.org/dictionary/english/toxic) 2020

"Meaning of poisonous in English" *Cambridge Dictionary* (https://dictionary.cambridge.org/dictionary/english/poisonous) 2020

"American Chemical Society National Historic Chemical Landmarks. Bakelite: The World's First Synthetic Plastic" *ACS* (http://www.acs.org/content/acs/en/education/whatischemistry/landmarks/bakelite.html) 2020

"Paul Hermann Müller: Swiss Chemist" The Editors of Encyclopaedia Britannica. *Encyclopaedia Britannica*. (https://www.britannica.com) 2020

"Synthetic Organic Chemicals: Definition & Examples" Danielle Reid. *Study.com* (https://study.com) 31 March 2017

"EPA Releases First Major Update to Chemicals List in 40 Years" EPA Press Office (https://www.epa.gov) 19th Feb 2019

"Identifying and Reducing Environmental Health Risks of Chemicals in Our Society" Robert Pool, and Erin Rusch. *The National Academies Press*. 2014

"Toxic chemicals released by industries this year" *Worldometer*. (https://www.worldometers.info) 2020

"Fourth National Report on Human Exposure to Environmental Chemicals" *Department of Health and Human Services, and Centers for Disease Control and Prevention*. (https://www.cdc.gov) 2009

"Using silicone wristbands to evaluate preschool children's exposure to flame retardants" Molly L. Kile et al. *Environmental Research*. Elsevier. 2016

"Biomonitoring Summary: Dichlorodiphenyltrichloroethane (DDT)" *Centers for Disease Control and Prevention*. (https://www.cdc.gov) 2017

"Global assessment of the state-of-the-science of endocrine disruptors" Terri Damstra et al. *World Health Organization*, (https://www.who.int) 2002

"State of the science of endocrine disrupting chemicals - 2012" Åke Bergman et al. INTER-*Organization Programme For The Sound Management Of Chemicals*. (https://www.who.int) 2012

"Estimating burden and disease costs of exposure to endocrine-disrupting chemicals in the European union." *The Journal of Clinical Endocrinology and Metabolism*. The Endocrine Society. 2015

"Early prenatal exposure to suspected endocrine disruptor mixtures is associated with lower IQ at age seven." Tanner EM et al. Environment International. Elsevier. 2020

"'It's killing us': why firefighters are battling to ban flame retardants" Jessica Glenza, and Lauren Aratani. *The Guardian. (*https://www.theguardian.com*)* May 24, 2019

"Impacts of Gut Bacteria on Human Health and Diseases" Yu-Jie Zhang et al. *International Journal of Molecular Sciences*. MDPI. 2015

"Effects of Intermittent Fasting on Health, Aging, and Disease" Rafael de Cabo, and Mark P. Mattson. *The New England Journal of Medicine*. Massachusetts Medical Society. 2019

"The effect of short-term fasting on liver and skeletal muscle lipid, glucose, and energy metabolism in healthy women and men" Browning, JD et al. *Journal Of Lipid Research*. American Society for Biochemistry and Molecular Biology. 2012

"The effect of intermittent energy and carbohydrate restriction v. daily energy restriction on weight loss and metabolic disease risk markers in overweight women" Harvie, Michelle et al. *British Journal Of Nutrition*. Cambridge University Press. 2013

"The effects of intermittent or continuous energy restriction on weight loss and metabolic disease risk markers: a randomized trial in young overweight women" Harvie, Michelle et al. *International Journal Of Obesity*. Nature Research. 2011

"Effects of intermittent feeding upon body weight and lifespan in inbred mice: interaction of genotype and age." Goodrick CL et al. *Mechanisms of Ageing and Development*. Elsevier. 1990

"Liver: Anatomy and Functions" *Johns Hopkins Medicine*. (https://www.hopkinsmedicine.org) 2020

"Restoration of Liver Mass after Injury Requires Proliferative and Not Embryonic Transcriptional Patterns." Hasan H. Otu et al. *The Journal of Biological Chemistry*. ASBMB. 2007

"The Complementary and Alternative Medicine for Endometriosis: A Review of Utilization and Mechanism" Sai Kong et al. *Evidence-Based Complementary and Alternative Medicine*. Hindawi. 2014

"Toxicological Function of Adipose Tissue: Focus on Persistent Organic Pollutants" Michele La Merrill et al. *Environmental Health Perspectives*. National Institute of Environmental Health Sciences. 2013

"Male versus female skin: What dermatologists and cosmeticians should know" S. Rahrovan et al. *International Journal of Women's Dermatology*. Elsevier. 2018

"Adiponectin expression in subcutaneous adipose tissue is reduced in women with cellulite." Emanuele E et al. *International Journal of Dermatology*. Wiley-Blackwell. 2011

"The 12 initial POPs under the Stockholm Convention" Stockholm Convention. (http://chm.pops.int) 2001

"Cellulite and its treatment." Rawlings AV. *International Journal of Cosmetic Science*. Wiley. 2006

"Serum Polychlorinated Biphenyls Increase and Oxidative Stress Decreases with a Protein-Pacing Caloric Restriction Diet in Obese Men and Women" Feng He, and Paul J. Arciero. *International Journal of Environmental Research and Public Health*. MDPI. 2017

"Cellulite: a cosmetic or systemic issue? Contemporary views on the etiopathogenesis of cellulite." Tokarska K et al. *Advances in Dermatology and Allergology*. Polish Society of Allergology 201

"Scientists Find a Natural Way to Clean Up Oil Spills, With a Plant-Based Molecule" Heather Hansman. Smithsonian Magazine. (https://www.smithsonianmag.com) July 29, 2015

"Algae as nutritional and functional food sources: revisiting our understanding" Mark L. Wells et al. *Journal of Applied Phycology*. Springer. 2017

"Microalgae for High-Value Products Towards Human Health and Nutrition." Barkia I, Saari N, and Manning SR. *Marine Drugs*. MDPI. 2019

"Microalgae Characterization for Consolidated and New Application in Human Food, Animal Feed and Nutraceuticals" Antonio Molino et al. *International Journal of Environmental Research and Public Health*. MDPI. 2018

"Antioxidant, Anticancer Activity and Phytochemical Analysis of Green Algae, *Chaetomorpha* Collected from the Arabian Gulf" Samina Hyder Haq et al. *Scientific Reports*. Nature Research. 2019

"Algae as promising organisms for environment and health" Emad A Shalaby. *Plant Signaling & Behavior*. Landes Bioscience. 2011

"Milk thistle in liver diseases: past, present, future." Abenavoli L et al. *Phytotherapy Research*. Wiley. 2010

"Silymarin/Silybin and Chronic Liver Disease: A Marriage of Many Years." Federico A et al. *Molecules*. MDPI. 2017

"Plants Consumption and Liver Health" Yong-Song Guan, and Qing He. *Evidence-Based Complementary and Alternative Medicine.* Hindawi. 2015

"Effect of herbal teas on hepatic drug metabolizing enzymes in rats" Pius P. Maliakal, and Sompon Wanwimolruk. *Journal of Pharmacy and Pharmacology.* Wiley. 2010

"The Diuretic Effect in Human Subjects of an Extract of *Taraxacum officinale* Folium over a Single Day" Bevin A. Clare et al. *Journal of Alternative and Complementary Medicine.* Hindawi. 2009

"A review of the pharmacological effects of Arctium lappa (burdock)." Chan YS et al. *Inflammopharmacology.* Springer. 2011

"Acute diuretic, natriuretic and hypotensive effects of a continuous perfusion of aqueous extract of *Urtica dioica* in the rat" Abdelhafid Tahri et al. *Journal of Ethnopharmacology.* Elsevier. 2000

"Nettle extract (*Urtica dioica*) affects key receptors and enzymes associated with allergic rhinitis" Randall S. Alberte. *Phytotherapy Research.* Wiley. 2009

"Clinical Effects of Regular Dry Sauna Bathing: A Systematic Review" Joy Hussain, and Marc Cohen. *Evidence-Based Complementary and Alternative Medicine.* Hindawi. 2018

"Far infrared radiation (FIR): its biological effects and medical applications" Fatma Vatansever, and Michael R. Hamblin. *Photonics & Lasers in Medicine.* De Gruyter. 2012

"Health benefit of vegetable/fruit juice-based diet: Role of microbiome" Susanne M. Henning et al. *Scientific Reports.* Nature Research. 2017

"Antibiotic Resistance Threats in the United States, 2013" Tom Frieden. Centers for Disease Control and Prevention. (https://www.cdc.gov) April 23, 2013

"Prevalence of inappropriate antibiotic prescriptions among US ambulatory care visits, 2010–2011" Fleming-Dutra, K et al. Centers for Disease Control and Prevention. *JAMA.* American Medical Association. May 2016

"Antimicrobial resistance: risk associated with antibiotic overuse and initiatives to reduce the problem" Carl Llor, and Lars Bjerrum. Therapeutic Advances in Drug Safety. SAGE. 2014

"Antibiotic stewardship in the intensive care unit" Charles-Edouard Luyt et al. *Critical Care.* BioMed Central. 2014

"Intestinal candidiasis and antibiotic usage in children: case study of Nsukka, South Eastern Nigeria" Ifeoma M Ezeonu et al. *African Health Sciences.* Makerere University Medical School. 2017

"Immune defence against *Candida* fungal infections." Mihai G. Netea et al. *Nature Reviews Immunology.* Nature Publishing Group. 2015

"Hidden Killers: Human Fungal Infections" Gordon D. Brown et al. *Science Translational Medicine.* AAAS. 2012

"Do Wellness Tourists Get Well? An Observational Study of Multiple Dimensions of Health and Well-Being After a Week-Long Retreat" Marc M. Cohen et al. *The Journal of Alternative and Complementary Medicine.* Mary Ann Liebert. 2017

"The health impact of residential retreats: a systematic review" Dhevaksha Naidoo, Adrian Schembri, and Marc Cohen. *BMC Complementary and Alternative Medicine*. BioMed Central. 2018

Chapter 13: Your Liver Is A Muscle

"Super Size Me" *Wikipedia* (https://en.wikipedia.org/wiki/Super_Size_Me) 2020

"The association of pattern of lifetime alcohol use and cause of death in the European Prospective Investigation into Cancer and Nutrition (EPIC) study" Manuela M Bergmann et al. *International Journal of Epidemiology*. Oxford University Press. 2013

Chapter 14: Negativity Kills Longevity

"The Mountain of Youth: What We Can Learn from Okinawa, Japan" Jocelyn Catenacci. *Juxtaposition Global Health Magazine*. (https://juxtamagazine.org) April 2, 2018

"First autopsy study of an Okinawan centenarian: absence of many age-related diseases." Bernstein AM et al. Journals of Gerontology Series A: Biological Sciences and Medical Sciences. Oxford Academic. 2004

"Positive attitude towards life and emotional expression as personality phenotypes for centenarians" Kaori Kato et al. *Aging (Albany NY)*. Impact Journals. 2012

"The cultural context of "successful aging" among older women weavers in a northern Okinawan village: the role of productive activity." Willcox DC et al. *The Journal of Cross-Cultural Gerontology*. Springer. 2007

"Aging gracefully: a retrospective analysis of functional status in Okinawan centenarians." Willcox DC et al. *The American Journal of Geriatric Psychiatry*. Elsevier. 2007

"Okinawans: Their Food, Good Health, Music, Clothes And Culture" Jeffrey Hays. *Facts and Details*. (http://factsanddetails.com) 2009

"Longevity and diet in Okinawa, Japan: the past, present and future." Miyagi S et al. *Asia-Pacific Journal of Public Health*. SAGE. 2003

"Healthy aging diets other than the Mediterranean: A Focus on the Okinawan Diet" Donald Craig Willcox et al. *Mechanisms of Ageing and Development*. Elsevier. 2014

"The Role of Positive Emotions in Positive Psychology: The Broaden-and-Build Theory of Positive Emotions" Barbara L. Fredrickson. *American Psychologist*. American Psychological Association. 2001

"Effect of Positive Well-Being on Incidence of Symptomatic Coronary Artery Disease" Lisa R. Yanek et al. The American Journal of Cardiology. Elsevier. 2013

"The neuroscience of placebo effects: connecting context, learning and health" Tor D. Wager, and Lauren Y. Atlas. *Nature Reviews Neuroscience*. Nature Research. 2018

"Academic Physicians Use Placebos in Clinical Practice and Believe in the Mind–Body Connection" Rachel Sherman, and John Hickner. *Journal of General Internal Medicine*. Springer. 2008

"Increasing placebo responses over time in U.S. clinical trials of neuropathic pain" Alexander Tuttle et al. *Pain*. Wolters Kluwer. 2015

"Arthroscopic partial meniscectomy versus sham surgery for a degenerative meniscal tear." Sihvonen R et al. *The New England Journal of Medicine*. Massachusetts Medical Society. 2013

"13 more things: The nocebo effect" *New Scientist*. (https://www.newscientist.com) 2nd September 2009

"Doomed" Woman Died On Schedule" *Herald Tribune*. (http://www.baltimoreorless.com) November 18. 1966

"Mysteries of the mind: Your unconscious is making your everyday decisions" Marianne Szegedy-Maszak. *ENGL 2210 World Literature II*. Auburn University (http://www.auburn.edu) 2005

"The Subconscious Mind of the Consumer (And How To Reach It)" Manda Mahoney. *Working Knowledge*. Harvard Business School. 13 Jan 2003

"General Education Board" *Wikipedia*. (https://en.wikipedia.org/wiki/General_Education_Board) 2020

"Stress In America TM 2019" *American Psychological Association* (APA). (https://www.apa.org) November 2019

"The Depression Cure" Stephen S. Ilardi. *Da Capo Press*. 2009

"The efficacy of light therapy in the treatment of mood disorders: a review and meta-analysis of the evidence." Golden RN et al. *The American Journal of Psychiatry*. APA Publishing. 2005

"Is Exercise a Viable Treatment for Depression?" James A. Blumenthal et al. *ACSMs Health & Fitness Journal*. American College of Sports Medicine. 2012

"How One Second Could Cost Amazon $1.6 Billion In Sales" Kit Eaton. *Fast Company*. (https://www.fastcompany.com) 15th March 2012

"Adolescent social media use and mental health from adolescent and parent perspectives." Barry CT et al. *Journal of Adolescence*. Elsevier. 2017

"#Sleepyteens: Social media use in adolescence is associated with poor sleep quality, anxiety, depression and low self-esteem." Woods HC, and Scott H. *Journal of Adolescence*. Elsevier. 2016

"No More Fomo: Limiting Social Media Decreases Loneliness And Depression" Melissa G. Hunt et al. *Journal of Social and Clinical Psychology*. Guilford Publications Inc. 2018

"Why You Should: Write Down Your Goals" Emina Dedic, and Gail Mathews. *Snow College*. (https://www.snow.edu) 2020

"Why Visual Teaching?" Timothy Gangwer, and Gloria C. Rzadko-Henry. *Visual Teaching Alliance for the Gifted & Talented*. (http://visualteachingalliance.com) 2020

"Time of conscious intention to act in relation to onset of cerebral activity (readiness-potential). The unconscious initiation of a freely voluntary act." Libet B et al. *Brain: A Journal of Neurology.* Oxford Press. 1983

"Metacognition of intentions in mindfulness and hypnosis" Peter Lush, Peter Naish, and Zoltan Dienes. *Neuroscience of Consciousness.* Oxford Academic. 2016

"Mindfulness training and systemic low-grade inflammation in stressed community adults: Evidence from two randomized controlled trials" Daniella K. Villalba et al. *PLOS One.* Public Library of Science. 2019

Chapter 15: Nourish The Skin You're In

"Vitamin E relieves most cystic breast disease; may alter lipids, hormones" Elizabeth Rasche González. *JAMA.* American Medical Association. 1980

"Plasma fatty acid profiles in benign breast disorders." Gateley CA et al. *British Journal of Surgery.* Wiley. 1992

"Underarm antiperspirants/deodorants and breast cancer" Philippa D Darbre. *Breast Cancer Research.* BioMed Central. 2009

"Antiperspirant use and the risk of breast cancer." Mirick DK, Davis S, and Thomas DB. *Journal of the National Cancer Institute.* Oxford University Press. 2002

"An earlier age of breast cancer diagnosis related to more frequent use of antiperspirants/deodorants and underarm shaving." McGrath KG. European Journal of Cancer Prevention. Lippincott Williams & Wilkins. 2003

"The Mortician's Mystery" Joel S. Finkelstein et al. *The New England Journal of Medicine.* Massachusetts Medical Society. 1988

"Victory for advocates on lead acetate: FDA agrees to ban toxic lead compound from hair dyes" Keith Gaby, and Tom Neltner. *Environmental Defense Fund.* (https://www.edf.org) October 30, 2018

"FDA Bans Lead-Based Neurotoxin from Consumer Hair Dyes" Monica Amarelo. *Environmental Working Group.* (https://www.ewg.org) October 30, 2018

"Europe Has Banned 1,300 Toxins From Beauty Products. The United States? Just 11." *Countable.* (https://www.countable.us) 3rd March 2020

"Prohibited & Restricted Ingredients in Cosmetics" *US Food & Drug Administration.* (https://www.fda.gov) 3rd November 2017

"The chemistry of cosmetics" Oliver Jones, and Ben Selinger. *Australian Academy of Science.* (https://www.science.org.au) 2019

"What are Phthalates?" Tox Town. *US National Library of Medicine.* (https://toxtown.nlm.nih.gov) 2017

"Contact dermatitis to methylisothiazolinone" Maria Antonieta Rios Scherrer et al. *Brazilian Annals of Dermatology.* Brazilian Society of Dermatology. 2015

"Methylisothiazolinone" Mari Paz Castanedo-Tardana, and Kathryn A Zug. *Dermatitis.* Wolters Kluwer. 2013

"Long-term repetitive sodium lauryl sulfate-induced irritation of the skin: an in vivo study." Branco N et al. *Contact Dermatitis.* Wiley. 2005

"Ethylene Oxide (EtO): Evidence of Carcinogenicity" *National Institute for Occupational Safety and Health*. (https://www.cdc.gov/niosh) 6th June 2014

"Safety Evaluation of Polyethylene Glycol (PEG) Compounds for Cosmetic Use" Hyun-Jun Jang et al. *Toxicological Research*. Korean Society of Toxicology. 2015

"No More Toxic Tub: Getting Contaminants Out Of Children's Bath & Personal Care Products" Heather Sarantis, Stacy Malkan, and Lisa Archer. The Campaign for Safe Cosmetics. (www.SafeCosmetics.org) March 2009

"Effect of Sunscreen Application on Plasma Concentration of Sunscreen Active Ingredients" Murali K. Matta et al. *JAMA*. American Medical Association. 2020

"Concentrations of the Sunscreen Agent Benzophenone-3 in Residents of the United States: National Health and Nutrition Examination Survey 2003–2004" Antonia M. Calafat et al. *Environmental Health Perspectives*. NIEHS. 2008

"Effect of Sunscreen Application Under Maximal Use Conditions on Plasma Concentration of Sunscreen Active Ingredients" Murali K. Matta et al. *JAMA*. American Medical Association. 2019

"The Trouble With Ingredients in Sunscreens" *Environmental Working Group*. (https://www.ewg.org) 2020

"Self-reported sunscreen use and urinary benzophenone-3 concentrations in the United States: NHANES 2003-2006 and 2009-2012" Rachel D Zamoiski et al. *Environmental Research*. Elsevier. 2015

"Toxicopathological Effects of the Sunscreen UV Filter, Oxybenzone (Benzophenone-3), on Coral Planulae and Cultured Primary Cells and Its Environmental Contamination in Hawaii and the U.S. Virgin Islands" C.A. Downs et al. *Archives of Environmental Contamination and Toxicology*. Springer. 2015

"Skincare Chemicals and Coral Reefs" *National Oceanic and Atmospheric Administration*. (https://oceanservice.noaa.gov) January 2020

"Sunscreen Use and Duration of Sun Exposure: a Double-Blind, Randomized Trial" Philippe Autier et al. *Journal of the National Cancer Institute*. Oxford University Press. 1999

"Small Amounts of Zinc from Zinc Oxide Particles in Sunscreens Applied Outdoors Are Absorbed through Human Skin" Brian Gulson et al. *Toxicological Sciences*. Oxford University Press. 2010

"Water fluoridation for the prevention of dental caries" Anne-Marie Glenny et al. *Cochrane Database of Systematic Reviews*. John Wiley & Sons, Ltd. 2015

"Patterns of dental caries following the cessation of water fluoridation." Maupomé G et al. *Community Dentistry and Oral Epidemiology*. Wiley. 2001

"Something in the water: is fluoride actually good for cities?" Ian Wylie. (https://www.theguardian.com) April 13, 2016

Chapter 16: Green Mean Cleaning Machine

"Getting Up to Speed: Ground Water Contamination" *Environmental Protection Agency* (https://www.epa.gov) 1993

"Household Cleaning Product-Related Injuries Treated in US Emergency Departments in 1990-2006" Lara B McKenzie et al. *Pediatrics*. American Academy of Pediatrics. 2010

Chapter 17: Smart Technology, Dumb Humans

"Health effects of Radiofrequency Electromagnetic Fields (RF EMF)" Alicja Bortkiewicz. *Industrial Health*. National Institute of Occupational Safety and Health. 2019

"France: New National Law Bans Wifi In Nursery School!" Annie Sasco. Environmental Health Trust. (https://ehtrust.org) Feb 19, 2015

"Cancer epidemiology update, following the 2011 IARC evaluation of radiofrequency electromagnetic fields (Monograph 102)" Anthony B.Miller et al. *Environmental Research*. Elsevier. 2018

"What Does the Research Tell Us About the Risk of Electromagnetic Radiation (EMR)?" Victor Leach, and Steven Weller. *Secretary of Oceania Radiofrequency Scientific Advisory Association*. (https://www.orsaa.org) 2017

"Planetary electromagnetic pollution: it is time to assess its impact" Priyanka Bandara, and David O Carpenter. *The Lancet*. Elsevier. 2018

"Effect of electromagnetic radiation of cell phone tower on foraging behaviour of Asiatic honey bee, Apis cerana F." Ritu Ranjan Taye et al. *Journal of Entomology and Zoology Studies*. Akinik Publications. 2017

"The effects of electromagnetic fields from power lines on avian reproductive biology and physiology: a review." Fernie KJ, and Reynolds SJ. *Journal of Toxicology and Environmental Health: Part B*. Taylor & Francis. 2005

"Worldwide decline of the entomofauna: A review of its drivers" Francisco Sánchez-Bayoa, and Kris A.G.Wyckhuys. *Biological Conservation*. Elsevier. 2019

"Scientists and doctors warn of potential serious health effects of 5G" Rainer Nyberg, and Lennart Hardell. *5G Appeal*. (https://www.5gappeal.eu) Launched on September 13, 2017

"Multifocal Breast Cancer in Young Women with Prolonged Contact between Their Breasts and Their Cellular Phones" John G. West et al. *Case Reports in Medicine*. Hindawi. 2013

"Habits of cell phone usage and sperm quality – does it warrant attention?" Ariel Zilberlicht et al. *Reproductive BioMedicine Online*. Elsevier. 2015

"Self-reporting of Symptom Development From Exposure to Radiofrequency Fields of Wireless Smart Meters in Victoria, Australia: A Case Series" Federica Lamech. *Alternative Therapies in Health and Medicine*. InnoVision Health Media. 2014

"Health Concerns associated with Energy Efficient Lighting and their Electromagnetic Emissions" Magda Havas. *Health Concerns Associated with Energy Efficient Lighting and Their Electromagnetic Emissions*." Scietific Committee on Emerging and Newly Indentified Health Risks (SCENIHR). 2008

"Utilization of Metal Lathe Waste as Material for the Absorption of Electromagnetic Radiation Based Orgonite" Anisya Lisdiana et al. *International Journal of Advances in Agricultural & Environmental Engineering*. IICBE. 2014

Chapter 18: Conscious Clothing

"Child labour in the textile & garment industry" Pauline Overeem, and Martje Theuws. *The Centre for Research on Multinational Corporations (SOMO).* (https://www.somo.nl) March 2014

"What the Rana Plaza Disaster Changed About Worker Safety" Nadra Nittle. *Racked.* (https://www.racked.com) April 13, 2018

"The Rana Plaza Accident and its aftermath" *International Labour Organisation.* (https://www.ilo.org) 2018

"The Current Health and Wellbeing of the Survivors of the Rana Plaza Building Collapse in Bangladesh: A Qualitative Study" Humayun Kabir et al. *International Journal of Environmental Research and Public Health.* MDPI. 2019

"Health vulnerabilities of readymade garment (RMG) workers: a systematic review" Humayun Kabir et al. *BMC Public Health.* BioMed Central. 2019

"Fast Fashion's Detrimental Effect on the Environment" Rashmila Maiti. Earth.Org (https://earth.org) Jan 29th 2020

"Waste Couture: Environmental Impact of the Clothing Industry" Luz Claudio. *Environmental Health Perspectives.* ISEE. 2007

"Textile dyeing industry an environmental hazard" Rita Kant. *Natural Science.* Scientific Research Publishing. 2012

"Dressed to Kill" Sydney Ross Singer, and Soma Grismaijer. Avery Publishing. 1995

"Risk Factors of Breast Cancer in Women in Guangdong and the Countermeasures" An-Qin Zhang et al. *Journal of Southern Medical University.* Nanfang yi ke da xue xue bao bian ji bu. 2009

"Patologias mamarias generadas por el uso sostenido y seleccion incorrecta del brassier en pacientes que acuden a la consulta de mastologia" Marcos Eduardo Quijada Stanovich et al. *Ginecologia y Obstetricia.* Últimas Publicaciones. 2011

"Bras linked to rise in breast cancer" Ilona Amos. *The Scotsman.* (https://www.scotsman.com) 26th May 2014

"Bra Wearing Not Associated With Breast Cancer Risk: A Population-Based Case-Control Study" Lu Chen, Kathleen E. Malone, and Christopher I. Li. *Cancer Epidemiology, Biomarkers & Prevention.* AACR. 2014

Chapter 19: Eco-Therapy

"The Health Benefits of the Great Outdoors: A Systematic Review and Meta-Analysis of Greenspace Exposure and Health Outcomes" Caoimhe Twohig-Bennett, and Andy Jones. *Environmental Research.* Elsevier. 2018

"Happiness is greater in natural environments" George MacKerron, and Susana Mourato. *Global Environmental Change.* Elsevier. 2013

"A Forest Bathing Trip Increases Human Natural Killer Activity and Expression of Anti-Cancer Proteins in Female Subjects" Q Li et al. Journal of Biological Regulators & Homeostatic Agents. Biolife. 2008

"Effect of forest bathing trips on human immune function" Qing Li. *Environmental Health and Preventive Medicine*. Springer. 2010

"Influence of Forest Therapy on Cardiovascular Relaxation in Young Adults" Juyoung Lee et al. *Evidence-Based Complementary and Alternative Medicine*. Hindawi. 2014

"Psychological Benefits of Walking through Forest Areas" Chorong Song et al. *International Journal of Environmental Research and Public Health*. MDPI. 2018

"Creativity in the Wild: Improving Creative Reasoning through Immersion in Natural Settings" Ruth Ann Atchley, David L. Strayer, and Paul Atchley. *PLOS One*. Public Library of Science. 2012

"Green Space and Health" Houses of Parliament: Parliamentary Office of Science and Technology. *POSTnote*. (https://www.parliament.uk) October 2016

"Effect Of A Short Period Whole Body Vibration With 10 Hz On Blood Biomarkers In Wistar Rats" Milena de Oliveira Bravo Monteiro et al. *African Journal of Traditional, Complementary and Alternative Medicines*. African Ethnomedicines Network. 2017

"Neighborhood greenspace and health in a large urban center" Omid Kardan et al. *Scientific Reports*. Nature Research. 2015

Chapter 20: Quit Your Job

"KFC founder Colonel Sanders didn't achieve his remarkable rise to success until his 60s" Richard Feloni. *Business Insider*. (https://www.businessinsider.com) June 25, 2015

Chapter 21: Get A Pet

"About Pets & People" Centers for Disease Control and Prevention. (https://www.cdc.gov) 2019

"Health Benefits of Pet Ownership" Kristina Solch. The Ohio State University: Veterinary Medical Center. (https://vet.osu.edu) 2016

"Association between life span and body condition in neutered client-owned dogs" Carina Salt et al. *Journal of Veterinary Internal Medicine*. Wiley. 2018

"Decoding Pet Food" Mark Kastel et al. *The Cornucopia Institute*. (https://www.cornucopia.org) November 2015

"Models of Inflammation: Carrageenan- or Complete Freund's Adjuvant-Induced Edema and Hypersensitivity in the Rat" Jill C. Fehrenbacher et al. *Current Protocols in Pharmacology*. Wiley. 2012

"Report on Carcinogens, Fourteenth Edition" Department of Health and Human Services. (https://ntp.niehs.nih.gov) November 3, 2016

"Ewg's Dirty Dozen Guide To Food Additives: Generally Recognized As Safe – But Is It?" Environmental Working Group. (https://www.ewg.org) November 12, 2014

Made in the USA
Middletown, DE
30 October 2023

41542244R00236